CRASH COURSE

Second Edition

Rheumatology and Orthopaedics

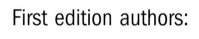

First edition authors:
Annabel Coote
Paul Haslam

CRASH COURSE

Second Edition

Series editor
Daniel Horton-Szar
BSc (Hons), MBBS (Hons), MRCGP
Northgate Medical Practice
Canterbury
Kent, UK

Faculty advisor
Annabel Coote
MBChB, MRCP
Specialist Registrar in
Rheumatology, Royal Hallamshire
Hospital, Sheffield, UK

Paul Haslam
MBChB, FRCS Ed, FRCS (Tr & Orth)
Consultant Orthopaedic Surgeon,
Doncaster Royal Infirmary,
Doncaster, UK

Rheumatology and Orthopaedics

Daniel Marsland

MBChB, MRCS(Eng)

ST2 Cardiothoracics, Royal Brompton and Harefield
NHS Trust, London, UK

Sabrina Kapoor

MBChB, BMedSC, MRCP (London)

Specialist Registrar in Rheumatology, Wythenshawe Hospital,
South Manchester University Hospital Trust, Manchester, UK

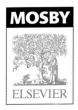

MOSBY
ELSEVIER

Edinburgh • London • New York • Oxford • Philadelphia • St Louis • Sydney • Toronto 2008

MOSBY
ELSEVIER

Commissioning Editor:	Alison Taylor
Development Editor:	Kim Benson
Project Manager:	Frances Affleck
Page design:	Sarah Russell
Icon illustrations:	Geo Parkin
Cover design:	Stewart Larking
Illustration management:	Merlyn Harvey

First edition 2004
Second edition 2008

ISBN: 978-0-7234-3471-9

British Library Cataloguing in Publication Data
A catalogue record for this book is available from the British Library

Library of Congress Cataloging in Publication Data
A catalog record for this book is available from the Library of Congress

Note
Knowledge and best practice in this field are constantly changing. As new research and experience broaden our knowledge, changes in practice, treatment and drug therapy may become necessary or appropriate. Readers are advised to check the most current information provided (i) on procedures featured or (ii) by the manufacturer of each product to be administered, to verify the recommended dose or formula, the method and duration of administration, and contraindications. It is the responsibility of the practitioner, relying on their own experience and knowledge of the patient, to make diagnoses, to determine dosages and the best treatment for each individual patient, and to take all appropriate safety precautions. To the fullest extent of the law, neither the Publisher nor the Authors assumes any liability for any injury and/or damage to persons or property arising out of or related to any use of the material contained in this book.

The Publisher

Printed in China

It has been estimated that musculoskeletal problems are responsible for one in four GP consultations. No matter what medical or surgical career you choose to follow, you are guaranteed to be exposed to patients with orthopaedic or rheumatological conditions. Despite this, teaching in these specialities can be neglected in the undergraduate curriculum.

As a medical student going home for Christmas you will be asked for an opinion on your mate's injured knee, your auntie's bunions and your father's sciatica. (All these scenarios happened to us!) Hopefully this book will prepare you for these embarrassing situations!

The book is designed to give medical students a head start on the wards and make the exciting world of orthopaedics and rheumatology fun and easy to learn. It is also of use to foundation doctors (and will help pass your workplace based competency assessments!), physiotherapists, occupational therapists and nurses.

We hope you enjoy the book, pass your exams, and then follow a career in orthopaedics or rheumatology.

Daniel Marsland
Sabrina Kapoor
Annabel Coote
Paul Haslam

More than a decade has now passed since work began on the *Crash Course* series. Medicine never stands still, and the work of keeping this series relevant for today's students is an ongoing process. This second edition builds upon the success of the preceding books and incorporates a great deal of new and revised material, keeping the series up to date with the latest medical research and developments in pharmacology and current best practice.

As always, we listen to feedback from the thousands of students who use *Crash Course* and have made further improvements to the layout and structure of the books. Each chapter now starts with a set of learning objectives, and the self-assessment sections have been enhanced and brought up to date with modern exam formats. We have also worked to integrate material on communication skills and gems of clinical wisdom from practising doctors. This will not only add to the interest of the text but will reinforce the principles being described.

Despite fully revising the books, we hold fast to the principles on which we first developed the series: *Crash Course* will always bring you all the information you need to revise in compact, manageable volumes that integrate pathology and therapeutics with best clinical practice. The books still maintain the balance between clarity and conciseness, while providing sufficient depth for those aiming at distinction. The authors are junior doctors who have recent experience of the exams you are now facing, and the accuracy of the material is checked by senior clinicians and faculty members from across the UK.

I wish you all the best for your future careers!

Dr Dan Horton-Szar
Series Editor

Acknowledgements

We thank:

The senior authors Annabel Coote and Paul Haslam.

Mr Stan Jones, consultant orthopaedic paediatric surgeon, Sheffield Children's Hospital, for supplying the paediatric radiology images and helping with the cerebral palsy section.

Mr Richard Gibson, consultant orthopaedic surgeon, Northern General Hospital, Sheffield, for supplying some of the trauma images.

Andy Hamer and Michael Snaith, the Faculty Advisors for the first edition.

Dr Rodney Amos for his help with the section on juvenile idiopathic arthritis.

Dr David Moore, consultant radiologist, Northern General Hospital, Sheffield, for supplying many of the orthopaedic images.

Dedication

To the Marslands for their support throughout my education and to the Durani family and my new wife Priyanka. **DM**

To Ash, Mum, Dad, Sanjay, Sandeep and grandma for their support and patience during the writing of this book. **SK**

To Timothy and Magnus. **AC**

To Audrey, Freddie, Mathew and Harry. **PH**

Contents

Glossary

Allodynia A painful response to a stimulus that does not usually cause pain.

Arthrodesis Joint fusion surgery.

Arthroplasty Joint replacement surgery.

Baker's cyst Synovial cyst found in the popliteal fossa, usually associated with knee arthritis (osteoarthritis or rheumatoid arthritis).

Bouchard's node A bony swelling of the proximal interphalangeal joint caused by osteoarthritis.

Boutonnière deformity A deformity of the finger seen in rheumatoid arthritis, characterized by flexion of the proximal interphalangeal joint and hyperextension of the distal interphalangeal joint.

Bursitis Inflammation of a bursa.

Cauda equina syndrome Compression of the central nerve roots in the spinal canal causing bladder and bowel disturbance and saddle anaesthesia.

Chondrocalcinosis The presence of calcium pyrophosphate crystals in cartilage.

Chondrosarcoma Slow growing malignant tumour of cartilagenous origin.

Codman's triangle X-ray appearance when a bone tumour elevates the periosteum.

Compartment syndrome Increasing pressure within a myofascial compartment exceeds capillary pressure resulting in compromised circulation to muscles and nerves within the compartment.

Crystal arthropathy Includes a range of diseases of the joint resulting from crystal deposition including gout and chondrocalcinosis.

Cytokine Intercellular messenger protein.

Dactylitis Swelling of a whole digit in the hand or foot, commonly found in the spondyloarthropathies and sometimes referred to as a 'sausage digit'.

Diaphysis Shaft of a long bone.

Developmental dysplasia of the hip (DDH) Failure of the acetabulum to develop normally resulting in subluxation or dislocation of the femoral head.

Dupuytren's contracture Contracture of the palmar fascia results in fixed flexion of the digits (most commonly the ring finger).

Enthesopathy Degeneration/inflammation of a tendon or ligament where it inserts into bone.

Epiphysis Part of bone between the physis and the joint.

Ewing's sarcoma Malignant tumour of connective tissue origin in children and young adults, typically affecting proximal long bones and the pelvis.

Flail chest Occurs when two or more consecutive ribs are fractured in two or more places. This results in a mobile segment which moves paradoxically with respiration and causes impaired ventilation.

Fracture Break in the continuity in the cortex of normal bone.

Ganglion Cystic lesion associated with a joint or tendon.

Glasgow Coma Score Objective measure of consciousness based on best eye opening, verbal and motor responses.

Haemarthrosis Blood in a joint.

Haemothorax Blood in the pleural cavity.

Hallux valgus Correct term for bunion deformity.

Heberden's node A bony swelling of the distal interphalangeal joint caused by osteoarthritis.

J sign Seen with lateral maltracking of the patella.

Keratoderma blenorrhagica A pustular skin rash, usually confined to the palms and soles, associated with reactive arthritis.

Kyphosis Excessive forward curvature of the spine.

Lachmann's test Test for anterior cruciate ligament rupture.

Lipoma Benign adipose tissue.

Livedo reticularis A reticular, purplish discoloration usually seen on the extensor surfaces of the legs.

Lymphoma Primary malignant tumour of lymphoid tissue.

Morton's neuroma Painful nerve lesion in the foot.

Open fracture A fracture associated with breach in the overlying epithelium and dermis allowing potential contamination of the fracture site with bacteria.

Osgood–Schlatter disease Traction apophysitis of the tibial tuberosity.

Osteochondritis dissecans Separation of subchondral bone and the overlying cartilage (usually affects the knee).

Osteochondroma (exostosis) Common benign bone tumour with a thick cartilagenous cap.

Osteoid osteoma Painful benign bone tumour which is self-limiting.

Osteomyelitis Infection within bone.

Osteosarcoma Aggressive malignant primary bone tumour.

Pannus Inflamed synovial tissue that erodes the articular cartilage in rheumatoid arthritis.

Pathological fracture Break in the continuity of the cortex of abnormal bone.

Perthes disease Segmental avascular necrosis of the femoral head.

Pes planus Flat foot.

Phalen's test Holding the wrist in palmar flexion reproduces the symptoms of carpal tunnel syndrome.

Physis Growth plate of a bone.

Pneumothorax Air within the pleural cavity.

Raynaud's phenomenon Pallor, coolness, numbness and discomfort of an extremity (commonly a digit) due to vasospasm.

Red flag signs Features of back pain that suggest sinister pathology.

Rheumatoid factor An antibody to the Fc fragment of immunoglobulin G (IgG) commonly found in rheumatoid arthritis.

Rheumatoid nodules Subcutaneous swellings occurring in patients with rheumatoid arthritis who test positive for rheumatoid factor.

Sarcoma Malignant neoplasm of connective tissue origin.

Schirmer's test A test used to measure tear production in patients with dry eyes.

Schöber test A measurement of flexion at the lumbar spine.

Sciatica Pain radiating down the posterior aspect of the leg below the level of the knee.

Sclerodactyly Fibrotic thickening of the skin over the fingers seen in systemic sclerosis.

Scoliosis Lateral deviation of the spine.

Shock Inadequate tissue perfusion and oxygenation due to acute circulatory failure.

Spinal claudication Spinal stenosis compressing the spinal cord results in pain and numbness in the back and legs. It is relieved by sitting forward.

Spinal shock Results from spinal injury causing temporary total loss of function distal to the level of the injury (different from neurogenic shock).

Spondylolisthesis Forward displacement of one vertebra on another.

Spondylolysis A defect in the pars interarticularis. May result in a spondylolisthesis.

Swan neck deformity A deformity of the finger seen in rheumatoid arthritis, characterized by flexion of the metacarpophalangeal joint, hyperextension of the proximal interphalangeal joint and flexion of the distal interphalangeal joint.

Synovitis Inflammation of the synovium.

Tarsal tunnel syndrome Painful condition of the foot in which the posterior tibial nerve is compressed in the tarsal tunnel.

Tenosynovitis Inflammation of the synovial lining of a tendon sheath.

Tension pneumothorax A one-way valve develops in the lung surface. This allows air into the pleural cavity during inspiration but closes during expiration. This results in compression of the mediastinal structures and requires immediate decompression.

Tinel's test Tapping over the median nerve in the wrist reproduces the symptoms of carpal tunnel syndrome.

Thomas' test A test for fixed flexion deformity of the hip.

Tophus A hard deposit composed of monosodium urate crystals occurring in or near the joints in chronic gout.

Trendelenburg test A test for weak hip abductors.

Valgus Angulation away from the midline.

Varus Angulation towards the midline.

Vasculitis Inflammation of the blood vessels.

Yellow flag signs Psychosocial aspects of back pain associated with a poor outcome.

THE PATIENT PRESENTS WITH

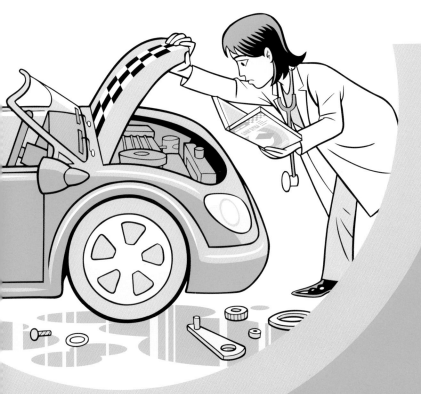

Regional pain

Objectives

In this chapter you will learn to:

- Recognize important features in the history and examination for back pain.
- Give a differential diagnosis for back pain including sinister causes and know how to investigate these.
- Recognize patterns of upper limb and neck pain in order to be able to make an accurate diagnosis.
- Understand the relevant anatomy of the knee and ankle and be able to list a differential diagnosis for pain.
- Know how to investigate regional pain in the spine, upper and lower limbs appropriately.

BACK, HIP AND LEG PAIN

One of the most common presentations to a GP is that of back, hip and/or leg pain. 80% of the population will have an episode of back pain at some time in their lives.

The patient may have one or any combination of the three symptoms. An important point to note is that many patients do not know where the hip joint is and most will point to the iliac crest or further posteriorly towards the sacroiliac joint and tell you this is their hip! Other misconceptions abound: one patient may tell you his sciatica is playing up or another that her slipped disc has 'popped out again'.

So when faced with such a patient the physician must decide, on the basis of the history and examination, whether the pain is from the back or the hip joint and if what the patient is telling you is correct!

Differential diagnosis

- Simple low back pain (see Ch. 21).
- Osteoarthritis (see Ch. 8).
- Hip.
- Spine.
- Prolapsed intervertebral disc (see Ch. 21).
- Rheumatoid or other inflammatory arthritis (see Chs 9 and 10).

- Vertebral crush fracture (see Ch. 12).
- Avascular necrosis of hip.
- Spinal stenosis/spondylolisthesis (see Ch. 21).
- Malignancy (see Ch. 20).
- Discitis (see Ch. 21).
- Abdominal causes (referred, e.g. pancreatitis/dissecting aortic aneurysm).
- Trochanteric bursitis.
- Paget's disease.

History focusing on back, hip and leg pain

There are essentially four different presentations (Fig. 1.1):

- Back pain.
- Back and leg pain.
- Hip pain with or without leg pain.
- Leg pain.

Back pain

Simple low back pain

Acute low back pain without radiation into the leg suggests simple low back pain—particularly if the patient gives a history of lifting or straining, and the pain is worse on movement and activity (so-called 'mechanical pain'). The pain is usually described as a band across the back and may be extremely severe.

Fig. 1.1 Patterns of pain around the back, leg and hip.

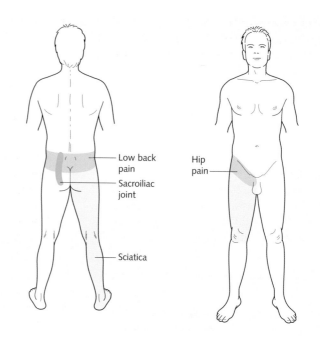

Signs of sinister back pain

Figure 1.2 shows 'red flag' signs that should alert the clinician to the possibility of serious spinal pathology. Malignancy such as spinal metastases is not uncommon. A history of fever might suggest discitis. Night sweats and weight loss are associated with malignancy and also tuberculosis.

Pain may radiate to the back from intra-abdominal pathology.

Red flag signs of sinister back pain
Age of onset <20 or >55 years
History of malignancy
Persistent, non-mechanical pain
Night pain
Fever/unexplained weight loss
Bladder/bowel dysfunction
Progressive neurology, abnormal gait, saddle anaesthesia

Fig. 1.2 Red flag signs of sinister back pain.

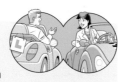

Beware of 'yellow flag' signs. These are based on psychosocial factors which can increase the chronicity of back pain. Examples include a patient's negative attitude that back pain is harmful and disabling. Ongoing compensation proceedings regarding a back injury, depression, social and financial problems, or an expectation that passive treatment such as bed rest is better than active treatment can also have adverse effects on prognosis.

Sciatica

True sciatica radiates down the back of the leg and into the foot. It may be of acute onset from a specific incident, and is typically constant with acute exacerbations lasting seconds. The nature of the pain is like an electric shock and can be very severe. It is aggravated in certain positions such as standing straight and by sneezing or coughing and relieved by bending forward with the knee flexed. Over time the pain usually settles.

Spinal stenosis

In spinal stenosis the patient typically has back pain, and the leg pain comes on after walking and is relieved by rest and leaning forward, so called spinal claudication.

Back and leg pain

Back and leg pain suggests that there is nerve root entrapment.

Facet joint osteoarthritis

Facet joint osteoarthritis of the spine can also radiate into the leg but the pain does not extend below the knee and is aching in character.

Hip pain with or without leg pain

True hip joint pain is felt in the groin and can radiate down the front of the thigh to the knee. The pain of an arthritic hip is of gradual onset, deep and gnawing. It can be unrelenting and persistent. Night pain may be present.

A fractured hip is a common emergency presentation in elderly patients. Usually there is a clear history of a fall but this is not always the case, particularly in confused patients.

Leg pain

Occasionally a prolapsed intervertebral disc presents with leg pain only (sciatica) without the back pain.

Loss of function/degree of disability

Patients will complain of limitation of certain activities, which may be recreational, work related or more basic activities of daily living.

It is important to know how much impact the disorder has on normal day-to-day living.

Back pain is the leading cause of sickness from work.

Associated symptoms

It is essential to ask about urinary or bowel disturbance in any patient with back pain. Incontinence of urine or faeces suggests a cauda equina syndrome needing urgent investigation and surgical decompression.

Numbness, pins and needles and weakness of the foot should be elicited in the history and suggest true sciatica.

Weight loss and a history of previous malignancy indicate possible malignancy.

Examination focusing on back, hip and leg pain

General examination

Look at the patient: weight loss, anaemia and general ill-health may suggest malignancy.

Look at the posture and gait:

- A stooped posture with flexion of the knee suggests sciatica.
- A frail old lady with a stooped posture may have osteoporotic fractures.

- A very stiff spine may be simple low back pain or ankylosing spondylitis.
- Fixed flexion of the hip with an antalgic or Trendelenburg gait is likely to be hip pathology. There may be a limb length discrepancy.
- Look for deformity of the spine, previous scars, wasting and any lower limb deformity.

Perform the Trendelenburg and Thomas tests as described in Chapter 27. These are tests aimed at examining the hip and, if positive, suggest hip pathology.

Palpation

- With the patient standing, palpate the spine and surrounding muscles for tenderness. In simple low back pain, often the area around the posterior superior iliac spine and sacroiliac joint is tender.
- The hip is too deep to palpate but feel around the greater trochanter for bursae.

Movement

- Assess movements of the spine. Diminished movement is likely if pathology is present. It may be impossible for the patient to comply because of pain.
- Hip movements will be reduced if an arthritic process is present. Usually internal rotation and abduction are the first to be lost.

Special tests

Straight leg raising will be diminished with a positive sciatic stretch test if the nerve root is irritated by a prolapsed disc or spinal stenosis.

A peripheral nervous system examination may show weakness and sensory loss in a single nerve root pattern.

Investigation of a patient with back, hip and leg pain

Blood tests

These are not always necessary but should be performed to exclude sinister causes in patients over 55 years of age or as guided by clinical suspicion.

Full blood count may reveal:

- Raised white cell count if infection is present such as in discitis.
- Anaemia in malignancy.

Biochemistry is required only to exclude abdominal causes and help confirm cases of malignancy.

- Erythrocyte sedimentation rate (ESR) and C-reactive protein (CRP) are elevated in infection and malignancy.
- Patients presenting with metastatic disease and an unknown primary need thorough investigation. Biopsy specimens should be taken at surgery.
- Alkaline phosphatase is elevated in Paget's disease.

Plain X-ray

This may show:

- Normal appearances in simple low back pain, prolapsed disc and even in malignancy or infection if early in the disease process (it is therefore not a good screening test and some departments have stopped routine spinal X-rays in young patients).

- Osteoarthritic changes in the hip and spine.
- A spondylolisthesis.
- Destruction of the vertebral body, classically the pedicle (winking owl sign) (Fig. 1.3), indicating malignancy.
- Fracture.
- Erosion of vertebral body around the disc due to infection.

Further special tests may be needed if there is doubt about the diagnosis or to plan surgery:

- Isotope bone scanning: hot spot in infection and malignancy.
- CT scanning: for looking at bony structures in detail, e.g. spondylolisthesis.
- Magnetic resonance imaging: useful for looking at soft tissue structures, including identification of disc prolapse and nerve root prior to surgery; and early detection of malignancy and infection.

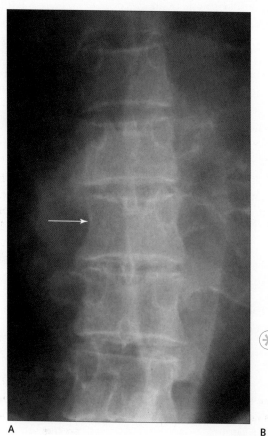

Fig. 1.3 Malignancy of the spine. The winking owl sign occurs when the pedicle is destroyed due to metastasis. The missing 'eye' represents bony destruction of the pedicle by tumour, so always look closely at the pedicles.

A

B

(✳) missing 'eye' represents bony destruction of the pedicle by tumour, therefore always look closely at the pedicles

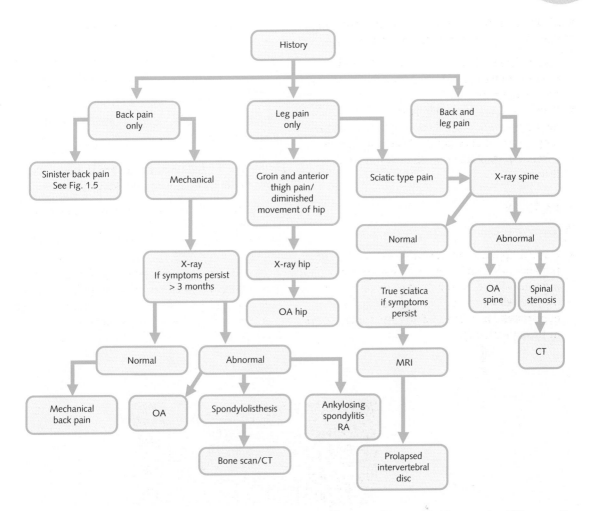

Fig. 1.4 Algorithm for the diagnosis and investigation of back, hip and leg pain. CT, computed tomography; MRI, magnetic resonance imaging; OA, osteoarthritis; RA, rheumatoid arthritis.

Algorithms for the diagnosis and investigation of back, hip and leg pain and for the investigation of sinister back pain are provided in Figures 1.4 and 1.5.

KNEE PAIN

Knee pain is a very common presenting complaint, accounting for over a third of all referrals to orthopaedic surgeons.

Differential diagnosis

- Osteoarthritis (see Ch. 8).
- Meniscal injuries (see Ch. 22).
- Ligament injury.
- Rheumatoid or other inflammatory arthritis (including crystal arthritis).
- Referred from hip or spine.
- Osteochondritis.
- Bursitis (see Ch. 24).
- Septic arthritis (see Ch. 16).
- Anterior knee pain/patellofemoral disorders.

History focusing on knee pain

The first thing to consider is the patient's age and occupation. A young athletic patient with a recent injury is unlikely to have rheumatoid arthritis (think of meniscal/ligamentous injuries). Similarly an elderly patient with gradual onset of pain over many years will most likely have an arthritic process.

7

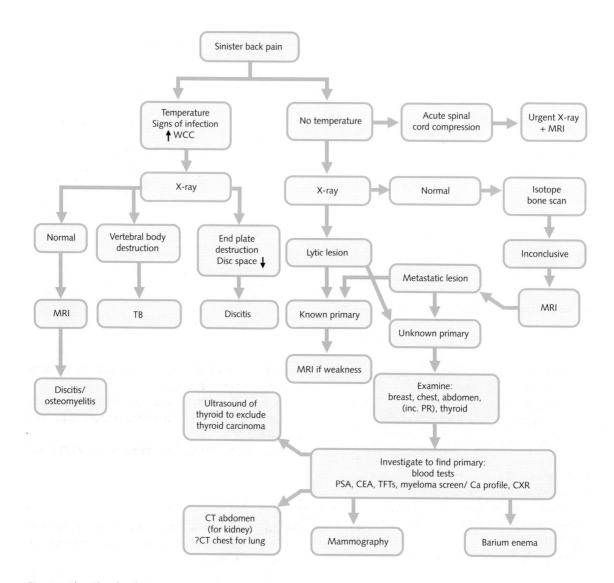

Fig. 1.5 Algorithm for the investigation of sinister back pain. Ca, calcium; CEA, carcinoembryonic antigen; CXR, chest X-ray; MRI, magnetic resonance imaging; PR, per rectum; PSA, prostate specific antigen; TFTs, thyroid function tests; WCC, white cell count.

The characteristics of the pain will give clues to the underlying diagnosis.

Site of pain

Pain can be generalized or localized.

Generalized pain ('all over') suggests an arthritic process affecting the whole joint. Large effusions such as after an injury or in sepsis also give a tense painful joint.

Localized pain depends on the site. Commonly painful areas around the knee are shown in Figure 1.6.

- Anterior: patellofemoral pain is felt here. Pain is felt at the front of the knee in prepatellar and infrapatellar bursitis as well as the obvious diagnosis of anterior knee pain.
- Medial or lateral: localized pain to either joint line could be osteoarthritis (particularly so in varus knees on the medial joint line) or from meniscal tears and collateral ligament sprains.
- Posterior pain is less common but could be related to a large Baker's cyst or bursitis.

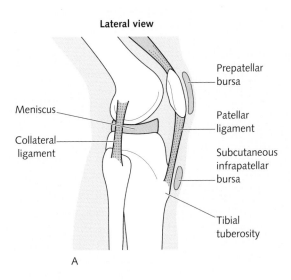
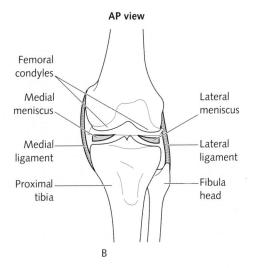

Fig. 1.6 Anatomical structures in the knee that cause pain.

- Pain down the back of the knee could be referred from the spine.
- Pain down the front of the thigh and into the knee suggests hip pathology.

The mode of onset is usually gradual, over a few weeks or months. If there is a sudden onset the most likely cause is an injury to the knee such as a meniscal tear or fracture. A history of spontaneous pain over days is most likely due to septic or crystal arthritis but could signal a flare-up of inflammatory conditions.

Pain and stiffness in the morning improving through the day suggest an inflammatory arthritis.

Pain originating from knee pathology rarely radiates but hip pain is commonly felt in the knee, particularly in children.

Nature of pain

Meniscal tear often gives a sharp stabbing pain.

Arthritic pain is usually a deep gnawing pain.

Constant pain that is not affected by activity is often a feature of anterior knee pain.

Aggravating/relieving factors

Arthritic pain is generally worse on activity and relieved by rest.

Classically patellofemoral pain is worse on walking up or down stairs.

Meniscal tears may give more trouble in deep flexion or when twisting.

In an acute crystal or septic arthritis the pain is intense and any movement exacerbates this considerably.

Pain from prepatellar bursitis is worse on kneeling.

Loss of function

Patients may have significant disability due to their knee pain. They may notice decreased movement or loss of full extension.

Athletic patients with a meniscal tear or cruciate ligament injury will tell you they don't trust the knee during certain sporting activities and may be unable to do them at all.

Deformity (see Ch. 5)

Patients with arthritis may notice that they are gradually becoming more 'bow-legged' or 'knock-kneed'. A windswept deformity (one valgus knee and one varus knee) is more common in rheumatoid arthritis (RA).

Associated symptoms

It is important to ask some closed questions when taking a history in a patient with knee pain.

Ask about any generalized symptoms of ill health such as a fever.

Any history of injury is important, as often a sportsman/woman will ignore a knee injury for many years prior to seeking help. The anterior cruciate ligament (ACL) may have been torn, so take a detailed history about what happened.

- Ask if the patient heard a 'snap'.
- Ask how long the swelling took to appear (very sudden swelling suggests ACL rupture).
- Ask whether the patient could play on (unlikely if significant injury occurred).
- A history of locking suggests meniscal injury or loose body.
- Giving way may be due to a ligamentous problem such as ACL rupture.

Past medical history

Of particular interest will be any previous operations or fractures to the knee, such as meniscectomy or arthroscopy.

Drug history

Ask about medications such as analgesics and non-steroidal anti-inflammatory drugs (NSAIDs).

Examination

As with any orthopaedic examination, the principles are look, feel and move.

Remember to examine the other knee as a comparison. This will give you an idea of how lax they are normally (this varies considerably) and how much movement they have.

Remember to examine the hip when examining the knee.

General inspection could reveal signs of rheumatoid arthritis.

Watch the patient walk into the room, look for an antalgic or Trendelenburg gait.

Inspection

- Look at the patient on standing, as any deformity will be more obvious. A varus deformity is more common than a valgus one.

- Look for previous scars around the knee, wasting (particularly quadriceps), swelling and erythema.
- Swelling can be localized, such as a prepatellar bursa (a boggy swelling in front of the knee) or more generalized, such as an effusion.

Palpation

- Palpate for an effusion as described in Chapter 27.
- Palpate for tenderness around the knee; joint line tenderness is common in a patient with a meniscal tear. A meniscal cyst may also be found.
- Palpate behind the knee for a bursa or Baker's cyst.
- Patellofemoral crepitus can be felt (and sometimes heard) on flexing and extending the knee in osteoarthritis.

Movement

- A locked knee results in lack of full extension but often flexion is normal. This can be quite subtle so compare with the other side.
- Fixed flexion deformity (common in osteoarthritis) also causes loss of full extension but the history is more gradual.
- Arthritis results in variable amounts of decreased flexion.
- See if any deformity is correctable.

Special tests (see page 199–201)

- Collateral ligament tears are apparent on abnormal opening up of the joint on the affected side.
- Anterior cruciate ligament laxity is demonstrated by positive Lachmann's and anterior drawer tests.
- Posterior cruciate ligament laxity is seen as a sag of the tibia at 90° and can be misdiagnosed as an ACL tear when performing the anterior drawer test (the abnormal forward movement of the tibia is due to its sagging back in the first place).
- Maltracking of the patella can be seen when observing the knee bending from flexion to extension (so-called J sign).
- Patella apprehension will be positive in a patient with previous dislocation.

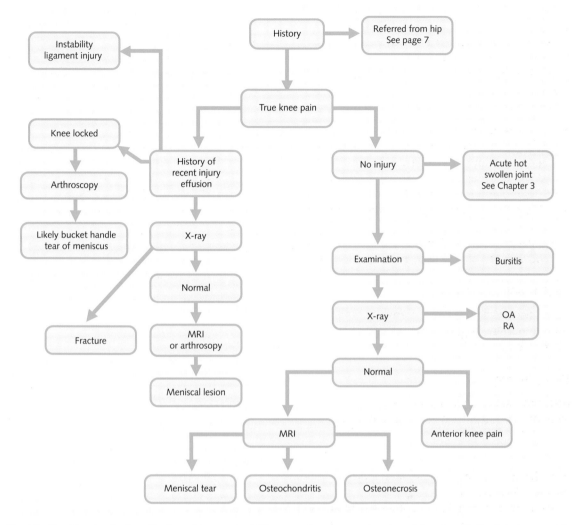

Fig. 1.7 Algorithm for the investigation of knee pain. MRI, magnetic resonance imaging; OA, osteoarthritis; RA, rheumatoid arthritis.

Investigations

Figure 1.7 provides an algorithm for the investigation of knee pain.

Blood tests

A full blood count (FBC) and measurements of ESR and CRP should be performed in suspected cases of infection and will show raised inflammatory markers and a high white cell count (WCC).

X-rays

X-ray images should be taken standing (joint space narrowing becomes more obvious) and include anteroposterior (AP), lateral and skyline views.

The X-ray may:

- Confirm rheumatoid arthritis or osteoarthritis.
- Show a fracture.
- Be normal.

Remember to consider an X-ray of the hip based on your history and examination findings.

Further imaging

This is only warranted under certain conditions:

- Magnetic resonance imaging (MRI): useful to confirm meniscal or ligamentous pathology.
- Computed tomography (CT): gives detailed information on bony structures; also useful to visualize patellar tracking.

- Isotope bone scanning: occasionally used if unsure about diagnosis. It will show 'hot spots' due to increased activity in many conditions including osteoarthritis, but also rarer causes such as osteomyelitis and bone tumours. It is a sensitive test but not specific. A normal bone scan is reassuring if one suspects sinister pathology.

Always send fluid obtained to microbiology for microscopy, culture and sensitivities (M, C + S) and ask the laboratory to look for crystals.

Aspiration

Aspiration of joint fluid is a very simple method of investigation and can give clues to the diagnosis. Look at the fluid obtained:

- Straw/yellow fluid: likely to be a simple effusion or possibly a crystal arthropathy.
- Green or dirty fluid: likely to be pus, and septic arthritis is likely.
- Blood: a haemarthrosis occurs after injury or occasionally in bleeding disorders or patients on warfarin. Blood and fat globules (a lipohaemarthrosis; Fig. 1.8) are present in fracture or ACL rupture.

Arthroscopy

Knee arthroscopy involves 'keyhole' surgery to look into the joint to see if there is any pathology.

Such exploratory operations used to be very common but now most surgeons will have a clear idea about the diagnosis before operating in such a way.

Often, based on clinical findings, the surgeon is sure of the diagnosis and will operate without the need for further investigations such as MRI scanning. This is particularly true in a locked knee.

ANKLE AND FOOT PAIN

Differential diagnosis

The differential diagnosis of pain in the ankle and/or foot is shown in Figure 1.9.

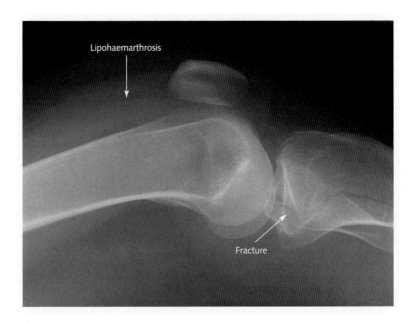

Fig. 1.8 A lipohaemarthrosis in the suprapatellar pouch (arrow) secondary to a tibial plateau fracture (arrow). A fluid level is seen as the fat 'floats' on the blood.

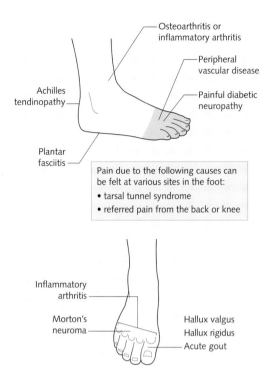

Fig. 1.9 Differential diagnosis of ankle and/or foot pain.

History

The following points should be covered when taking a history from patients with ankle or foot pain:

Site and chronological pattern of pain
(see Fig. 1.9)

- Recurrent self-limiting pain suggests crystal arthropathy (e.g. gout).
- Chronic pain with soft-tissue swelling suggests inflammation or infection.

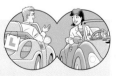

It is important to enquire what impact pain in the ankle or foot has on a patient's function and lifestyle. Achilles tendinopathy can ruin the career of an athlete, but may interfere little with the activities of a patient who leads a more sedentary lifestyle.

Presence of associated symptoms

- Back or knee pain suggest that the pain may be referred.
- Coldness and pallor of the foot may be due to peripheral vascular disease.
- Paraesthesiae or 'burning' pain can occur with Morton's neuroma, painful diabetic neuropathy or tarsal tunnel syndrome.

Detailed past medical history

- Plantar fasciitis is associated with spondyloarthropathies, so ask about a history of psoriasis or inflammatory bowel disease.
- Primary osteoarthritis (OA) is rare in the ankle or subtalar joints, so OA at these sites is usually secondary to previous ankle instability or fracture.
- Diabetes mellitus may be complicated by a painful neuropathy.
- Smoking, hypertension and diabetes mellitus are risk factors for peripheral vascular disease.

Presence of any precipitating factors

- Repetitive trauma due to running, jumping or other athletic activities can predispose to Achilles tendinopathy or plantar fasciitis ('policeman's heel').
- A recent illness or initiation of diuretic therapy may trigger an acute attack of gout.

Examination

The ankle and foot should be inspected during weight-bearing as well as in the neutral position. Some clinical signs are more obvious when the patient is standing.

Inspection

Inspection of the foot and ankle may reveal the following signs:

- Callus under metatarsophalangeal (MTP) joints (common in rheumatoid arthritis).

- Valgus deformity at the first MTP joint (hallux valgus).
- Erythematous swelling of a joint (acute gout or inflammatory arthritis).
- Swelling in the region of the Achilles tendon (Achilles tendinopathy).
- Ischaemic changes due to peripheral vascular disease.
- Plaques of psoriasis.

Palpation

Palpation of the foot and ankle should assess the following:

- Swelling: is it bony or soft?
- Joint tenderness.
- Tenderness of the plantar fascia and Achilles tendon.
- Tenderness between the metatarsal heads and/or the nodular swelling of a Morton's neuroma.
- Tenderness over the posterior tibial nerve posterior to the medial malleolus (common in tarsal tunnel syndrome).
- Strength of the peripheral pulses.

Movement

Movement of the foot and ankle should be compared to that on the opposite side. Passive dorsiflexion of the ankle will exacerbate the pain of Achilles tendinopathy. Restriction of movement and crepitus of the first MTP joint is seen with hallux rigidus.

Examination of other joints

This must include the knee, hip and lumbar spine.

Neurological examination

Neurological examination of the lower limbs is essential if there is any suspicion that the pain might be referred from the lumbar spine. Sensation should be tested. Diabetic neuropathy will cause sensory loss in a stocking distribution, whereas in Morton's neuroma it is localized to the borders of adjacent toes. Tarsal tunnel syndrome usually causes numbness in the sole of the foot.

Investigations

Blood tests

- The ESR and CRP will be elevated in most cases of inflammatory arthritis and crystal arthropathy.
- Serum uric acid levels are usually raised during acute attacks of gout.
- The finding of a positive rheumatoid factor in a patient with synovitis is suggestive of rheumatoid arthritis.

Radiological investigations

- Plain X-rays may show signs of an inflammatory or degenerative arthritis.
- Ultrasonography can identify abnormalities of the Achilles tendon and Morton's neuromas.
- Magnetic resonance imaging can also be used to assess tendons and neuromas. MRI of the lumbosacral spine is the investigation of choice in patients with ankle or foot pain that is thought to be due to nerve root compression.

Synovial fluid examination

Synovial fluid examination under polarized light microscopy should be performed if there are any pointers to a crystal arthropathy, such as acute erythema, pain and swelling in the first MTP joint, midfoot or ankle.

Nerve conduction studies

These are useful in confirming the diagnosis of tarsal tunnel syndrome or peripheral neuropathy.

NECK AND/OR UPPER LIMB PAIN

Differential diagnosis

Figures 1.10–1.13 give the differential diagnoses that should be considered when patients present with neck, shoulder, elbow, or wrist and hand pain.

Remember that pain in any bone or joint can be due to trauma, sepsis or malignancy.

Differential diagnosis of neck pain

Mechanical neck pain
Cervical spondylosis
Cervical disc prolapse
Cervical discitis
Metastatic vertebral deposits
Referred pain from:
• Local structures (e.g. thyroiditis, cervical lymphadenopathy)
• Distant structures (e.g. ischaemic heart disease, subphrenic abscess)

Fig. 1.10 Differential diagnosis of neck pain.

Differential diagnosis of shoulder pain

Rotator cuff pathology (impingement, tendinopathy or tear)
Capsulitis
Arthritis of the acromioclavicular joint
Arthritis of the glenohumeral joint
Bicipital tendinopathy
Polymyalgia rheumatica
Referred pain from
• Neck pathology
• Cardiac ischaemia
• Pancoast's tumour
• Intra-abdominal pathology (e.g. subphrenic abscess)

Fig. 1.11 Differential diagnosis of shoulder pain.

Differential diagnosis of elbow pain

Lateral epicondylitis (tennis elbow)
Olecranon bursitis
Crystal arthropathy
Osteoarthritis
Inflammatory arthritis
Medial epicondylitis (golfer's elbow)
Referred pain from the neck or shoulder

Fig. 1.12 Differential diagnosis of elbow pain.

Differential diagnosis of pain in the hand and wrist

Osteoarthritis
Carpal tunnel syndrome
Tenosynovitis
Inflammatory arthritis
Crystal arthropathy
Ulnar nerve entrapment
Raynaud's phenomenon
Complex regional pain syndrome
Referred pain from the cervical spine, shoulder or elbow

Fig. 1.13 Differential diagnosis of pain in the hand and wrist.

Complex regional pain syndrome

This is also referred to as reflex sympathetic dystrophy, algodystrophy, or Sudeck's atrophy. It is not common, but can affect any part of the musculoskeletal system. It is included in this section, as the distal forearm and hand are most often involved. The key features are of pain, hypersensitivity and autonomic disturbances, which can affect the integrity of the skin.

History

The following points should be covered when taking a history from a patient with neck or upper limb pain:

Onset of pain

• Subacute in polymyalgia rheumatica or crystal arthropathy.
• Gradual in osteoarthritis.

History of recent trauma or strenuous activity

• A fall on an outstretched hand, particularly in an elderly person, may result in a Colles fracture or rotator cuff tear.
• Trauma can trigger complex regional pain syndrome.
• Unaccustomed repetitive upper limb use, such as painting a ceiling, may provoke rotator cuff tendinopathy or lateral epicondylitis.

The presence of any other precipitating factors

• Raynaud's phenomenon is provoked by cold weather.
• Acute gout may be precipitated by the introduction of drugs that affect the serum urate level.

Site of pain

• The site of pain may give a clue to its origin. Figure 1.14 shows how the site of shoulder pain varies with the cause.
• Carpal tunnel syndrome causes pain in the radial three and a half digits.

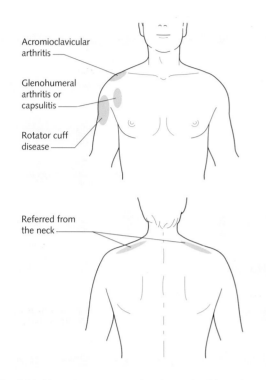

Acromioclavicular arthritis

Glenohumeral arthritis or capsulitis

Rotator cuff disease

Referred from the neck

Fig. 1.14 Many structures can give rise to shoulder pain. These diagrams show how the site of pain varies with the origin.

Movements that aggravate the pain

- Shoulder pain due to rotator cuff pathology will be exacerbated by abduction of the shoulder.
- Shoulder pain that is referred from the neck will be exacerbated by neck movements.

Presence of associated symptoms

- Stiffness is found in inflammatory conditions such as inflammatory arthritis or polymyalgia rheumatica.
- Referral of neck pain to the upper limbs or the presence of paraesthesiae may be due to cervical nerve root irritation.
- Weakness or clumsiness of the lower limbs or urinary symptoms may result from cervical cord compression.
- Dizziness may occur as a result of vertebral artery compression in severe degenerative disease.
- Paraesthesiae usually accompany pain in median or ulnar nerve entrapment.

- A painful response to stimuli that do not usually cause pain (e.g. light touch) is called allodynia and occurs in complex regional pain syndrome.
- Fever, weight loss and general malaise raise the possibility of sepsis, malignancy or inflammatory conditions such as polymyalgia rheumatica.
- Some symptoms will give a clue to the presence of disease that may be causing referred pain (e.g. haemoptysis in a patient with a Pancoast's tumour).

A suggested algorithm for the examination and investigation of patients with neck and/or upper limb pain is shown in Figure 1.15.

Examination

Inspection

Inspection of the affected joint and surrounding area is important. This may reveal:

- Loss of the normal cervical lordosis due to cervical spondylosis or muscle spasm.
- Wasting of the shoulder muscles from chronic rotator cuff tendinopathy.
- Shiny, erythematous swelling of the elbow or wrist due to acute gout or pseudogout.
- Heberden's or Bouchard's nodes in osteoarthritis.
- Synovial swelling of the small hand joints or tendon sheaths in rheumatoid arthritis.
- Rheumatoid nodules.
- Plaques of psoriasis.
- Gouty tophi.
- Wasting of the thenar or hypothenar muscles resulting from median or ulnar nerve compression respectively.
- Ischaemic changes in the digits due to Raynaud's phenomenon.
- Changes in skin colour, with atrophy and reduced hair growth as features of complex regional pain syndrome.

Palpation

As well as accurately identifying tender structures, palpation also helps in the assessment of swelling. Hard, bony swelling as seen in osteoarthritis should be distinguished from the softer boggy, synovial swelling of inflammatory arthritis. Inflamed tendon

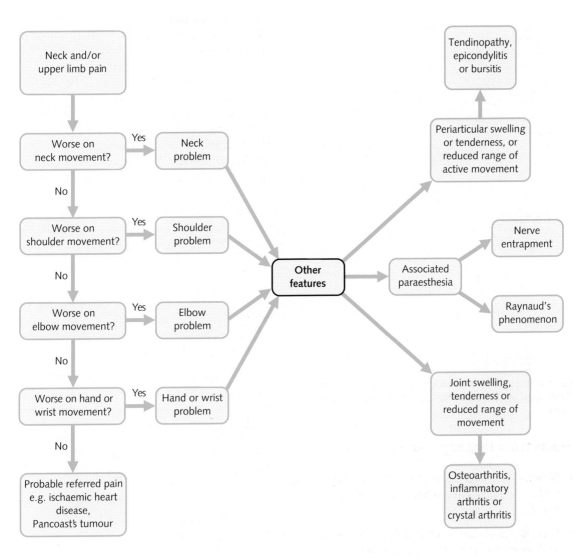

Fig. 1.15 Algorithm for the diagnosis of neck and/or upper limb pain.

sheaths in the hand or wrist may feel thickened or nodular and palpation may produce crepitus.

Assessment of joint movement

Assessment of joint movement is valuable in a hunt for the source of pain.

- In the shoulder, a reduction in passive and active movement suggests arthritis or capsulitis of the joint. A reduction in active movement, with normal passive movement, suggests a rotator cuff problem.
- Movement of the elbow in lateral epicondylitis will probably be normal, but resisted

dorsiflexion of the wrist will exacerbate the pain.

Examination of other body systems

Neurological examination of the cranial nerves and all four limbs is essential in a patient with neck pain and any neurological symptoms. Cervical radiculopathy and cord compression should be excluded. Motor and sensory function of the median and ulnar nerves should be assessed in cases of hand and wrist pain (Fig. 1.16). Tinel's and Phalen's tests may be abnormal in carpal tunnel syndrome (see Fig. 25.3, p. 182).

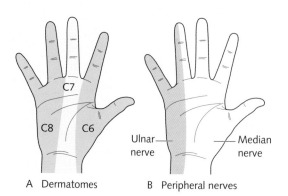

A Dermatomes   B Peripheral nerves

Fig. 1.16 Nerve entrapment in the upper limb can cause pain, paraesthesiae or sensory loss in the hand. The digit(s) affected give a clue as to which nerve is involved.

Examination of the cardiovascular, respiratory and abdominal systems may reveal a source of referred pain.

Investigations

The choice of investigations depends on the clinical examination findings. In some cases, the diagnosis is obvious from examination and further investigation is not required. For example, a 75-year-old man who complains of pain in his digits and has squaring of his first carpometacarpal joint and Heberden's nodes has osteoarthritis. Plain X-rays will confirm the diagnosis, but will not alter his management in any way.

Blood tests

- ESR and CRP may be raised in inflammatory, infectious or malignant conditions.
- The finding of a positive rheumatoid factor in a patient with synovitis is suggestive of rheumatoid arthritis.
- Serum uric acid is likely to be raised in cases of gout.

Synovial fluid examination

- Polarized light microscopy may detect urate or calcium pyrophosphate crystals.

- Microscopy and culture should be performed if there is any suspicion of infection.

Radiological investigations

X-rays

Plain X-rays may show signs of:

- Degenerative or inflammatory arthritis.
- Calcification due to tendinopathy.
- Periosteal reaction due to enthesitis.
- Bony metastasis.

X-rays are of little value in cervical spondylosis. There is poor correlation between the severity of radiographic signs and symptoms. Many people develop radiographic signs of spondylosis with increasing age, yet never suffer from neck pain.

Ultrasound scans

Ultrasound scanning can demonstrate thickening and oedema of tendon sheaths in tenosynovitis.

MRI and CT scans

These are useful in the following circumstances:

- Imaging the cervical cord and nerve roots.

- Detecting rotator cuff inflammation or degeneration.

Isotope bone scans

Isotope bone scans show increased tracer uptake in areas of accelerated bone turnover, such as inflammation, infection, malignancy or fracture. The finding of a 'hot spot' should be followed by MRI or CT scanning.

Nerve conduction studies

These can help to exclude cervical radiculopathy in patients with neck pain and upper limb paraesthesiae. Those with abnormal nerve conduction should proceed to an MRI or CT scan. Reduced nerve conduction velocities are seen in median and ulnar nerve entrapment.

Widespread musculoskeletal pain

Objectives

In this chapter you will learn to:

- List the causes of widespread musculoskeletal pain.
- Recognize how pain and stiffness due to inflammatory disease varies in severity throughout the day.
- Select appropriate investigations for the assessment of patients with widespread musculoskeletal pain.

Differential diagnosis

Patients sometimes present with widespread musculoskeletal pain. The differential diagnosis is shown in Figure 2.1.

The age, sex and race of the patient will give some guide to the likely diagnosis. For example, polymyalgia rheumatica (PMR) rarely affects people under the age of 60 years, fibromyalgia and systemic lupus erythematosus (SLE) are more common in women than in men and osteomalacia is more prevalent in Asian than in Caucasian populations.

Paraneoplastic rheumatic syndrome

This is a rare, but important, cause of musculoskeletal pain. Patients with lymphoma, leukaemia or other malignancies sometimes present with rheumatic symptoms. These can mimic inflammatory polyarthritis or PMR.

History

A thorough history should be taken, covering the following points:

Onset of pain

A relatively sudden onset (over 1–2 days) is common in PMR and can occur in inflammatory arthritis. A more gradual onset (over days to weeks) is more typical of the other diagnoses shown in Figure 2.1.

Timing of pain

As a rule, pain that is worse in the mornings and improves throughout the day is more likely to be inflammatory in origin.

Site of pain

Patients may find it hard to distinguish whether the pain is arising from their muscles or joints. In fibromyalgia, pain originates from the muscles and soft tissues, but many patients will complain that it is their joints that are hurting. Pain in the region of the shoulder and pelvic girdles is typical of PMR.

Presence of stiffness

Patients with musculoskeletal pain due to any cause may complain of stiffness. Significant stiffness that is maximal in the mornings and lasts for more than 30 minutes suggests inflammatory arthritis, SLE or PMR.

Associated symptoms

- Temporal headaches or jaw claudication are suggestive of giant cell arteritis associated with PMR.
- A history of skin rashes, mouth ulcers or Raynaud's phenomenon raises the possibility of SLE.

The differential diagnosis of widespread musculoskeletal pain

Inflammatory polyarthritis
Fibromyalgia
Systemic lupus erythematosus
Polymyalgia rheumatica
Metabolic bone disease (osteomalacia, hypercalcaemia)
Paraneoplastic rheumatic syndrome

Fig. 2.1 The differential diagnosis of widespread musculoskeletal pain.

- Psychiatric problems, such as anxiety and depression, can be features of fibromyalgia or SLE.
- Abdominal pain and confusion can occur in hypercalcaemia.

Examination and investigation

A suggested algorithm for the examination and investigation of patients with widespread musculoskeletal pain is shown in Figure 2.2.

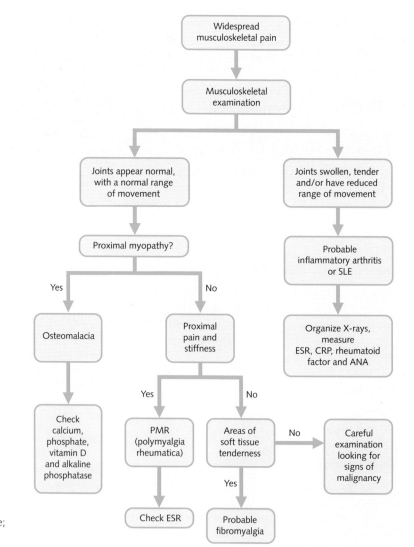

Fig. 2.2 Algorithm for the investigation of widespread musculoskeletal pain.
ANA, antinuclear antibody;
CRP, C-reactive protein;
ESR, erythrocyte sedimentation rate;
PMR, polymyalgia rheumatica;
SLE, systemic lupus erythematosus.

Examination

Examination can help make the decision as to whether the pain is arising from the joints, muscles or soft tissues. The joints should be examined for signs of inflammation. Power in all four limbs should be measured and the soft tissues palpated for areas of tenderness.

Examination of other systems is also important. The presence of livedo reticularis and a facial rash would suggest SLE, whilst the discovery of hepatomegaly and lymphadenopathy would raise the suspicion of malignancy.

Investigation

Investigations should be guided by the examination findings. It is important to remember that they may be normal in the early stages of disease and should be repeated if symptoms persist. For example, the radiological signs of inflammatory arthritis may take months to appear.

Blood tests

- The ESR is likely to be raised in cases of PMR, inflammatory arthritis, SLE or malignancy.
- Serum calcium levels may be low in osteomalacia.
- Parathyroid hormone levels should be checked in the presence of hypercalcaemia to exclude hyperparathyroidism.
- Serum alkaline phosphatase may be elevated in osteomalacia. It can also rise in response to inflammation.
- An immunology screen, including measurement of antinuclear and anti-double-stranded DNA antibodies and immunoglobulin levels, will be abnormal in active SLE.
- Rheumatoid factor is found in the serum of up to 90% of patients with rheumatoid arthritis.

Radiological investigations

X-rays of the small joints may show the erosive changes of inflammatory arthritis. Radiographs of the long bones and pelvis should be taken if the patient has risk factors for osteomalacia, such as reduced sunlight exposure or intestinal malabsorption. Looser's zones may be seen.

Other radiological tests (e.g. chest X-ray, abdominal ultrasound scan) may be necessary if there is any suspicion of malignancy.

An acute hot swollen joint

Objectives

You should be able to:

- Give a list of differential diagnoses for a hot swollen joint.
- Take a history from a patient picking out relevant details.
- Understand how to investigate a hot swollen knee.

Differential diagnosis

- Septic arthritis.
- Crystal synovitis.
  —Gout
  —Pseudogout.
- Inflammatory arthritis (rheumatoid arthritis or seronegative spondyloarthropathy).
- Transient synovitis.
- Haemarthrosis.

The phrase 'acute hot swollen joint' implies that the patient has presented as an emergency with rapid onset of symptoms and a large painful effusion.

History focusing on the acute hot swollen joint

Pain

Patients with acute gout or septic arthritis classically have very severe pain. However, it is difficult to differentiate these conditions from other causes of hot swollen joints as the majority of patients will present with intense pain that is worse on movement.

Patient age and sex

All of the above conditions could present in the adult patient, whereas only septic arthritis, reactive arthritis and possibly inflammatory arthritis are likely causes in children.

Gout is more common in men, and rheumatoid arthritis is more common in women.

Which joint?

Certain joints are more commonly affected by specific disorders (Fig. 3.1):

- Gout commonly affects the first metatarsophalangeal (MTP) joint of the foot.
- Pseudogout is common in the knee and wrist.
- Multiple joint involvement points to an inflammatory disorder such as rheumatoid arthritis (RA) or juvenile idiopathic arthritis (JIA).

Is the patient ill?

Fever, night sweats, rigors and general flu-like symptoms suggest likely infection but it is possible to have the same symptoms in an acute 'flare-up' of an inflammatory arthropathy.

Previous history

This is likely in gout as 90% of patients with an acute attack will have recurrent episodes.

It is unlikely in septic arthritis unless the patient has a predisposing factor such as sickle cell disease (see Ch. 18).

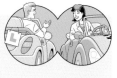

Be careful. Patients with known inflammatory or crystal arthritis can present with joint infection and due to the effects of immunosuppressant drugs may not mount the usual inflammatory response. As such the joint may not have the typical features associated with infection.

Fig. 3.1 Likely diagnosis for each joint in a patient presenting with an acute hot swollen joint.

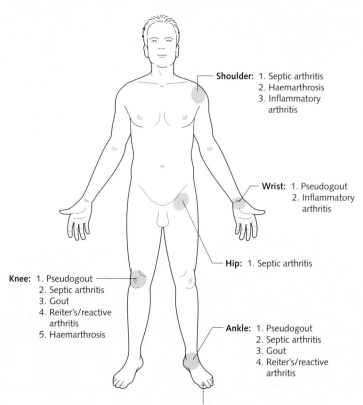

Shoulder: 1. Septic arthritis
2. Haemarthrosis
3. Inflammatory arthritis

Wrist: 1. Pseudogout
2. Inflammatory arthritis

Hip: 1. Septic arthritis

Knee: 1. Pseudogout
2. Septic arthritis
3. Gout
4. Reiter's/reactive arthritis
5. Haemarthrosis

Ankle: 1. Pseudogout
2. Septic arthritis
3. Gout
4. Reiter's/reactive arthritis

First metatarsophalangeal joint: 1. Gout

Associated symptoms

Patients with an inflammatory disorder may have systemic features of the disease process such as sacroiliac joint pain in ankylosing spondylitis or painful metacarpophalangeal (MCP) joints in RA.

Eye symptoms can occur in:

- Reiter's syndrome (conjunctivitis).
- Rheumatoid arthritis (keratoconjunctivitis).
- Juvenile idiopathic arthritis (uveitis).

Patients with a history of recent sexually transmitted disease or diarrhoea are likely to have Reiter's syndrome.

Also consider gonococcal arthritis in patients with a history of sexually transmitted diseases (STDs).

A recent viral illness can result in a reactive arthritis.

Past medical history

Gout is linked with increased cell turnover and therefore any illness can predispose to it due to increase in breakdown products.

Patients with malignancy having chemotherapy are particularly prone to gout due to vast numbers of cells being 'killed' (see Ch. 14).

As mentioned in Chapter 18, certain conditions also predispose to joint infection, e.g. intravenous drug use (IVDU).

Patients with a bleeding disorder (such as haemophilia) or on warfarin are at risk of developing an acute haemarthrosis (bleeding into a joint). These patients can present in such a way with an acutely swollen tender joint.

Drug history

Diuretics and low dose aspirin can increase uric acid levels, predisposing to gout.

Patients on steroids or other immunosuppressants are at increased risk of infection.

Social history

Alcohol excess predisposes to gout and high purine diets also contibute.

Examination of a patient with an acute hot swollen joint

General

- Most patients presenting in such a way will look unwell, be uncomfortable and may be agitated.
- A pyrexia suggests infection but mildly elevated temperatures can be present in gout and inflammatory arthritis.
- The patient should be examined for general signs of inflammatory arthritis.
- Patients with gout may have gouty tophi; these are commonly found on extensor surfaces of the elbow and fingers.

The joint

- The knee is the most commonly affected joint overall.

- Any affected joint will have a tense effusion and be exquisitely tender to any passive movement.
- A full examination of the joint is unnecessary and impossible!
- A thorough examination of other joints should be performed to make sure the patient has a monoarthritis (i.e. no other joints are involved).

Investigation of a patient with an acute swollen joint

An algorithm for the investigation of a patient with an acute swollen joint is shown in Figure 3.2.

Blood tests

The aim of initial investigation is to confirm or exclude septic arthritis. Do not rely on blood tests alone which may be normal.

- A raised white cell count (WCC) suggests infection but can be raised due to inflammatory causes.
- Inflammatory markers C-reactive protein (CRP) and erythrocyte sedimentation rate (ESR) can be raised in all the conditions listed above,

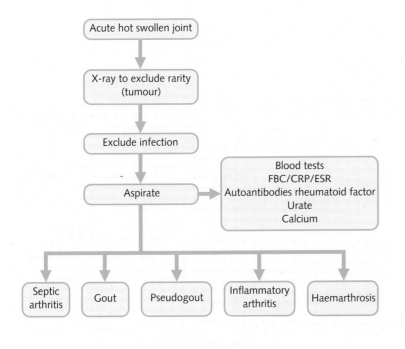

Fig. 3.2 Algorithm for the investigation of an acute hot swollen joint. CRP, C-reactive protein; ESR, erythrocyte sedimentation rate; FBC, full blood count.

25

particularly septic arthritis and inflammatory arthritis.

Normal inflammatory markers cannot completely exclude infection.

- Serum urate may be elevated, normal or low in patients with acute gout.
- Serum calcium should be checked as pseudogout can be caused by hyperparathyroidism.
- If haemarthrosis is suspected a clotting screen should be performed and patients on warfarin should have their international normalized ratio (INR) checked.

X-rays

Plain X-rays of the affected joint may show:

- Normal appearances.
- Chondrocalcinosis (found in pseudogout due to calcium deposition in menisci).
- Bony erosions associated with gout or inflammatory arthritis.

Of all the investigations the most important is aspiration of the joint.

Aspiration/synovial fluid analysis

- A superficial joint such as the knee is simple to aspirate, particularly when there is a tense effusion.
- Deeply situated joints such as the hip require ultrasound or X-ray guidance.
- In every case fluid aspirated must be sent to microbiology for urgent microscopy, culture and sensitivity (usually written as M, C and S). In addition to this the technician should look for crystals.
- The general appearance of the aspirate should be described (see Chs 1 and 30).

Ultrasound

Ultrasound scanning is useful to detect an effusion, particularly in the hip.

A child with a limp

4

Objectives

You should be able to:

- Give a list of the most likely differential diagnoses according to the age of the child.
- Understand what to look for on examination of the neonate, infant and child.
- Investigate a child with a limp to rule out serious conditions.
- Differentiate between an ill and a well child.

Differential diagnosis

- Septic arthritis.
- Irritable hip.
- Developmental dysplasia of the hip (DDH).
- Perthes disease.
- Slipped upper femoral epiphysis (SUFE).
- Osteomyelitis.
- Occult trauma.
- Neuromuscular causes.
- Juvenile idiopathic arthritis.
- Malignancy (very rare).

History focusing on the child with a limp

There is a big difference between an infant aged 15 months and an adolescent aged 15 years. Infants will not give an accurate history and if very unwell may be distressed and uncooperative. The majority of children do, however, give a good history.

Age

The most important factor in assessing a child with a limp is the age of the child. Figure 4.1 shows the likely differential diagnosis depending on the age of the child.

Sex

The sex of the child can also give clues to the diagnosis; for example, Perthes disease is much more common in boys than in girls.

Is the child ill?

To answer this question the general state of the child must be noted. Systemically unwell children will show little interest in play or food and simply will not be themselves. Fever, rigors and night sweats should be noted as well as duration of symptoms. An unwell child suggests infection or juvenile idiopathic arthritis (JIA).

Pain

Most children limp because of pain.

Any child complaining of knee pain must be suspected of having hip pathology.

The history in Perthes disease is often of a vague gradual onset of pain and limp.

More sudden onset of pain is more likely due to trauma or infection.

The classic history for a slipped upper femoral epiphysis is often a background of hip pain for weeks followed by sudden increase in pain.

Transient synovitis of the hip gives pain in the groin and mimics septic arthritis.

Occasionally sinister causes of pain (such as bone tumours) present with gradually increasing pain (including night pain) not relieved by simple analgesia.

Painless limp

- Late-presenting DDH presents with a limp and leg length discrepancy.

Fig. 4.1 Diagnosis by age in a child with a limp.

Diagnosis by age in a child with a limp	
All ages	Infection (septic arthritis or osteomyelitis) Juvenile idiopathic arthritis
Infant (1–3 years)	Late-presenting developmental dysplasia of the hip (DDH) Irritable hip Neuromuscular Occult trauma (including non-accidental injury)
Childhood (3–11 years)	Perthes disease Irritable hip Neuromuscular Slipped upper femoral epiphysis (SUFE) Non-accidental injury (NAI)
Adolescence (12–16 years)	SUFE Infection

- Neuromuscular disorders such as cerebral palsy result in poor gait due to muscle imbalance rather than pain.
- Cerebral palsy can present as developmental delay but milder forms can present later in childhood as the weakness becomes more apparent.
- Muscular dystrophy can also present with gradual onset of weakness and limp.

Associated symptoms

History of injury may be elicited in occult trauma but in non-accidental injury (NAI) this will not be forthcoming.

Multiple joint aches and pains suggest juvenile arthritis.

A recent history of upper respiratory tract infection (URTI) or otitis media is often found in patients with transient synovitis.

In JIA the eyes can be involved as part of the systemic effects of the disease. If left untreated blindness can result.

Past medical history

Any previous history of Perthes disease or slipped upper femoral epiphysis (SUFE) is very important as these patients are at increased risk of developing disease in the opposite hip.

Family history

A family history of Perthes disease and DDH also leads to an increased risk.

Examining a child with a limp

General

Systemic features of ill-health such as pyrexia, drowsiness and irritability should be noted and will point towards infection as the cause.

Multiple joint problems may be obvious initially, suggesting juvenile idiopathic arthritis.

Neuromuscular disorders may be obvious or detected on neurological examination.

Inspection

Gait
- An antalgic gait is present in painful conditions such as Perthes or irritable hip.
- A Trendelenburg gait (see Ch. 27) is present in a toddler with late DDH.
- Neuromuscular disorders give a variety of patterns of gait abnormality.
- A worrying sign is a child too ill or in too much pain to weight-bear.

Standing
- An abnormal single large posterior skin crease is present in DDH.
- In slipped upper femoral epiphysis or infection, the hip is often held in an abnormal position of external rotation and flexion (Fig. 4.2).

Further inspection could reveal scars, swelling or erythema.

- Perthes disease results in loss of abduction and flexion. Complete loss of abduction is a worrying sign in Perthes as this may indicate subluxation of the joint.
- In septic arthritis any movement gives extreme pain.

Investigating a child with a limp

Figure 4.3 provides an algorithm for the investigation of a child with a limp.

Blood tests

Markedly raised white cell count (WCC), erythrocyte sedimentation rate (ESR) and C-reactive protein (CRP) are present in infection but these inflammatory markers can also be mildly increased in synovitis or JIA.

Very rare causes of abnormal blood tests include leukaemia. Creatinine kinase is raised in muscular dystrophy.

X-rays

A plain X-ray is often unnecessary in the younger child, particularly in cases of transient synovitis.

A hip radiograph may show:

- A dislocated hip.
- Perthes disease.
- A slipped upper femoral epiphysis.
- Evidence of infection (remember X-rays are initially normal).
- A fracture.

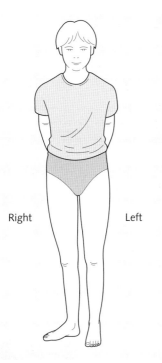

Right Left

Fig. 4.2 External rotation deformity: child with externally rotated right leg in slipped upper femoral epiphysis.

Fixed flexion

If the Thomas test is positive (a fixed flexion deformity) suspect significant pathology such as advanced Perthes, DDH or SUFE.

Limb length discrepancy

- A short leg is typical of DDH.
- Apparent shortening (see Ch. 27) will be present if there is any fixed flexion deformity.

Palpation

Palpate any tender areas for effusion, warmth and localized pain.

Tenderness over the tibial tubercle is likely to be due to Osgood–Schlatter disease.

The hip joint cannot be palpated because it is a deep joint

Palpation around the knee will reveal joint line tenderness in conditions such as osteochondritis or, in older children, meniscal tears.

Movement

- Loss of hip movements indicates pathology.
- DDH results in loss of abduction compared with the other side.

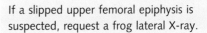
If a slipped upper femoral epiphysis is suspected, request a frog lateral X-ray.

If you are sure the problem is from the knee then anteroposterior (AP) and lateral knee X-rays should be performed and may show:

- Osgood–Schlatter disease.
- Osteochondritis dissecans.
- A fracture.

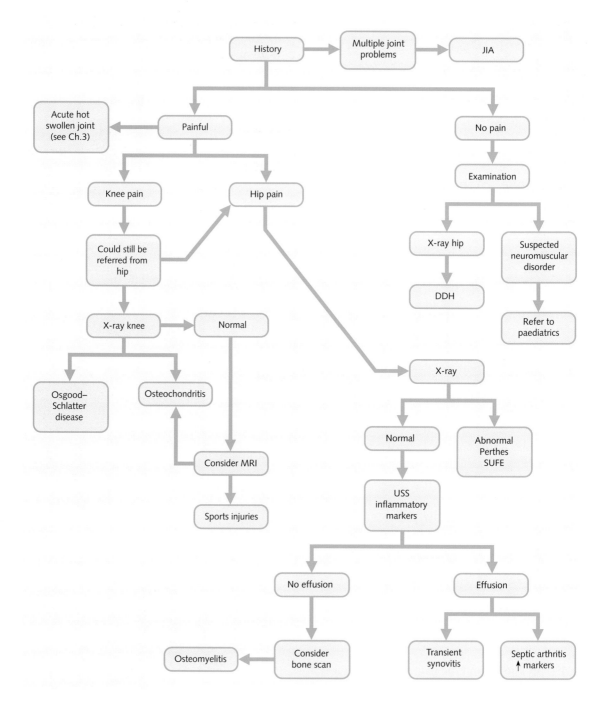

Fig. 4.3 Algorithm for the investigation of a child with a limp. DDH, developmental dysplasia of the hip; JIA, juvenile idiopathic arthritis; SUFE, slipped upper femoral epiphysis; USS, ultrasound scan.

Ultrasound

Ultrasound is a very useful investigation for suspected joint problems, particularly of the hip, which is deeply situated.

The scan will show an effusion in:

- Septic arthritis.
- Transient synovitis.
- Perthes disease (early).

Isotope bone scanning

If hot, this is likely to be significant and possible causes are:

- Osteomyelitis—the scan will also show any seeding of infection.
- Malignancy.

Magnetic resonance imaging (MRI)

MRI is not a first-line investigation in children but is useful in:

- Diagnosis of knee disorders (see Ch. 22).
- Bone and soft tissue tumours.
- Osteomyelitis.

Definition

A deformity is due to an abnormal alignment or appearance of bone, joint or soft tissues.

A deformity can be correctable (able to return to original position) or fixed.

- Valgus deformity—bent away from the midline.
- Varus deformity—bent towards the midline.

Valgus and varus deformities of the knee are illustrated in Figure 5.1.

Causes of deformity

There are many causes of deformity and rather than list all of them the different causes have been listed as three groups, as follows:

1. Soft tissue:
   —Scarring
   —Swelling
   —Wasting
   —Overgrowth, e.g. Dupuytren's contracture.
2. Bone:
   a. Congenital
   b. Acquired:
      —Previous fracture
      —Infection
      —Tumours
      —Metabolic bone disease, e.g. sabre tibia in Paget's disease
      —Growth plate injury.
3. Joint:
   —Contracture (e.g. Volkmann's ischaemic contracture)
   —Muscle imbalance (e.g. polio)

   —Chronic arthritis (varus knee in osteoarthritis).

History focusing on deformity

Patients present with deformities for different reasons:

- Pain (usually associated with arthritic conditions).
- Disability (e.g. shortening of limb).
- Appearance (e.g. scoliosis).

Deformities in children are usually noted by the parents and often these patients have normal variations of growth and simply need reassurance (see Ch. 15).

It is important to recognize whether the deformity is due to a generalized disease process or only affects one limb.

An important initial question would be to ask if any other joints or limbs are involved.

Congenital deformities

Congenital deformities usually present at birth and are noted at delivery, although some will now be picked up on antenatal scanning.

An obstetric, birth and family history (the deformity could be present in siblings or either parent) should be noted.

Patients (or parents, if a child) will usually tell you they have 'had it since birth'.

If this is the case ask what has changed to make the patient seek help now.

The deformity may have progressed or become painful.

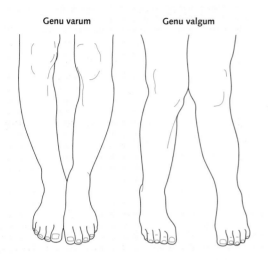

Genu varum   Genu valgum

Fig. 5.1 Genu varum and genu valgum.

Cerebral palsy produces variable clinical deformities as the child grows.

Late presentation of developmental dysplasia of the hip (DDH; see Ch. 15) can occur, in which case the child will present with a limp.

Acquired deformities

Post-fracture, injury or sepsis

As a general rule deformities resulting from injuries are unilateral (i.e. you usually only injure one limb) and deformities from arthritis are bilateral (e.g. hand disease in rheumatoid arthritis).

This is usually progressive unilateral deformity following a specific injury.

Patients can often 'manage' very well with severe deformity until many years after an injury and then present with pain as secondary osteoarthritis becomes symptomatic.

Painful deformities

A painful deformity suggests an arthritic process but the patient is much more likely to present with pain before deformity becomes apparent. Typical deformities are varus knees and Heberden's nodes in osteoarthritis.

Paget's disease can also present with painful deformity.

Painless deformity

Painless deformity is common with neurological causes (such as ulnar claw hand) or in Dupuytren's disease.

Such conditions affecting the hand can cause significant disability due to loss of function.

Following a cerebrovascular accident (CVA) a patient has deformity due to muscle spasticity.

Loss of function

There is a wide variation in the effects of the deformity on function. Simple things such as being unable to wear a pair of shoes because of toe deformities can cause significant disability. Patients with severe Dupuytren's disease have difficulty washing their face (sometimes poking themselves in the eye!).

Appearance

Often patients simply complain about the appearance of the deformity.

Scoliosis causes a prominent rib hump which is unsightly, and as most patients are of adolescent age significant distress results. If very severe, spinal deformity can result in chest complications due to decreased expansion.

One of the most common deformities seen is hallux valgus (bunions) and patients may 'only' complain that they have difficulty finding shoes to fit (not a good reason to operate)!

Associated symptoms

Generalized joint swelling and pain with deformity suggest inflammatory arthropathy.

Progression of deformity

The timing of events is important. Patients may have had the deformity for some years and present because there has been sudden progression or interference with day-to-day activities.

Examination of a patient with a deformity

There are features common to all deformities but the majority involve assessment of a limb or digit as described in Chapter 27.

Is the deformity correctable?

A deformity can be fixed or mobile.

- A mobile deformity will return to its original position when stressed. Only joint deformities can be mobile; an example is early varus deformity in osteoarthritis of the knee.
- A fixed deformity will not return to the original position. Most deformities are fixed. An example of a fixed deformity is a malunited tibial fracture.

Is there an associated condition?

Examine the whole patient to look for any generalized conditions associated with deformities such as an inflammatory arthritis.

- A patient with rheumatoid arthritis (RA) may have several typical deformities (usually in the hand).
- Patients with psoriatic arthropathy often present with very severe hand deformities (arthritis mutilans).
- A patient with cerebral palsy needs regular assessment, as deformity due to muscle imbalance can lead to fixed deformity (see Ch. 15, Fig 15.8) and secondary bone changes.

Common joint deformities

We will now look at each joint, looking for common deformities.

Hand

Examination of the hand may show:

- Thickened palmar fascia with fixed flexion deformity of the proximal interphalangeal (PIP) and metacarpophalangeal (MCP) joints (most commonly of the little and ring fingers), indicating Dupuytren's disease (Fig. 5.2).
- Heberden's nodes in osteoarthritis.
- Ulnar drift of the MCP joint, boutonnière deformity and swan-neck deformity, indicating rheumatoid arthritis.
- Ulnar claw hand.

Elbow

The most important deformities at the elbow are cubitus valgus and cubitus varus (Fig. 5.3) and they are usually secondary to childhood fractures (supracondylar fracture of the elbow).

Shoulder

- A dislocated shoulder results in an abnormal contour (see Ch. 22).
- A winged scapula results from a long thoracic nerve palsy and the scapula is lifted off the chest wall on pushing forward.

Spine

- A torticollis (muscle spasm of the sternocleidomastoid muscle) causes the head to turn to the affected side.
- A kyphosis is a flexion deformity of the spine (Fig. 5.4).

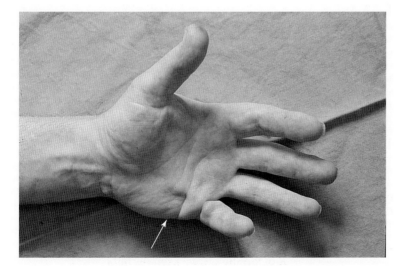

Fig. 5.2 Dupuytren's contracture of the palmar fascia (from Klippel J H, Dieppe P A (eds) 1998 Rheumatology, 2nd edn. Mosby, London).

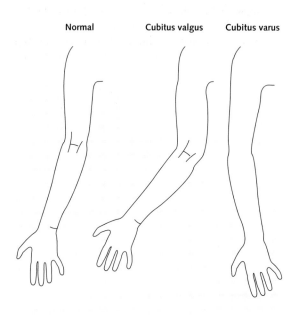

Fig. 5.3 Normal angle of the elbow, cubitus valgus and cubitus varus.

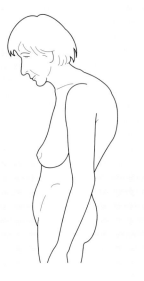

Fig. 5.4 A thoracic kyphosis.

- A scoliosis is a lateral and rotational curvature of the spine.

Hip

- Hip conditions may present with leg length discrepancy.

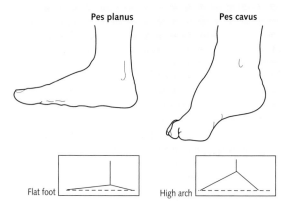

Fig. 5.5 Features of pes planus and pes cavus.

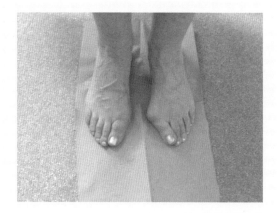

Fig. 5.6 Hallux valgus (bunions): right post- and left pre-operation. Note that the great toe is also pronated.

- Fixed flexion of the hip gives patients an abnormal posture with the knee flexed and they often stoop to the affected side.

Knee

The knee is one of the most common sites for obvious clinical deformity.

- Varus or valgus knees can be constitutional (inherited) or secondary to degenerative change.
- Fixed flexion deformity of the knee results in loss of full extension and commonly occurs in osteoarthritis.

Foot and ankle

Deformities of the foot and ankle are also common (Figs 5.5 and 5.6). Common deformities of the fore-foot are shown in Figure 29.14 (p. 202).

Investigation of a deformity

The majority of simple deformities need little or no investigation.

- Blood tests. If inflammatory arthropathy is suspected check erythrocyte sedimentation rate (ESR), C-reactive protein (CRP), rheumatoid factor (RhF), autoantibodies.
- Abnormal biochemistry is present in Paget's disease (see Ch. 12).

- X-rays. The joint or limb involved will usually require X-ray examination.
- Nerve conduction studies are useful in assessing deformity secondary to peripheral nerve injury, e.g. ulnar claw hand.
- Computed tomography (CT) scans are sometimes used to reconstruct complex deformities (3-D CT reconstruction).

A limb swelling

Objectives

You should be able to:

- Give a list of differential diagnoses for a limb swelling.
- Take a focused history from a patient with a limb swelling.
- Examine and describe a limb swelling.
- Know how to investigate a limb swelling.
- Recognize sinister features of a limb swelling.

Differential diagnosis

It is helpful to consider differential diagnoses in relation to the anatomical location.

- Skin or subcutaneous:
  —Rheumatoid nodule
  —Lipoma
  —Bursitis
  —Neurofibroma
  —Cyst.
- Joint:
  —Joint effusion
  —Ganglion
  —Baker's cyst.
- Bone:
  —Bone tumour
- Muscle/deep soft tissues:
  —Sarcoma.

Patients commonly present with lumps, bumps and swellings. The majority of these are benign, but it is important not to overlook very rare tumours presenting in this way.

History focusing on a swelling

The following points are important:

Duration of symptoms
How long has the patient had the lump or swelling, and when did the patient first notice it?

Increase in size
Has it increased in size recently or grown rapidly? Tumours may present in this way.

Solitary or multiple
Does the patient have more than one lump or swelling and if so where? Neurofibromata or rheumatoid nodules are often multiple.

Variability
Does the swelling come and go and if so over what period? Classically a ganglion will disappear and then recur.

Is it painful?
A tense effusion will be painful, as may bursitis. Deep pain related to a bony or soft tissue mass may be sinister. The majority of such lesions are not painful.

Loss of function
Does the swelling or lump inhibit the patient in any way. Swellings around the hand can be a nuisance to patients and those on the foot can rub when shoes are worn.

Associated symptoms

Usually there will be none.

The general health of the patient should be ascertained with weight loss, fatigue and poor health being sinister symptoms.

Occasionally large swellings or masses can compress vessels or nerves, e.g. osteochondroma.

Patients presenting with joint swelling may have other symptoms related to the underlying disease process, such as pain in the joint if arthritic.

A patient may have painless joint swelling as a presenting feature of a more generalized inflammatory condition. It is important therefore to ask about other joints such as those in the hand.

A patient with a Baker's cyst may have pain in the knee.

Occupational history

Patients who kneel frequently, such as carpet fitters, are very prone to developing prepatellar bursitis.

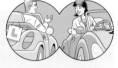

Patients will often think that their swelling is a cancer. Ask them if they are worried about it and if you are sure it is nothing to worry about (as the vast majority are) then tell them! Often patients don't mind having a small lump such as a lipoma or ganglion and just need reassurance.

Examination focusing on a swelling

The affected area or joint should be examined and also the local lymph nodes.

The following points relate to a swelling or mass rather than a joint effusion, which should be obvious on clinical examination.

When examining a lump or swelling the following points should be elicited.

Site
Which limb is affected and where is the lesion?

Size
Sinister pathology should be suspected in any lump larger than 5 cm.

Skin

- Is the lesion within the skin, in the subcutaneous tissue or deep to the fascia? Painful deep lesions are suspicious and need investigation.

- Is the skin normal over the lesion, inflamed or abnormal?

Consistency
Is the lesion soft, firm or hard? A lipoma is often described as firm.

Diffuse or discrete
Some swellings are large without clear margins and appear to merge with the surrounding structures, whereas others are more easily palpable.

Surface
Is the surface of the lesion smooth or irregular?

Mobile or fixed
A discrete mass may be fixed to the underlying structures, like a ganglion, or more mobile, e.g. a lipoma.

Fluctuance
Fluctuant lesions contain fluid, such as a Baker's cyst.

Pulsatile
Pulsatile and expansile lesions are vascular aneurysms.

Transillumination
Fluid-filled or soft lesions (e.g. lipoma) will transilluminate when tested with a pen torch if the fluid is clear.

The patient presenting with joint swelling only

This has been covered in Chapters 2 and 3. Occasionally a patient will present with swelling of a single large joint and this can be the onset of a generalized condition such as rheumatoid arthritis.

Therefore examine other joints such as the hand (if rheumatoid arthritis is suspected) or the spine (if ankylosing spondylitis).

Investigation of a patient with a swelling

We will consider joint swelling as a separate condition from a discrete swelling or mass.

Joint swelling (effusion)
Exclude infection (see Ch. 3).

Blood tests should be carried out, including rheumatoid factor and autoantibodies to look for inflammatory arthritis.

X-rays may show osteoarthritis/rheumatoid arthritis or be normal.

Synovial fluid analysis is performed for gout and pseudogout.

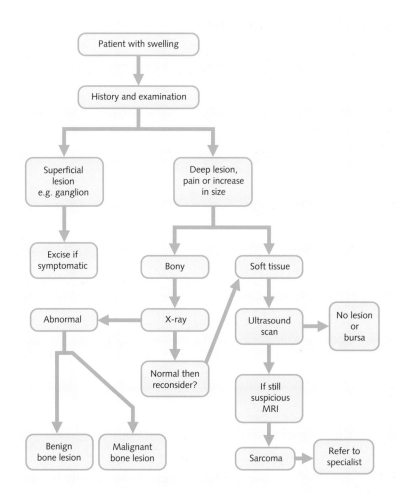

Fig. 6.1 Algorithm for the investigation of a limb swelling. MRI, magnetic resonance imaging.

A limb swelling or lump

Further investigation may be unnecessary.

For example, a patient has a cystic lesion on the volar aspect of the wrist, which comes and goes and is fixed to deep structures. The lesion is firm, smooth and transilluminates. This patient has a ganglion and this can be confirmed by aspirating jelly-like fluid.

Further investigation is necessary if there is doubt about a diagnosis.

- If bony pathology is suspected an X-ray of the affected limb should be performed. A benign or malignant bony lesion may be found.

- A deeply situated soft tissue lesion may be a sarcoma and if so needs further investigation.
- An initial ultrasound scan may be useful to confirm the presence of a mass and whether it is fluid filled or solid.
- However, an MRI scan with contrast gives detail regarding the exact nature of the lesion.
- If doubt still exists, the patient should be referred to a specialist sarcoma service and the next step would be a biopsy.
- An algorithm for the investigation of a limb swelling is given in Figure 6.1.

An incidental bone lesion on X-ray

It is quite common for patients to present with bony lesions on X-ray. These are usually incidental findings (the X-ray was taken for another reason such as minor trauma and an abnormality is found) and cause great concern to patients.

Examples include a chest X-ray taken for respiratory disease showing a lesion in the clavicle or a pelvic X-ray taken for hip disease showing metastatic prostate carcinoma.

Differential diagnosis of a lesion on X-ray

Benign lesions are quite common.

Primary bone malignancy is extremely rare.

Secondary bone tumours are common in the elderly.

Infection can present as a bone lesion.

Benign tumours/disorders

- Osteochondroma.
- Osteoid osteoma.
- Enchondroma.
- Bone cysts.
- Fibrous dysplasia.

Malignant tumours

- Primary:
  —Osteosarcoma
  —Ewing's sarcoma
  —Chondrosarcoma.
- Secondary—metastatic deposit:
  —Breast
  —Lung
  —Prostate
  —Renal
  —Thyroid
  —Bowel.
- Haemopoietic diseases:
  —Myeloma
  —Lymphoma.

Infection

- Osteomyelitis.

Metabolic bone disease

- Paget's disease.

Describing bone lesions on X-ray

Practise describing bone defects and lesions whenever possible.

1. Name and age of patient.
2. Site—which bone and where in the bone:
   - The lesion can be in the diaphysis (shaft), metaphysis (cancellous bone between the growth plate and shaft) or epiphysis (between the growth plate and the joint).
   - The lesion can primarily affect either the cortex or medulla of the bone.
3. Appearance:
   - The lesion can be lytic (e.g. breast metastasis) (Fig. 7.1), sclerotic (e.g. prostate metastasis), mixed or calcified (enchondroma).

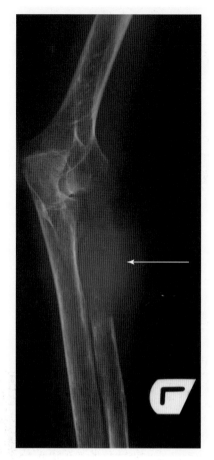

Fig. 7.1 Lytic lesion (proximal radius) is suggestive of malignancy.

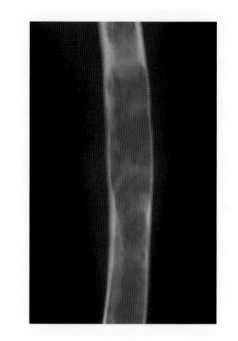

Fig. 7.2 Fibrous dysplasia (from Klippel J H, Dieppe P A (eds) 1998 Rheumatology, 2nd edn. Mosby, London).

6. What is the lesion doing to the bone?
   - Cortical destruction is typical of a malignant process.
   - Cortical thinning does occur in benign disease due to expansion.

History of incidental X-ray finding

When the patient returns following the X-ray the following points must be elicited in the history, looking for clues as to the diagnosis.

Age of patient

Certain lesions such as bone cysts are more common in children, and other benign bone lesions such as enchondroma usually occur in young adults.

Overall, primary malignant tumours are very rare and metastatic bone disease is a disease of the elderly.

Pain

Although the patient may not have offered pain as a symptom initially, when a lesion is discovered the patient must be asked if the area is painful. The

- Ground glass (fibrous dysplasia) (Fig. 7.2).
- Abnormal bony architecture, e.g. post-osteomyelitis.
4. Zone of transition:
   - A well-defined border between the lesion and the normal bone suggests a benign slow-growing lesion (it is clearly demarcated).
   - A broad, irregular or indistinct zone of transition where the change from abnormal to normal is poorly defined suggests a malignant process (Fig. 7.3).
5. What is the bone doing in response?
   - A significant periosteal reaction with Codman's triangle (see Fig. 22.4, p. 159), onion skinning and sunray spicules (Fig. 7.4) is a feature of malignancy.
   - Infection can also cause a periosteal reaction.

44

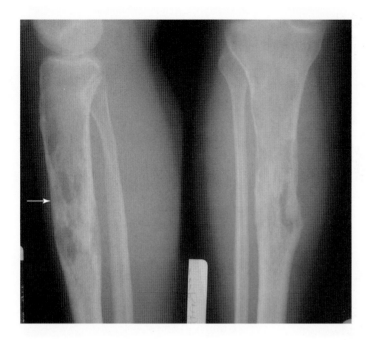

Fig. 7.3 A poorly defined zone of transition suggests malignancy.

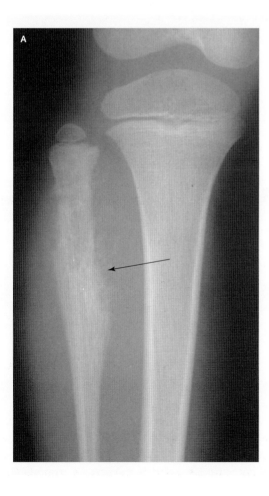

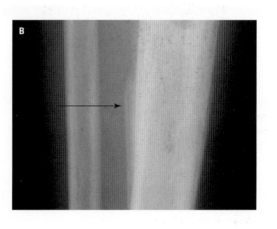

Fig. 7.4 Primary bone tumour showing: (A) sunray spicules; (B) onion skinning.

patient may have ignored any pain or just put it down to 'arthritis playing up'.

Pain that is severe and does not respond to simple analgesia, particularly if night pain is a feature, suggests a malignant process.

Swelling

Benign lesions are more likely to present with swelling, particularly osteochondroma, a lesion commonly found around the knee.

Malignant tumours may have pain and swelling but it is rare for a bone tumour to present with swelling only.

General health

General features of ill-health such as tiredness, weight loss, poor appetite and fever suggest a systemic illness such as malignancy, haemopoietic disorders or infection.

Primary bone malignancy is unlikely to present with widespread features of malignancy as patients will usually present with pain and swelling before these general features have developed.

It is important to ask about any other areas of pain in the musculoskeletal system, particularly if considering widespread metastatic disease.

Past medical history

A previous history of carcinoma is extremely important when dealing with such a patient. The lesion should be treated as a metastatic lesion until proven otherwise.

Breast malignancy can be dormant for many years prior to re-presenting with metastases.

Examination focusing on a patient with an X-ray abnormality

Site

Different lesions are more common in certain locations, for example enchondromas are more common in the hand.

Secondary bone metastases tend to be found in the central skeleton.

Limb examination

Examination of the affected limb will usually be normal.

Tenderness, redness and swelling would be present in:

- Impending or actual fracture associated with a bone metastasis.
- Osteomyelitis.
- Osteoid osteoma.
- Malignant primary bone tumour.

Malignant secondaries or bone lesions from haemopoietic diseases rarely show any external features.

Generalized

In secondary malignancy with unknown primary, it is important to examine:

- Breast (for carcinoma).
- Chest (for lung tumours).
- Abdomen (for renal or bowel tumours and evidence of haemopoietic disease such as liver and spleen enlargement).
- Per rectum (PR) (prostate).
- Thyroid (for carcinoma).

Investigation of a bone lesion on X-ray

The X-ray

It is important to obtain two views taken at 90° to one another and to obtain full-length views of the entire bone (to ensure there are no further lesions along the same bone).

Most benign lesions need no further investigation and repeat X-rays after 6 months are useful to ensure the bone lesion does not change in appearance and develop any sinister features.

Further investigation

Further investigation is only necessary if there is doubt about the diagnosis or to confirm or exclude malignancy.

It is not uncommon for patients to present with a lesion on X-ray to find they have metastatic disease from an unknown primary. Make sure this news is broken in the right way, preferably once all the information is available and with relatives and nursing staff present.

Blood tests

- A full blood count (FBC) may show anaemia of chronic disease.
- Liver function tests (LFTs) could be deranged if liver metastases are present.
- The calcium profile is often raised in generalized malignancy, and alkaline phosphatase is raised in Paget's disease.
- C-reactive protein (CRP) and erythrocyte sedimentation rate (ESR) are raised in infection or malignancy.
- A very high ESR suggests myeloma. It is confirmed with serum electrophoresis and urinary Bence Jones proteins.
- Prostate-specific antigen (PSA) is elevated in prostate malignancy.
- Carcinoembryonic antigen (CEA) is elevated in bowel carcinoma.

Isotope bone scan

This is a very useful tool to detect further lesions in malignancy or to see if a lesion is active (i.e. hot on bone scan). Infection will show up 'hot' as will malignant lesions.

Of the benign lesions only osteoid osteoma will show increased uptake.

Computed tomography (CT)

CT is used to confirm osteoid osteoma.

Magnetic resonance imaging (MRI)

MRI can detect early metastatic lesions before X-ray features are apparent.

It is also used to define the extent of malignant bone tumours and can help to distinguish between benign and malignant lesions.

Biopsy

It can be very difficult to be certain of the diagnosis in some cases. A biopsy will prove whether the tumour is benign or malignant and exclude infection as the cause.

Altered sensation and weakness

You should be able to:

- Recognize patterns of neurological pain from the history and examination.
- Give a differential diagnosis for neurological symptoms affecting the upper and lower limbs.
- Know common investigations used to investigate neurological conditions.

Neurological symptoms occur when there is a nerve lesion. Patients may complain of numbness, pins and needles, electric shock type pain, burning, hypersensitivity, pain, and weakness. The pattern of these symptoms will help diagnose which nerve is causing the problem.

Differential diagnosis

- Carpal tunnel syndrome.
- Ulnar nerve entrapment.
- Morton's neuroma.
- Tarsal tunnel syndrome.
- Post surgery, e.g. superficial radial nerve neuroma.
- Spinal pathology
  —Disc prolapse
  —Osteoarthritis
  —Cervical rib
  —Malignancy.
- Nerve tumours, e.g. neurofibroma, schwannoma.
- Medical causes, e.g. multiple sclerosis.
- Peripheral neuropathy, e.g. alcoholism, diabetes mellitus, drugs, vitamin B12 deficiency.
- Complex regional pain syndrome.

History

The following points should be covered:

Site

Global or specific.

Very important in determining which nerve is affected (see examination section).

Onset of symptoms

- Acute onset usually occurs with disc prolapse where pain may be the main feature.
- Gradual onset where there is gradual increase in nerve compression, e.g. spinal stenosis.
- May occur after trauma, e.g. carpal tunnel syndrome after distal radius fracture.
- Accidental laceration to a nerve during surgery can result in a painful neuroma and is most common at the elbow (ulnar nerve) and wrist (superficial radial nerve).

Nature of symptoms

Exacerbating features
Sneezing and coughing often exacerbate symptoms of leg pain with disc prolapse.

Relieving features
- Patients with carpal tunnel syndrome often get night pain which is relieved by hanging their hand down off the bed.
- Patients with lumbar spinal stenosis suffer pain, and numbness in their legs after walking short distances (spinal claudication) which is relieved by sitting forward.

Associated features
- Loss of bowel or bladder function in patients with back pain should be treated as cauda equina syndrome until proven otherwise.
- Check for constitutional features such as weight loss, malaise, or haemoptysis (lung cancer) if malignancy is suspected. Pancoast's tumour can present with shoulder symptoms.

- Patients with undiagnosed diabetes mellitus may have weight loss, polyuria and polydipsia associated with peripheral neuropathy.

Past medical history

The following can predispose to nerve lesions:

- Pregnancy can predispose to carpal tunnel syndrome (see page 181 for other predisposing conditions).
- Malignancy.
- Previous surgery.
- Trauma.
- Osteo and rheumatoid arthritis.
- SLE.

Drug history

Some chemotherapy agents can cause peripheral neuropathy.

Social history

Manual jobs may trigger ulnar or carpal tunnel symptoms.

Alcohol.

Family history

Neurofibromatosis (Von Recklinghausen's disease).

Examination

Knowledge of myotomes and dermatomes will help determine the level of a spinal cord lesion. For peripheral nerve lesions know the sensory distribution and motor function. Some special tests may reproduce nerve symptoms such as tapping a nerve (Tinel's test). Café au lait spots are characteristic of neurofibromatosis.

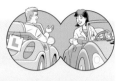

Patients with severe carpal tunnel syndrome will often be having sleepless nights. They look tired, unhappy and even depressed. It is important not to underestimate the effect this has and take this into consideration when planning treatment. Simple splints may allow them a good night's sleep.

Investigation

Plain radiographs of the spine will show osteophytes causing nerve root compression. MRI provides very detailed soft tissue images and is commonly used to investigate spinal pathology such as a disc prolapse. Ultrasound can diagnose a Morton's neuroma. Nerve conductions studies are used routinely to confirm carpal tunnel syndrome and can be used to diagnose other peripheral nerve lesions.

DISEASES AND DISORDERS

Osteoarthritis

Objectives

You should be able to:

- Define and classify osteoarthritis (OA).
- List the causes of secondary OA.
- Outline the pathological processes in the development of OA .
- Describe the clinical features of OA.
- Describe the X-ray features of OA.
- Understand the basic conservative and surgical treatments for OA.

Definition

Osteoarthritis (OA) is a non-inflammatory disorder of synovial joints characterized by articular surface wear and formation of new bone (attempts at repair). It is also known as degenerative joint disease and characterized by joint pain, stiffness and swelling of joints.

Incidence

Osteoarthritis is the most common joint disease, affecting up to 85% of the population at some time in their lives. It is often asymptomatic and the true prevalence of symptomatic OA in the western world is around 20%.

Pathology and aetiology

Histologically the weight-bearing cartilage surface degenerates and eventually wears away completely, exposing the subchondral bone, which becomes eburnated (Fig. 9.1). Cysts occur because of microfracture of the articular surface and new bone laid down (sclerosis) in the surrounding bone. Disorganized new bone is produced at the margins of joints (osteophytes) as the disease progresses. In addition to this, the synovial lining becomes thickened and inflamed, often producing excess synovial fluid (an effusion).

These changes explain the four cardinal features seen on X-ray of joint space: narrowing, sclerosis, cysts and osteophytes.

Osteoarthritis is described as primary where no underlying cause is found or secondary where there is a clear predisposing factor.

Primary osteoarthritis has many aetiological factors but the exact cause is not known. A variety of genetic and environmental factors are implicated in causing osteoarthritis. This type of arthritis is more common in women and increases with age.

In secondary osteoarthritis a cause is clearly identified and these are shown in Figure 9.2.

Clinical features

The presenting complaints of patients with osteoarthritis are variable. The patient is usually systemically well and complains of pain which is usually aching or burning in nature and localized to the joint but may be referred to the joint below.

The history is often of gradually increasing, asymmetrical joint pain over several years, the level of which is variable but can be severe. The pain is

53

Early changes

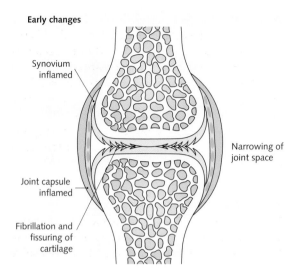

Synovium inflamed

Narrowing of joint space

Joint capsule inflamed

Fibrillation and fissuring of cartilage

Changes secondary to loss of cartilage

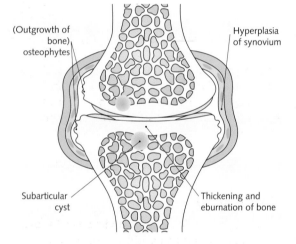

(Outgrowth of bone) osteophytes

Hyperplasia of synovium

Subarticular cyst

Thickening and eburnation of bone

Fig. 9.1 Pathological changes in osteoarthritis.

worse after activity and relieved by rest, and as the disease progresses night pain can be a feature. Occasionally patients present with rapidly destructive OA, which can mimic a septic or inflammatory arthritis.

Classically pain in the hip can be referred to the knee.

Secondary causes of osteoarthritis

Congenital/developmental

Developmental dysplasia of the hip
Perthes disease
Slipped upper femoral epiphysis

Acquired
Trauma:
• Fractures involving joint surfaces
• Fractures causing significant deformity
• Ligamentous injury causing joint instability
Infection—septic arthritis
Avascular necrosis
Inflammatory arthritis, e.g. rheumatoid arthritis
Neuropathic—Charcot joints
Metabolic, e.g. Paget's disease
Iatrogenic—post-surgery, e.g. meniscectomy

Fig. 9.2 Secondary causes of osteoarthritis.

Patients can present with only one or multiple joint involvement.

Other symptoms include swelling, deformity (bow legs—varus knee), stiffness and weakness (usually secondary to wasting). Patients will also complain they are unable to do certain activities, which may be recreational or more basic activities of daily living (for example, patients with severe osteoarthritis of the hip are unable to put on socks or cut their own toenails).

Almost any synovial joint can be affected by osteoarthritis, most commonly the knee, hip, hands (often the first carpometacarpal joint), fingers (distal interphalangeal (DIP) joints) but also the spine, shoulder, elbow and wrist (Figs 9.3 and 9.4).

The examination begins as the patient enters the room.

• Look for a limp, use of a stick and how reliant the patient is on relatives for simple tasks such as undressing for examination.
• Deformity may be obvious but also note previous scars, redness, swelling and wasting of muscles on inspection.
• Palpate for an effusion, joint line tenderness and crepitus (cracking noise can be heard in severe cases).
• The range of movement of the particular joint will be diminished and there may be fixed deformity.
• The joints above and below should be examined.

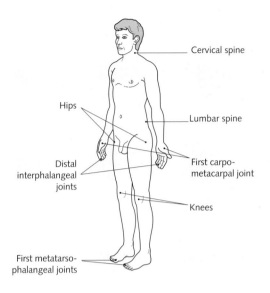

Fig. 9.3 Joints commonly affected by osteoarthritis.

Cervical spine

Hips

Lumbar spine

Distal interphalangeal joints

First carpo-metacarpal joint

Knees

First metatarso-phalangeal joints

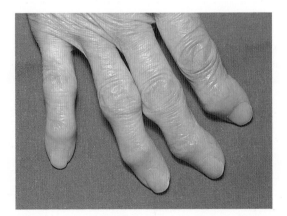

Fig. 9.4 Osteoarthritis of the hand, showing Herberden's nodes at the distal interphalangeal joints and Bouchard's nodes at the proximal interphalangeal joints (from Haslett C, Chilvers E R, Boon N A et al (eds) 2002 Davidson's principles and practice of medicine, 19th edn. Churchill Livingstone, Edinburgh).

Classic features of osteoarthritis include Herberden's nodes of the DIP joint and a Baker's cyst behind the knee.

Diagnosis and investigation

In many cases the diagnosis is clear from the history and clinical examination, and apart from a plain X-ray further investigation may be unnecessary.

Blood tests may be required to exclude septic or inflammatory arthritis in atypical cases if the treating doctor is not certain of the diagnosis.

X-rays will usually show decreased joint space, sclerosis, subchondral cysts and osteophytes (Fig. 9.5).

Management

There is no cure for osteoarthritis and treatment is aimed at relieving pain and maintaining function. The treatment for osteoarthritis can be conservative or surgical.

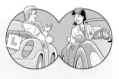

A detailed social history is very important in patients who have osteoarthritis. Ask about occupation, activities of daily living and hobbies. What is their normal mobility? These type of questions help to assess patients' quality of life and how their condition affects them.

Conservative

- Initially lifestyle advice including weight loss, regular exercise and avoidance of impact loading activities is given. Non-steroidal anti-inflammatory drugs such as diclofenac are good in the early stages providing the patient does not have a history of peptic ulceration. Other regular analgesia such as codeine and paracetamol should be prescribed if required.
- Physiotherapy improves gait and function of an affected limb, and simple measures such as a walking stick reduce pain on walking.
- Glucosamine is widely taken by the population at large but the small beneficial effect shown in some studies is probably a placebo effect.
- Injections of corticosteroids are useful for temporary relief, especially in patients unfit for surgery; however, there is a small risk of infection. New treatments such as hyaluronic

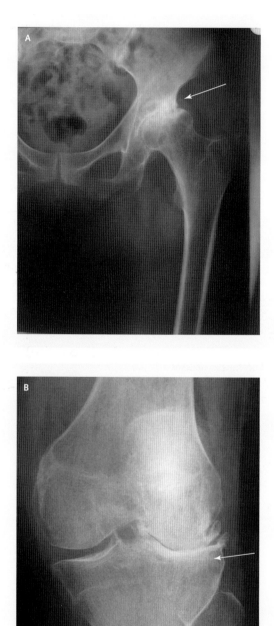

acid derivatives given by injection are expensive and not yet proven.

Surgical

Surgical treatments for osteoarthritis depend on the age of the patient, the joint involved and the level of pain and disability experienced. This is dealt with in more detail in Chapter 20.

The decision to operate can be difficult to make, as all surgery has risks and complications. Surgery may help when the patient says, 'I cannot cope any longer with the pain.'

Fig. 9.5 Features of osteoarthritis on X-ray: (A) hip; (B) knee.

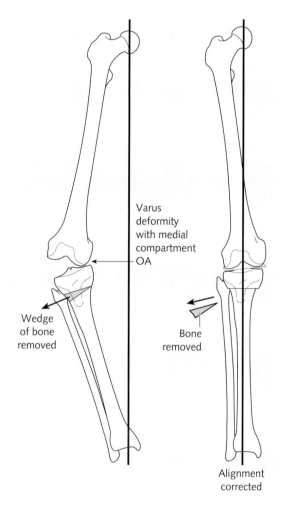

Varus deformity with medial compartment OA

Wedge of bone removed

Bone removed

Alignment corrected

Fig. 9.6 Osteotomy of the knee.

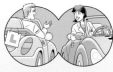

Arthroplasty surgery is not risk free and patients should be told that although the pain should improve, the joint will never function like a normal joint. Surgery can also have serious complications including infection and thromboembolism which in a small percentage of patients may be fatal. This must be explained during the consent process.

There are five things a surgeon can do to a joint:

1. Debride and washout. This is usually done for osteoarthritis of the knee and gives temporary relief in some patients although there is little evidence to support this.
2. Joint replacement (arthroplasty). This is most commonly of the hip or knee. It gives excellent pain relief in 90% of patients for at least 10 years.
3. Joint fusion. The two sides are removed and fused together. This is most commonly used around the foot and ankle; good pain relief is achieved provided fusion occurs but obviously movement is lost.
4. Joint excision. This is less commonly used nowadays. It is still used occasionally in the first metatarsophalangeal (MTP) joint and where other methods have failed (e.g. hip—Girdlestone's procedure).
5. Realignment surgery. Increased load passing through a joint because of a deformity often leads to osteoarthritis. The surgeon can realign the limb by breaking the bone above or below the joint, removing a wedge of bone and correcting the deformity. The most common site for this procedure is the knee. The patient will usually have a varus deformity of the knee (bow legs). The tibia is realigned to redistribute the load more evenly, slowing the progression of osteoarthritis. See Figure 9.6.

Further reading

Miller M D 2004 Review of orthopaedics, 4th edn. WB Saunders, Philadelphia

Solomon L, Warwick D, Nayagan D (eds) 2001 Apley's system of orthopaedics and fractures, 8th edn. Hodder Arnold, London

Orthoteers website: http://www.orthoteers.co.uk

Objectives

You should be able to:

- Understand the role that cytokines play in the pathogenesis of rheumatoid arthritis (RA).
- Describe the usual distribution of joint inflammation in RA.
- Recognize the common hand deformities caused by RA.
- Understand that RA causes systemic symptoms in addition to joint pain.
- List the causes of anaemia in RA.
- Describe the four main radiological signs of RA.
- Recognize the importance of the multidisciplinary team in the care of patients with RA.
- Name some disease-modifying antirheumatic drugs used in the treatment of RA.

Definition

Rheumatoid arthritis (RA) is a common inflammatory condition. It is characterized by polyarticular arthritis and follows a chronic course, resulting in significant disability. RA is a multi-system disease and is associated with a reduction in life expectancy.

RA has a major impact on patients' lives. After 20 years, 80% of patients are disabled. Life expectancy is reduced by between 3 and 18 years.

Incidence and prevalence

RA affects females more commonly than males. Most studies show a female-to-male excess of between two and four times. The annual incidence in the UK is 0.1–0.2/1000 in males and 0.2–0.4/1000 in females. RA prevalence in Europeans and North American Caucasians is close to 1%.

Aetiology

The aetiology of RA has not been explained. It appears to be multifactorial, with both genetic and environmental factors having an important influence.

Genetic factors

Genetic factors contribute approximately 50% to the aetiology. The inheritance of certain human leucocyte antigen (HLA) genes increases RA susceptibility and severity. HLA-DR4 is particularly important.

Environmental factors

Environmental influences on the development of RA are not well understood. People have examined the effects of various infections, occupations and lifestyle factors, but no links have been found.

Immunological abnormalities

In rheumatoid arthritis, the immunological mechanisms that usually protect the body by fighting infections and destroying malignant cells target normal tissue, resulting in joint damage. T-lymphocytes play a key role in the initiation of inflammation in RA (Figs 10.1–10.3).

The activated cells produce cytokines (intercellular messenger proteins), e.g. tumour necrosis factor-α (TNF-α), interleukin-1 (IL-1). These cytokines have many actions, including those shown in Figure 10.4.

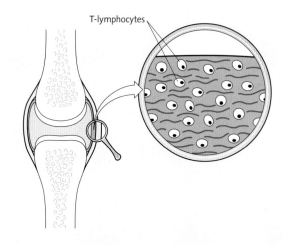

Fig. 10.1 T-lymphocytes (predominantly T-helper cells) accumulate in the synovium.

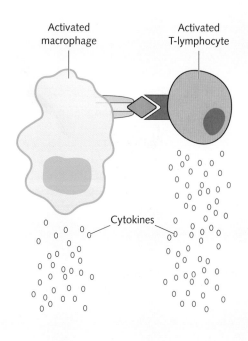

Fig. 10.3 T-lymphocytes with appropriate receptors interact with the macrophages and both cell types become activated.

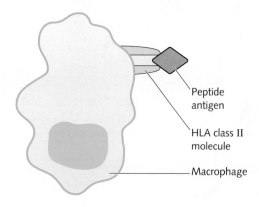

Fig. 10.2 Synovial macrophages (antigen-presenting cells) express peptide antigens on their cell surfaces in association with human lymphocyte antigen (HLA) class II molecules.

Actions of cytokines
Stimulation of inflammation
Attraction of other immune cells
Excess synovial fluid production
Cartilage destruction
Bone resorption
Stimulation of B-lymphocyte differentiation and maturation
Increased antibody production, including production of rheumatoid factor

Fig. 10.4 Actions of cytokines.

Rheumatoid factor is found in the serum of approximately 80% of patients with RA. High levels are associated with more severe disease and the presence of extra-articular features.

Pathology

The main pathological abnormality in RA is synovitis. As inflammatory cells infiltrate the synovium, it proliferates. Chronically inflamed tissue (pannus) extends from the joint margins, and erodes the articular cartilage (Fig. 10.5). Extensive erosion of cartilage and bone, with concomitant involvement of ligaments and joint capsules, leads to joint deformity.

Subcutaneous rheumatoid nodules are found in up to 20% of patients. They usually accompany severe disease and are possibly due to small vessel

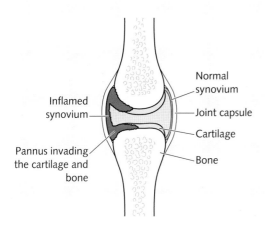

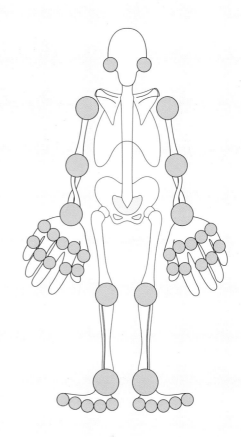

Fig. 10.5 Diagram of a synovial joint. One side is healthy, the other shows the pathological changes of RA.

vasculitis. Histology reveals a central area of fibrinoid necrosis surrounded by fibroblasts.

Clinical features

RA can develop at any time of life from infancy to old age. The peak age of onset is in the fourth and fifth decades. Symptoms usually begin gradually, developing over weeks or months. However, some people experience an acute onset.

The clinical features of RA can be divided into:

Fig. 10.6 The joints most commonly affected by RA.

- Articular features.
- Extra-articular features:
  —Systemic
  —Periarticular
  —Affecting distant organs.

Articular features of RA

The usual presenting symptoms of rheumatoid arthritis are joint pain, stiffness and swelling. Stiffness is usually noticed on waking in the morning and tends to improve as the day progresses. The duration of this early-morning stiffness is a useful marker of disease activity. RA predominantly targets small and medium joints in a symmetrical fashion (Fig 10.6), but sometimes other patterns of joint involvement are seen.

Monoarthritis
Occasionally, a patient presents with a monoarthritis of a larger joint such as the knee or shoulder.

Palindromic rheumatism
Synovitis appears to move rapidly from one region to another. Inflammation of one or more joints begins acutely, lasts for hours or days and then settles quickly. Patients experience recurrent attacks and many go on to develop typical RA.

Pain and stiffness lead to varying degrees of functional loss. Even in the early stages of the disease, patients can struggle with everyday tasks such as dressing and turning on taps because of active synovitis. In established RA, joint destruction results in further limitations.

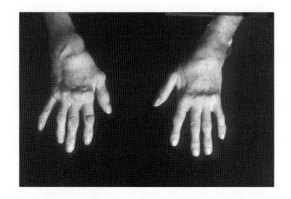

Fig. 10.7 The hands of a patient with RA. Note the synovitis of the wrists, metacarpophalangeal and proximal interphalangeal joints.

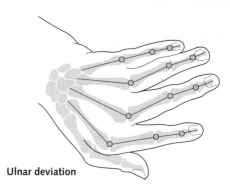

Fig. 10.8 Ulnar deviation.

Patients usually feel extremely frustrated by their loss of function. It is important that doctors listen sympathetically to their concerns and help them to find solutions. For example, the secretary who struggles to type because of her wrist pain may benefit from input from an occupational therapist and some wrist splints.

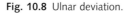

Fig. 10.9 Boutonnière and swan-neck deformities.

Synovitis causes 'boggy' joint swelling. The skin overlying an affected joint is usually warm and red due to increased local blood flow. On palpation, the swelling is tender and has a similar consistency to that of a grape.

The effects of RA on specific joint regions

The rheumatoid hand and wrist The hands and wrists are almost always involved in RA (Fig. 10.7). Synovitis typically occurs in the wrists, metacarpophalangeal (MCP) and proximal interphalangeal (PIP) joints, sparing the distal interphalangeal (DIP) joints. This inflammation can weaken the ligaments and tendons, producing well-recognized deformities.

Ulnar deviation of the fingers results from metacarpophalangeal joint synovitis (Fig. 10.8). Subluxation of the metacarpophalangeal joints can occur, with the proximal phalanges drifting in an ulnar and volar direction.

Boutonnière and swan-neck deformities of the digits are due to proximal interphalangeal joint synovitis and laxity and/or contractures of the extensor and flexor apparatus (Fig. 10.9). The boutonnière deformity is characterized by PIP flexion and DIP hyperextension. With swan-neck deformity there is MCP flexion, PIP hyperextension and DIP flexion.

Radial deviation of the wrist occurs to compensate partly for ulnar deviation of the fingers. Subluxation of the wrist results in prominence of the ulnar styloid.

The foot Forefoot synovitis and damage are common in rheumatoid arthritis. The proximal phalanges sublux dorsally and the metatarsal heads become eroded and displaced towards the floor. They can be easily palpated through the sole of the foot and

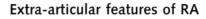

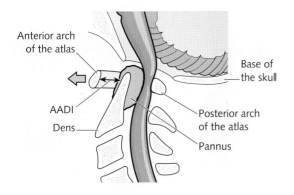

Anterior arch
of the atlas

Base of
the skull

AADI

Dens

Posterior arch
of the atlas

Pannus

Fig. 10.10 In normal adults, the distance between the anterior arch of the atlas and the dens (anterior atlanto-dental interspace, or AADI) should not exceed 3 mm. The diagram shows forward subluxation of the atlas on the axis. The spinal cord is compressed between pannus around the dens and the posterior arch of the atlas.

make weight-bearing very uncomfortable. Patients often feel as though they are 'walking on marbles'. Hindfoot involvement can also cause problems, with subtalar arthritis. Patients with established disease develop valgus deformities here.

The cervical spine Inflammation and erosive disease, affecting the uncovertebral joints and stabilizing ligaments of the first two cervical vertebrae, can result in atlantoaxial subluxation. The atlas slips forward on the axis, reducing the space around the spinal cord (Fig. 10.10). This produces neck pain that radiates to the occiput. Upper motor neuron damage resulting in a spastic quadriparesis is a rare complication.

Damage to the articulation between the occiput and atlas may allow the odontoid peg to move upwards, through the foramen magnum. This can threaten the cervical cord and brainstem, sometimes resulting in sudden death after minor jolts to the head and neck.

It is important to take lateral flexion X-rays of the cervical spine in RA patients requiring a general anaesthetic. The anaesthetist must be aware of any cervical instability so that precautions can be taken during intubation.

Extra-articular features of RA

Periarticular features

In addition to joint inflammation, patients with RA often experience other musculoskeletal problems.

Rheumatoid nodules Rheumatoid nodules are firm subcutaneous swellings that tend to develop in areas affected by pressure or friction, such as the fingers, elbows and Achilles tendon. They are seen in patients who test positive for rheumatoid factor. Nodulosis at any site can be complicated by infection.

Tenosynovitis and bursitis Tendon sheaths and bursae are lined with synovium. This can become inflamed in RA, resulting in tenosynovitis and bursitis. The flexor tendons of the fingers are often affected by tenosynovitis. The olecranon and subacromial bursae are common sites of bursitis.

Carpal tunnel syndrome Synovitis can cause entrapment of peripheral nerves. Median nerve compression resulting in carpal tunnel syndrome is common.

Systemic features of RA

As well as causing joint pain and swelling, active RA makes people feel generally unwell. The inflammation can result in systemic symptoms such as fever, weight loss and lethargy. These can be prominent, particularly in people with acute-onset RA, in whom infection and malignancy are important differential diagnoses.

When patients with RA first present, they have often felt fatigued for several months. They find it reassuring to hear that that systemic symptoms are common and usually improve when the joint inflammation is treated.

The effects of RA on distant organs

RA can affect many body systems (Fig. 10.11). Extra-articular disease can be serious and is associated with an increase in mortality.

Anaemia Anaemia of RA can be due to:

- Anaemia of chronic disease.
- Autoimmune haemolysis.
- Felty's syndrome.

Fig. 10.11 Extra-articular manifestations of RA.

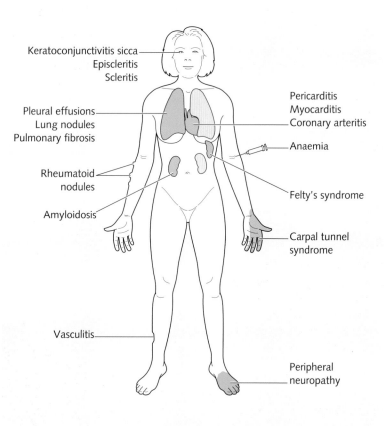

Keratoconjunctivitis sicca
Episcleritis
Scleritis

Pericarditis
Myocarditis
Coronary arteritis

Pleural effusions
Lung nodules
Pulmonary fibrosis

Anaemia

Rheumatoid nodules

Felty's syndrome

Amyloidosis

Carpal tunnel syndrome

Vasculitis

Peripheral neuropathy

Drugs used in the treatment of RA can also induce anaemia. Non-steroidal anti-inflammatory drugs can cause iron deficiency as a result of chronic blood loss from gastrointestinal inflammation. Disease-modifying antirheumatic drugs sometimes produce anaemia via bone marrow suppression.

Felty's syndrome Felty's syndrome is the association of RA with splenomegaly and leucopenia. It usually occurs in patients who are rheumatoid factor positive. The leucopenia leads to frequent bacterial infections. Lymphadenopathy, anaemia and thrombocytopenia can also occur.

Rheumatoid lung disease Although pulmonary disease is common in RA, it does not always produce symptoms. Males are more frequently affected than females.

Pleural effusions can occur early in the disease, sometimes preceding the arthritis. Rheumatoid factor can be detected in the fluid, which is a transudate. Lung nodules are found in patients who are seropositive and usually have subcutaneous nodules.

They rarely cause symptoms, but can cavitate or become infected. Pneumonitis can lead to pulmonary fibrosis.

Cardiac disease Pericardial inflammation is common in RA, but rarely symptomatic. Pericardial effusions can occur. Myocarditis is a rare manifestation of RA. Coronary arteritis is also rare and usually occurs as part of a generalized vasculitis.

Eye disease Keratoconjunctivitis sicca affects at least 10% of patients with RA. Eyes are dry because of reduced tear production and the cornea and conjunctiva can become damaged. Episcleritis and scleritis are less common. Both cause redness and often pain of the eye. Severe scleritis can rarely result in spontaneous scleral perforation, so needs treating aggressively.

Amyloidosis Secondary amyloidosis develops as a result of chronic inflammation. Many organs can be infiltrated, including the kidneys, heart, liver and gastrointestinal tract. Proteinuria due to renal disease is the commonest manifestation of amyloidosis in RA. Prognosis is poor.

Vasculitis Vasculitis occasionally complicates RA. It predominates in patients who are seropositive for rheumatoid factor and have severe disease. Common clinical features include leg ulcers and peripheral neuropathy. Rarely, there is involvement of coronary or cerebral vessels which leads to cardiac or cerebral ischaemia.

Investigations

The following investigations are useful:

Blood tests

Full blood count may show anaemia of chronic disease, thrombocytosis secondary to inflammation or leucopenia of Felty's syndrome.

Erythrocyte sedimentation rate, C-reactive protein and plasma viscosity are usually raised in the presence of synovitis and they are useful markers of response to treatment.

Rheumatoid factor is found in the serum of 70–90% of RA patients, but is often not detectable during the first few months of the disease. Those patients who lack the antibodies are sometimes described as having 'seronegative rheumatoid arthritis'. It is important to remember that rheumatoid factor is also found in at least 1% of the normal population. Patients with positive rheumatoid factor are more likely to have systemic involvement and have a worse prognosis.

Another serological test is now available to help with the diagnosis of rheumatoid arthritis. Anti-CCP (cyclic citrullinated peptide) antibodies can be present in patients who are rheumatoid factor negative and are felt to indicate a worse prognosis. They are not associated with systemic features.

Patients with joint pain are often told that they have RA on the basis of a positive rheumatoid factor alone. Rheumatoid factor can be present in 'healthy' people. The diagnosis of RA should only be made after interpreting the findings of a detailed clinical history and examination, and the results of all investigations.

Radiological investigations

Plain X-rays should be obtained to look for signs of RA (Fig. 10.12). These tend to be seen first in the small joints of the hands and feet (Figs 10.13 and 10.14).

Radiological changes are often not apparent when patients first present with RA. In patients with normal X-rays, but persistent symptoms, it is useful

The four main radiological signs of RA

Soft tissue swelling
Periarticular osteoporosis
Juxta-articular erosions
Narrowing of joint space

Fig. 10.12 The four main radiological signs of RA.

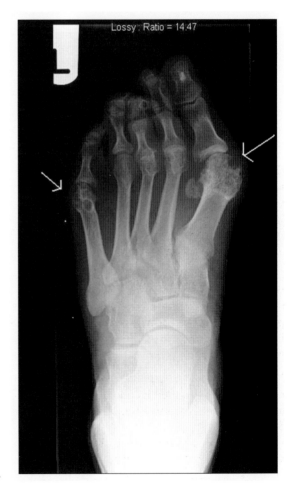

Fig. 10.13 Periarticular osteopenia and erosions of the metatarsophalangeal (MTP) joints

to repeat the X-rays after several months. Erosions can be detected sooner using ultrasound or magnetic resonance imaging.

The tests discussed above are always useful in the investigation of patients with possible RA. However, different clinical presentations often require additional investigations.

Management

Patients with RA should be cared for by a multidisciplinary team. Figure 20.8 (p. 147) lists the operations commonly performed on patients with RA. Figure 10.15 lists the professionals involved in the care of RA patients and gives details of the roles they play.

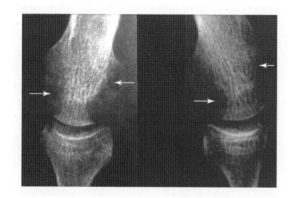

Fig. 10.14 Large erosions of two MCP joints.

Drug treatment

There are two main aims of drug treatment in RA:

- Reduction of symptoms.
- Prevention of damage by control of disease.

Non-steroidal anti-inflammatory drugs (NSAIDs)

NSAIDs can improve joint pain and stiffness, but have no effect on disease activity or progression. If a patient does not respond to one NSAID, it is worth trying another.

Corticosteroids

Corticosteroids can swiftly improve pain and swelling in RA. Low doses of oral prednisolone are often used to control symptoms early in the disease before DMARDs (see below) become effective. Corticosteroids can be given intra-articularly to treat local synovitis and are sometimes given via the intramuscular or intravenous route for a generalized flare of rheumatoid arthritis.

Disease-modifying antirheumatic drugs (DMARDs)

DMARDs are capable of suppressing disease activity and may slow progression of erosive joint damage. Some DMARDs suppress the immune system; others inhibit cell replication. However, for many of these drugs, the mechanism of action is not completely understood.

Professionals involved in the care of RA patients and the roles they play	
Professional	**Role**
Rheumatologist	Monitoring of disease activity Prescription and monitoring of drug therapy Identification and management of complications Referral to other specialists when necessary Coordination of team
Orthopaedic surgeon	Replacement of damaged joints Surgical synovectomy
Physiotherapist	Use of physical therapies to combat inflammation (e.g. ice, warmth) Prescription of exercises to maintain and improve muscular strength and range of joint movement
Occupational therapist	Splinting of acutely inflamed joints Advice on how to function whilst putting as little stress as possible on the joints (joint protection) Provision of aids and appliances to assist with activities of daily living
Podiatrist	Assessment of footwear and advice on choosing suitable shoes Provision of insoles to improve the mechanics of deformed feet Prevention and treatment of skin lesions, such as calluses and ulcers

Fig. 10.15 Professionals involved in the care of RA patients and the roles they play.

Some disease-modifying drugs and their potential side-effects

DMARD	Possible side-effects
Azathioprine	Gastrointestinal (GI) upset Bone marrow suppression
Cyclophosphamide	Bone marrow suppression Increased risk of malignancy Infertility
Ciclosporin	Renal impairment Hypertension Bone marrow suppression
Gold	Rash Proteinuria Bone marrow suppression
Hydroxychloroquine	Retinal damage
Leflunomide	Hypertension GI upset Bone marrow suppression
Methotrexate	GI upset Oral ulcers Raised liver enzymes Pneumonitis Bone marrow suppression
D-penicillamine	Rash Proteinuria Bone marrow suppression
Sulfasalazine	GI upset Raised liver enzymes Bone marrow suppression

Fig. 10.16 Some disease-modifying drugs and their potential side-effects.

DMARDs are slow-acting and take several weeks to produce a clinical effect. If a patient does not respond adequately to one DMARD, a second can be added or substituted.

Like many drugs, DMARDs can cause minor side-effects, including nausea, headache and rashes (Fig. 10.16). More serious complications such as bone marrow suppression, abnormal liver function and renal impairment are rarer, but well recognized. It is therefore important to monitor patients receiving DMARD therapy. The monitoring protocol depends on the drug prescribed. For example, a patient taking methotrexate should have a full blood count and tests of liver and renal function performed at intervals of 4–8 weeks.

Biological therapies

Biological therapies that target inflammatory mediators in RA are now widely used. Three agents that are currently available inhibit TNF-α. Etanercept is a soluble TNF-α receptor, and infliximab and adalimumab are monoclonal antibodies against TNF-α. These drugs produce good clinical results but are expensive and carry an increased risk of infection. The National Institute of Clinical Excellence (NICE) have issued strict guidelines for the use of these drugs in the UK. Disease activity scoring systems are employed to demonstrate that the biological drugs are producing good clinical responses. There is some evidence to suggest that patients who do not respond to one anti-TNF agent may respond if they are switched to another.

Drugs that manipulate other cytokines are in various stages of development. Rituximab is a monoclonal antibody against B cells which is used in the treatment of RA when anti-TNF therapy has failed. Abatacept is a T cell co-stimulation modulator.

Further reading

Cooper N J 2000 Economic burden of rheumatoid arthritis: a systematic review. *Rheumatology* **39**: 28–33

Gordon D A, Hastings D E 2003 Clinical features of rheumatoid arthritis. In: Hochberg et al (eds) Rheumatology, 3rd edn. Mosby, London, p 765–780

Moreland L W, Emery P 2003 TNF-inhibition in the treatment of rheumatoid arthritis. Taylor & Francis, London

O'Dell J R 2001 Combinations of conventional disease modifying anti-rheumatic drugs. *Rheum Dis Clin North Am* **27**: 415–426

Spondyloarthropathies

Definition

The term 'spondyloarthropathy' (SPA) (or 'spondyloarthritis') describes a group of related and often overlapping inflammatory joint disorders (Fig. 11.1). The SPAs are characterized by enthesitis as well as synovitis, and occur in patients who are seronegative for rheumatoid factor. For this reason, they are sometimes referred to as 'seronegative spondyloarthropathies'. An enthesis is the insertion of a tendon, ligament or capsule into bone.

Aetiology

All types of SPA are genetically associated with HLA-B27, a major histocompatibility complex (MHC) class 1 antigen. HLA-B27 is more closely linked with some SPAs than others. It is most prevalent in ankylosing spondylitis, affecting 85–95% of these patients. The antigen is carried by approximately 10% of healthy Caucasians.

The true aetiology of the SPAs is unknown. Infection is thought to be important. Bacterial DNA and proteins have been detected in joints affected by reactive arthritis (see below) and it is thought that infection may play a role in the development of other SPAs. It is possible that bacteria trigger an immune reaction in genetically predisposed people. There is an association with inflammatory bowel disease, which may be explained by an increase in the permeability of the gut to pathogens.

Pathology

The entheses are the key sites of inflammation in SPA. Initial inflammation and erosions are followed by fibrosis and ossification, which can result in ankylosis of joints. In ankylosing spondylitis (AS), the outer fibres of the vertebral discs become inflamed where they attach to the corners of the vertebral bodies. Erosions cause squaring of the vertebrae, and ossification leads to formation of syndesmophytes (bony bridges). The sacroiliac joints are commonly affected and often become fused. Synovitis is another feature of the SPAs. Peripheral joints tend to be more commonly involved in psoriatic and reactive arthritis than in enteropathic arthritis and AS.

Pathological changes are not always confined to the musculoskeletal system. Cardiac and pulmonary abnormalities can occur.

ANKYLOSING SPONDYLITIS

Clinical features

The prevalence of ankylosing spondylitis (AS) amongst Caucasians is 0.5–1%. It is three times more common in men than in women and tends to be more severe in men. It usually develops in early adulthood, with the peak age of onset being in the mid-20s. Presentation after the age of 45 years is rare.

Clinical features can be divided into two groups:

- Musculoskeletal.
- Extraskeletal.

Musculoskeletal features

Most symptoms in AS are due to spinal and sacroiliac disease. The typical patient presents with a gradual onset of lower back pain and stiffness. Symptoms are worse early in the morning and after long periods of rest. They usually improve with exercise. Involvement of the thoracic spine and enthesitis at the costochondral junctions may cause chest pain. Disease of the costovertebral joints can reduce chest expansion and restrict breathing.

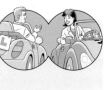

Lower back pain is common and usually due to mechanical or degenerative problems. It is important to consider the possibility of spinal inflammation, particularly when assessing young patients with troublesome back pain. Always ask about the presence of morning stiffness.

In the early stages of the disease, patients may have few clinical signs. The sacroiliac joints are often tender and pain can be reproduced by applying physical stress to the joints. This can be achieved by

The spondyloarthropathies
Ankylosing spondylitis
Psoriatic arthropathy
Reactive arthritis
Reiter's syndrome
Enteropathic arthritis

Fig. 11.1 The spondyloarthropathies.

applying pressure on the anterior superior iliac spines whilst the patient is lying supine.

Mobility of the lumbar spine is reduced. The Schober test is used to assess forward flexion in this region of the spine (see Fig. 11.2). With a pen, a mark is made on the skin at the lumbosacral joint, level with the dimples of Venus. A second mark is made 10 cm above. The patient bends forward with the legs straight and attempts to touch the floor. The distance between the two marks should increase by at least 5 cm.

Some patients with AS have an abnormal Schober test, but are able to touch their toes because of good hip flexion.

Most patients with AS experience exacerbations and remissions. In those with severe disease, the spine becomes progressively stiffer and posture deteriorates (Fig. 11.3). The normal lumbar lordosis is lost and the thoracic and cervical spines become increasingly kyphotic. The resulting stooped posture further restricts chest expansion and causes the abdomen to protrude. It is sometimes referred to as the 'question-mark posture'. Spinal disease can be complicated by atlantoaxial subluxation and fractures.

The peripheral joints are involved less commonly than the axial skeleton in AS. Inflammation tends to target medium/large joints such as the shoulders, hips or knees. Pain and tenderness due to enthesitis

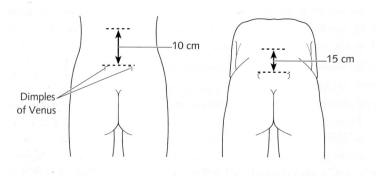

Fig. 11.2 The Schober test.

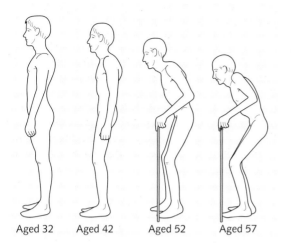

Aged 32   Aged 42   Aged 52   Aged 57

Fig. 11.3 Deterioration of posture in AS.

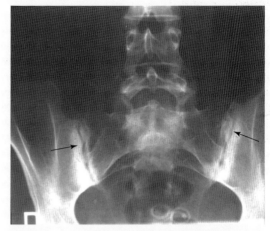

Fig. 11.4 Radiograph showing bilateral sacroiliitis.

can occur at many sites. Achilles tendonitis and plantar fasciitis are common examples of this.

Extraskeletal features

Systemic
Systemic features such as anorexia, fever, weight loss and fatigue trouble some patients, particularly early in the disease.

Extraskeletal features can be thought of as the four As.

Acute anterior uveitis Acute anterior uveitis (also called iritis) occurs in approximately one-third of patients with AS and does not correlate with the disease activity in the spine. The eye becomes red and painful and vision is blurred. It can be treated with steroid eye drops.

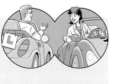

Patients suffering from any spondyloarthropathy should be warned of the risk of uveitis and told to seek medical help if they develop a painful, red eye.

Aortic incompetence/Ascending aortitis This occurs less frequently and usually late in the disease.

Apical lung fibrosis This is another late feature of AS.

Amyloidosis This is a rare complication.

Investigations

Blood tests

- A full blood count may reveal an anaemia of chronic disease.
- Erythrocyte sedimentation rate (ESR) and C-reactive protein (CRP) are often raised during active phases of the disease.
- Serological tests for rheumatoid factor are negative.
- Genotyping for HLA-B27 is expensive and unnecessary for diagnosis, which can be made on clinical and radiological findings.

Radiological investigations

X-rays are useful in the diagnosis of AS. An antero-posterior view of the pelvis will show the sacroiliac joints. These appear normal initially, but later sclerosis and erosions are seen, sometimes progressing to complete fusion (Fig. 11.4). Views of the lumbar spine may show squaring of the vertebrae and formation of syndesmophytes (Fig 11.5). These are due to ossification of the longitudinal ligaments and produce a bamboo appearance. Radiographs taken at other sites of enthesitis may show erosions, for example at the insertion of the plantar fascia or Achilles tendon. MRI scans of the sacroiliac joints and spine enable inflammation to be seen at an earlier stage and may help in deciding which patients will benefit from aggressive treatment.

71

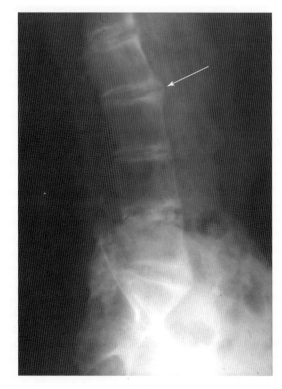

Fig. 11.5 Lateral radiograph showing syndesmophyte formation in the lumbar spine of a patient with advanced AS.

Management

Patients with AS should be cared for by a multidisciplinary team (see Fig. 10.15).

Physiotherapy

This is the most important element in the management of AS. Each patient should follow a long-term exercise programme with the aim of maintaining normal posture and physical activity. Hydrotherapy is also beneficial.

Drug treatment

Drug treatment can help to minimize pain and stiffness. Non-steroidal anti-inflammatory drugs (NSAIDs) can be effective (probably should not recommend regular use in view of cardiovascular side-effects). Indometacin is a particularly popular choice. Many disease-modifying antirheumatic drugs (DMARDs) have been tested in AS. There is little evidence to support their use, but sulfasalazine is sometimes used in an attempt to gain control of peripheral joint synovitis. Anti-TNF (tumour necro-sis factor) drugs are now being used for severe AS and seem quite promising.

Surgery

There are several indications for surgical intervention in AS. Joint replacement surgery is often performed in patients with hip involvement. Spinal osteotomy can help improve posture when severe spinal curvature interferes with forward vision. Cervical fusion is sometimes required for atlantoaxial subluxation.

REACTIVE ARTHRITIS

Reactive arthritis is an aseptic arthritis that develops after an anatomically distant infection. It mainly affects young adults and the triggering infection is usually of the gastrointestinal or genitourinary tract.

Remember that *Salmonella* and *Neisseria* can cause a true septic arthritis, so it is important to exclude this.

Clinical features

Symptoms start a few days to a few weeks after the infection. The onset is sometimes acute with high fever and fatigue.

Musculoskeletal features of reactive arthritis

The arthritis is typically asymmetrical and oligoarticular. It tends to target the large weight-bearing joints, fingers and toes. Dactylitis is often seen. This is involvement of an entire finger or toe, creating what is often called a 'sausage digit' . Enthesitis is common and some patients experience pain in the sacroiliac region.

Extraskeletal features of reactive arthritis

Patients with reactive arthritis can develop the uveitis and cardiac problems seen in AS, as well as other extra-articular features.

Conjunctivitis

This is sterile and can be unilateral or bilateral.

Urethritis

Sterile inflammation in the urogenital tract can cause symptoms of frequency, dysuria and sometimes urethral discharge. Cervicitis or prostatitis can occur.

Skin and mucosal lesions

Circinate balanitis can accompany urethritis. Some patients with reactive arthritis develop a sterile pustular rash on the palms of the hands and soles of the feet. This looks similar to pustular psoriasis and is called keratoderma blenorrhagica. Erythema nodosum is another recognized association.

Reiter's syndrome

The term 'Reiter's syndrome' is used to describe the triad of arthritis, urethritis and conjunctivitis in a patient with dysentery.

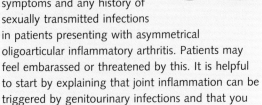

You must enquire about the presence of genitourinary symptoms and any history of sexually transmitted infections in patients presenting with asymmetrical oligoarticular inflammatory arthritis. Patients may feel embarassed or threatened by this. It is helpful to start by explaining that joint inflammation can be triggered by genitourinary infections and that you routinely ask patients these questions.

Clinical course of reactive arthritis

The symptoms of reactive arthritis vary in severity and usually last for weeks to months. Relapses are common and often occur several years later. At least 60% of patients have two or more attacks. Permanent joint damage can occur, but is rare.

Investigations

- Full blood count, erythrocyte sedimentation rate (ESR) and C-reactive protein (CRP) show a similar picture to that of AS.

- Serological tests including antibodies against *Salmonella*, *Campylobacter*, *Chlamydia* and *Neisseria* may help identify the organism responsible for the infection.

- Synovial fluid from any affected joints should be examined and a Gram stain and culture performed. Cultures are negative in reactive arthritis, but it is important to exclude septic arthritis.

- A cervical swab, midstream specimen of urine and stool sample should be obtained for bacterial culture.

- X-rays are initially normal. Later, fluffy periostitis may be seen in the calcaneus, digits or pelvis. Plantar spurs are common, but erosions are rare. Sacroiliitis and typical AS changes develop in some patients.

Management of reactive arthritis

As in AS, NSAIDs can help. Local corticosteroid injection can help enthesitis or synovitis. Sulfasalazine, azathioprine or methotrexate may be useful for persistent, severe disease.

Septic arthritis must be excluded before using corticosteroids.

Antibiotic therapy should be given if an organism is isolated. This probably has little influence on the disease course, but will help stop the spread of infection.

ENTEROPATHIC ARTHRITIS

Arthritis occurring in association with inflammatory bowel disease (IBD) is known as enteropathic arthritis. It occurs in approximately 10–20% of patients with Crohn's disease or ulcerative colitis.

Clinical features

Peripheral arthritis

A peripheral arthritis that is asymmetrical and mono- or oligoarticular can develop. It worsens when the severity of the bowel disease increases and improves if affected bowel is surgically removed.

Spondylitis and sacroiliitis

These are not related to the activity of the bowel inflammation and often predate the onset of Crohn's disease or ulcerative colitis.

Enthesopathy

This can accompany axial or peripheral joint disease.

Investigations

X-rays show typical spinal changes of AS. The peripheral arthritis causes few radiological changes.

Management

Treatment of the IBD is the main priority and will help the arthritis. Drugs, such as corticosteroids and sulfasalazine should improve both the bowel and joint disease.

NSAIDs often aggravate gastrointestinal symptoms in IBD. They should be used with caution and replaced with other forms of analgesia if poorly tolerated.

PSORIATIC ARTHROPATHY

Psoriatic arthropathy (PsA) is an inflammatory arthritis associated with psoriasis. Psoriasis occurs in 1–3% of the population, and approximately 10% of those affected develop psoriatic arthritis. It is particularly common in patients with nail involvement (Fig. 11.6) and affects men and women with a similar frequency.

Clinical features

Psoriatic arthritis may precede the diagnosis of psoriasis and does not correlate with the severity of the skin lesions. Five different patterns of joint disease are seen (Fig. 11.7).

Patients present with joint pain, stiffness and sometimes swelling. Dactylitis and enthesitis are common features. Involvement of a distal interphalangeal (DIP) joint is usually associated with pitting or onycholysis of the nail. Arthritis mutilans is extremely destructive and, fortunately, uncommon. Reabsorption of bone at the metacarpals and phalanges causes telescoping of the digits. They appear shortened but can be passively extended to their original length. Psoriatic spondylitis tends to cause milder symptoms than classical AS, and sacroiliitis is often asymmetrical and asymptomatic. The uveitis and cardiac lesions seen in other SPAs can occur.

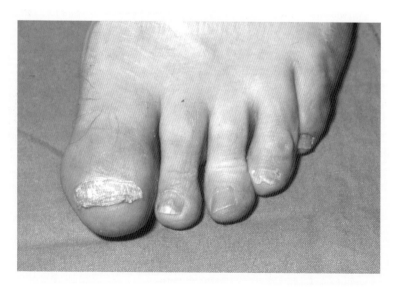

Fig. 11.6 Psoriatic nail pitting.

Patterns of joint disease in psoriatic arthritis
Distal arthritis involving the distal interphalangeal (DIP) joints
Asymmetrical oligoarthritis
Symmetrical polyarthritis indistinguishable from rheumatoid arthritis (RA)
Spondylitis
Arthritis mutilans

Fig. 11.7 Patterns of joint disease in psoriatic arthritis.

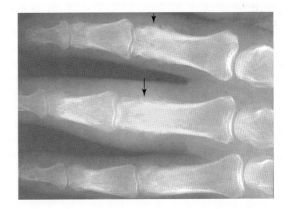

Fig. 11.8 Radiograph showing fluffy periosteal reaction and erosive changes in the digits of a patient with psoriatic arthritis.

Some patients present with articular features of psoriatic arthritis, but no history of skin disease. Careful inspection of areas such as the scalp and natal cleft may reveal small patches of psoriasis.

Investigations

Blood tests

Full blood count, ESR and CRP show a similar picture to that of AS. Rheumatoid factor is usually absent.

Radiological investigations

The radiological changes of PsA are asymmetrical and target the small joints of the hands and feet, particularly the DIP joints (Fig. 11.8). X-ray changes include:

- Erosions with proliferation of adjacent bone.
- Reabsorption of the terminal phalanges.
- Pencil-in-cup deformities.
- Periostitis.
- Ankylosis.
- New bone formation at entheses.

- Sacroiliitis is found in up to 30% of cases and is usually asymmetrical.

Management

Peripheral joint arthritis and spinal disease in PsA are treated in the same way as in RA and AS respectively. Physiotherapy, NSAIDs and DMARD therapy are all commonly used. Anti-TNF treatment is now widely used and has shown promising results.

Prognosis

The prognosis of PsA is usually good. Joint function is well preserved in most cases, but in some, a chronic, progressive, deforming arthritis may develop.

Further reading

Calin A, Taurog J D 1998 The spondyloarthritides. Oxford University Press, Oxford

Gladman D D 2002 Current concepts in psoriatic arthritis. *Curr Op Rheumatol* **14**: 361–366

Khan M A 1997 Spondyloarthropathies: Editorial review. *Curr Op Rheumatol* **9**: 281–283

Connective tissue diseases

Objectives

In this chapter you will learn:

- To recognize the clinical features of systemic lupus erythematosus (SLE).
- Which autoantibodies are associated with SLE.
- How to regognize, investigate and treat inflammatory muscle disease.
- The differences between limited cutaneous and diffuse cutaneous systemic sclerosis.
- The wide variety of ways in which patients with systemic vasculitis can present.

There is no strict definition of a connective tissue disease. The term is usually used to describe multi-system, inflammatory diseases that are associated with immunological abnormalities. There is overlap between these disorders, which share many clinical features (Fig. 12.1).

SYSTEMIC LUPUS ERYTHEMATOSUS

Definition

Systemic lupus erythematosus (SLE) is an inflammatory disease that can involve almost any organ or system of the body.

Prevalence

SLE has a worldwide prevalence of 10–50 per 100 000. It affects women at least 10 times more frequently than it affects men, and is more common in Asian and Afro-Caribbean people than in Caucasians.

Aetiology

There are genetic, environmental and hormonal contributions to its aetiology. SLE can be induced by drugs, such as minocycline or hydralazine. Drug-induced lupus tends to be mild, spares the kidneys and settles when the offending drug is withdrawn.

Pathology

Immune function in SLE is abnormal, with abnormal cell-mediated immunity, B-cell hyperactivity

and impaired immune complex clearance from tissues. A wide variety of autoantibodies have been described. The coagulation system may be abnormal and vasculopathy is frequent.

Clinical features

SLE usually develops between 15 and 40 years of age. The clinical features are diverse and the severity of the disease varies over time. Initial symptoms may be mild and rather vague, but it is the exacerbations of SLE and resultant tissue damage that cause significant ill-health. Severe lupus flares can result in life-threatening problems, including renal failure or cerebral vasculitis. Factors that may trigger flares of SLE are listed in Figure 12.2.

Non-specific features

Fatigue, malaise, fever and weight loss are common in SLE. The fatigue can be quite disabling and is difficult to treat.

Hypothyroidism is more common in SLE than in the general population and should be considered in patients with severe lethargy.

Musculoskeletal features

Approximately 90% of patients with SLE experience arthralgia or arthritis, usually polyarticular. The arthritis is not erosive and the symptoms are usually

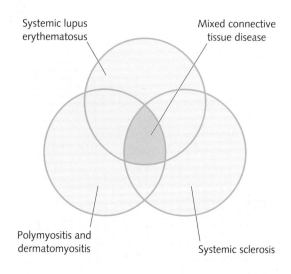

Fig. 12.1 Some members of the connective tissue disease family have overlapping features.

Factors capable of triggering flares of SLE
Overexposure to sunlight
Oestrogen-containing contraceptive therapy
Infection
Stress

Fig. 12.2 Factors capable of triggering flares of SLE.

more dramatic than the signs. If deformity occurs, it is due to tenosynovitis and fibrosis, rather than cartilage or bone erosion. Jaccoud's arthropathy is the name given to this deformity in the hands, as it resembles the deformity of rheumatic fever.

Myalgia is a common symptom of SLE. Avascular necrosis of bone can occur, as can osteoporosis, but they are usually a consequence of corticosteroid treatment, rather than of the disease itself. Septic arthritis is a rare, serious, outcome.

Dermatological features

There are many cutaneous manifestations of lupus. Photosensitivity is common (c. 60%) The characteristic 'butterfly' rash develops over the nose and cheeks (Fig. 12.3). Discoid lupus (demarcated, pigmented or atrophic plaques) can develop with no systemic features (Fig. 12.4).

Hair loss reflects disease activity and alopecia may develop. Mucosal ulceration may affect the

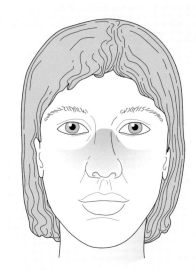

Fig. 12.3 The classic 'butterfly' rash of SLE.

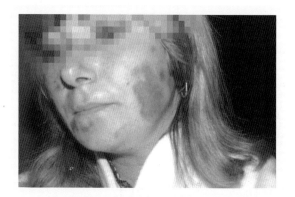

Fig. 12.4 Lesions of discoid lupus.

nose, mouth and vagina. Cutaneous vasculitis in SLE can present with urticarial lesions, livedo reticularis, palpable purpura and splinter haemorrhages.

Cardiovascular features

Serositis is common in SLE and pericarditis is the commonest cardiac manifestation. Myocarditis may accompany myositis and can present with arrhythmias or cardiac failure. Libman–Sacks endocarditis is due to non-infective vegetations and seldom causes clinical problems.

At least one-third of patients with SLE suffer from Raynaud's phenomenon. Vasospasm, usually provoked by the cold, causes peripheral ischaemia.

78

This can be seen in the digits, tip of the nose and ear lobes, which become pale and numb, before turning blue. The final phase is of redness and flushing due to eventual vasodilatation. Vasculitis presents with skin rashes or ulcers and can rarely affect internal organs, such as the lungs and brain.

Pulmonary features

Amongst the pulmonary features of lupus, pleurisy and pleural effusions are common. Acute pneumonitis can mimic pneumonia. Chronic pneumonitis causes pulmonary fibrosis. Pulmonary hypertension is rare.

Renal features

Glomerulonephritis is the commonest cause of lupus-related death in patients with SLE. Nephritis does not cause clinical symptoms until there is significant renal damage. It is therefore important to monitor patients' blood pressure and check their urine for protein, red cells and casts, so that renal disease can be detected early.

Neurological features

SLE can involve the central nervous system, cranial and peripheral nerves, producing a wide range of clinical features. These include headaches, psychiatric problems, seizures, neuropathies and chorea. Headaches are common and often migrainous. Psychiatric symptoms such as anxiety, depression and psychosis are also well-recognized effects of lupus.

Haematological features

Lymphopenia is usual in active SLE. It is sometimes difficult to distinguish whether other cytopenias, such as leucopenia and thrombocytopenia, are due to high disease activity or bone marrow suppression by drugs. Anaemia can be due to chronic inflammation or to autoimmune haemolysis, which affects at least 5% of lupus sufferers.

Gastrointestinal (GI) features

Aseptic peritonitis can present with abdominal pain and nausea, with or without ascites. Mild hepatosplenomegaly and vasculitis affecting the mesenteric vessels are other possible GI manifestations.

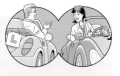

It is important to consider SLE as a possible cause of arthralgia, particularly in young women. Always ask about the presence of symptoms such as skin rashes, photosensitivity, oral ulcers, headaches, depression, Raynaud's phenomenon and pleurisy.

Overlap with other diseases

It is common for patients with SLE to develop secondary Sjögren's syndrome or the antiphospholipid antibody syndrome (see below).

Investigations

Serological tests

SLE is characterized by the presence of serum autoantibodies against nuclear components (see Fig. 12.5).

Other tests

- A full blood count should be performed regularly to screen for anaemia, leucopenia and thrombocytopenia.
- The urine should be checked with a dipstick that detects blood and protein to look for signs of nephritis.
- Urea, creatinine and electrolyte levels should also be monitored.
- The erythrocyte sedimentation rate (ESR) will rise during a flare of SLE (Fig. 12.6), but may sometimes be high when the patient feels quite well. The C-reactive protein (CRP) tends to remain normal unless infection, synovitis or serositis is present.
- Complement levels (C3 and C4) are usually depressed in active SLE.
- Coombs' test will be positive in patients with autoimmune haemolytic anaemia.
- Skin biopsy shows deposition of IgG and complement at the dermal–epidermal junction in patients with rashes (lupus 'band' test).
- Renal biopsy is sometimes performed to aid diagnosis or to establish prognosis in patients with abnormal renal function.

Fig. 12.5 Autoantibodies associated with SLE.

Autoantibodies associated with SLE	
Autoantibodies found in SLE	**Comments**
Antinuclear antibodies (ANA)	Detected in >95% of patients Not specific for SLE
Anti-Ro and anti-La antibodies	Associated with secondary Sjögren's syndrome and pulmonary fibrosis Mothers are at risk of having babies with neonatal SLE and congenital heart block
Anti-double-stranded DNA (dsDNA) antibodies	Very specific for SLE A good marker of disease activity
Antihistone antibodies	Often positive in drug-induced SLE
Antiphospholipid and anticardiolipin antibodies	May be positive

Indicators of high disease activity in SLE
Raised ESR High anti-DsDNA titres Low C3 and C4 complement levels

Fig. 12.6 Indicators of high disease activity in SLE.

Always consider SLE as a possible diagnosis in a patient with multisystem symptoms, particularly if the patient has a raised ESR and normal CRP.

Management

General measures

Education about SLE is essential. Patients are best advised to avoid factors that can precipitate lupus flares (see Fig. 12.2). They should wear long-sleeved clothes and use complete sunblock in any sunny weather. Infections should be promptly treated.

Pharmacological treatment

The choice of drug therapy in SLE depends on the severity and nature of the disease.

Mild SLE

Patients with symptoms such as arthralgia, lethargy or a faint rash may respond to non-steroidal anti-inflammatory drugs (NSAIDs) and/or antimalarial drugs, such as hydroxychloroquine.

Moderate SLE

Patients with more severe clinical features, such as serositis, severe arthritis, nephritis, autoimmune haemolytic anaemia, thrombocytopenia and neurological or psychiatric problems often require treatment with corticosteroids. Steroid sparing agents such as azathioprine, methotrexate or mycophenolate mofetil can be used.

Severe SLE

Flares of SLE that cause severe renal, neurological or haematological problems should be treated with cytotoxic drugs combined with corticosteroids. Cyclophosphamide is very effective. Tacrolimus and mycophenolate mofetil are alternatives.

Adjunctive treatment

Hypertension due to nephritis should be treated aggressively. Intravenous immunoglobulin infusions may help immune thrombocytopenia or neutropenia. Antiplatelet drugs or warfarin are required for patients with antiphospholipid antibody syndrome (see below). Anticonvulsants may be required in CNS disease.

Prognosis

The outlook for patients with SLE is improving. 5-year survival is at least 90%. When deaths do occur, they are usually a consequence of lupus nephritis, although some are due to serious infections precipitated by cytotoxic drugs.

Fig. 12.7 The major features of APS.

The major features of APS	
Venous thrombosis	Deep vein thrombosis and pulmonary emboli—most common Other veins can be affected (e.g. inferior vena cava, pelvic, renal, portal and hepatic veins)
Arterial thrombosis	Cerebral ischaemia (stroke, transient ischaemic attacks) Peripheral ischaemia
Fetal complications	Spontaneous abortions—often in the 3rd trimester Premature births
Thrombocytopenia	Not severe enough to cause haemorrhage

THE ANTIPHOSPHOLIPID SYNDROME

Definition

The antiphospholipid syndrome (APS) is characterized by recurrent vascular thrombosis, fetal loss and thrombocytopenia associated with persistently elevated levels of antiphospholipid antibodies. Antiphospholipid antibody production can complicate other autoimmune diseases, especially SLE. In these circumstances, patients are said to have secondary antiphospholipid syndrome.

Incidence

APS was first described 20 years ago. It is increasingly being recognized as a cause of thrombosis, but its incidence and prevalence are still unclear.

Pathology

The two main antiphospholipid antibodies are lupus anticoagulant and anticardiolipin antibodies. Their role in thrombosis is currently being investigated. They appear to induce a procoagulant state by binding to antigens on endothelial cells. Placental infarction is thought to be the mechanism behind fetal loss.

Clinical features

The major features of antiphospholipid syndrome are shown in Figure 12.7. Patients can develop additional clinical features (see Fig. 12.8).

Investigations

The diagnosis is based on the detection of anti-cardiolipin antibodies or a positive lupus anti-

Associated clinical features of APS
Livedo reticularis
Leg ulcers
Cardiac valve abnormalities (e.g. aortic and mitral regurgitation)
Chorea
Epilepsy
Migraine
Haemolytic anaemia

Fig. 12.8 Associated clinical features of APS.

coagulant assay. Anticardiolipin antibodies bind to cardiolipin or β_2 glycoprotein-1. The lupus anticoagulant assay measures the ability of antiphospholipid antibodies to prolong clotting tests such as the activated partial thromboplastin time (APTT). Serological tests for syphilis (e.g. Venereal Disease Research Laboratory (VDRL)) are often false biological positives. Thrombocytopenia may occur.

Management

General advice

The following steps are advisable:

- Avoidance of the oral contraceptive pill.
- Avoidance of smoking.
- Treatment of hypertension, hyperlipidaemia or diabetes mellitus.

Asymptomatic patients

Current recommendations are that patients with no history of thrombosis should be treated with low-dose aspirin.

Venous or arterial thrombosis

Patients with antiphospholipid syndrome should be anticoagulated in the usual way. However, it is recommended that anticoagulation is lifelong, because there is a risk of recurrent thrombosis. Prophylactic therapy with warfarin, aiming for an international normalized ratio (INR) of 2.5–3.0 is recommended.

Recurrent fetal loss

Warfarin should be stopped before conception because it is teratogenic. Subcutaneous heparin should be given throughout pregnancy.

SJÖGREN'S SYNDROME

Definition

Sjögren's syndrome is a chronic autoimmune disease, characterized by inflammation of exocrine glands. The salivary and lacrimal glands are predominantly affected, resulting in dryness of the eyes and mouth. Sjögren's syndrome can be primary or secondary (associated with other diseases). Causes of secondary Sjögren's syndrome are shown in Figure 12.9.

Prevalence

The prevalence of Sjögren's syndrome is 1–3%. It is nine times commoner in women than men.

Aetiology

The aetiology is unknown. The primary disease has a strong genetic association with HLA-DR3. It is thought that some environmental factor (probably a virus) may trigger Sjögren's syndrome in people with a genetic susceptibility.

Pathology

All organs affected by Sjögren's syndrome are infiltrated by lymphocytes. In the salivary glands, this

Diseases associated with secondary Sjögren's syndrome
RA
SLE
Systemic sclerosis
Polymyositis
Primary biliary cirrhosis
Chronic active hepatitis

Fig. 12.9 Diseases associated with secondary Sjögren's syndrome.

results in duct dilatation, acinar atrophy and interstitial fibrosis. There is marked activation of B-cells, resulting in increased immunoglobulin production.

Clinical features

Sjögren's syndrome predominantly affects people in the fourth and fifth decades. The main symptoms are ocular or oral.

Ocular symptoms

Reduced tear secretion results in the destruction of the corneal and conjunctival epithelium (keratoconjunctivitis sicca). Patients complain that their eyes feel dry, sore or gritty and they are usually red. Bacterial conjunctivitis is common.

Oral symptoms

Xerostomia (dryness of the mouth) leads to difficulties in swallowing dry food or talking for long periods. On examination of the oral cavity, the mucosa is dry, there is very little saliva and the tongue may be fissured. Dental caries is often seen and oral candidiasis is common. Intermittent parotid swelling affects at least half of patients with primary Sjögren's syndrome (Fig. 12.10), but is less common in secondary disease.

Other symptoms of exocrine dysfunction

Secretion from other exocrine glands may be diminished, producing a variety of clinical effects. For example, vaginal dryness can cause dyspareunia and lack of GI mucus secretion can result in oesophagitis or gastritis. There is an association with autoimmunity (e.g. thyroid disease).

Systemic features

Primary Sjögren's syndrome is a systemic disease and many patients develop extraglandular manifestations.

- Constitutional features include fatigue, weight loss and fever.
- Arthritis is episodic, non-erosive and very similar to the joint disease seen in SLE.
- Raynaud's phenomenon affects up to 50% of patients.
- Interstitial lung disease is mild and often subclinical.

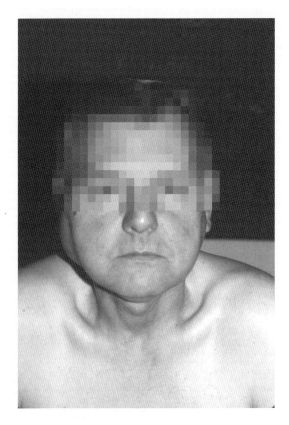

Fig. 12.10 Parotid swelling in Sjögren's syndrome.

- Interstitial nephritis can lead to renal tubular acidosis or nephrogenic diabetes insipidus.
- Vasculitis affects approximately 5% of patients and usually causes cutaneous lesions: purpura and ulcers.
- Neurological features vary widely. Peripheral neuropathies result from small vessel vasculitis. Cranial neuropathies, hemiparesis, seizures and movement disorders can also occur.
- Lymphomas, usually B-cell, are commoner in patients with Sjögren's syndrome than in the general population. They develop in the salivary glands, reticuloendothelial system, GI tract, lungs or kidneys.

Investigations

Schirmer's test

Schirmer's test is used to demonstrate reduced tear production. One end of a strip of filter paper is placed beneath the lower eyelid. The length of paper soaked by tears is measured after 5 minutes. Wetting of less than 5 mm suggests reduced secretion.

Rose Bengal staining

This is used to detect keratoconjunctivitis sicca. Rose Bengal is a dye that stains damaged corneal and conjunctival epithelium. This is seen clearly on slit-lamp examination.

Salivary flow rate monitoring

Salivary flow rate can be monitored with an isotope scan. This measures the rate at which a radiolabelled dye is taken up and excreted by the salivary glands. Both uptake and excretion are delayed in Sjögren's syndrome.

Labial gland biopsy and histology

Biopsy and histology of the labial glands from behind the lower lip is a very useful test. Lymphocytic infiltration can be seen.

Blood tests

- The ESR is usually high.
- A mild normocytic anaemia is common.
- Immunoglobulin levels are very high.
- Anti-Ro and anti-La antibodies, rheumatoid factor and antinuclear antibodies (ANA) are often found.

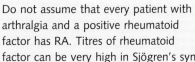

Do not assume that every patient with arthralgia and a positive rheumatoid factor has RA. Titres of rheumatoid factor can be very high in Sjögren's syndrome and patients with primary Sjögren's syndrome are often misdiagnosed as having RA.

Management

Treatment of Sjögren's syndrome is topical and symptomatic. Tear substitutes such as hypromellose eye drops help to lubricate the eyes. Occlusion of the canaliculi can help to block the drainage of tears and keeps the conjunctiva moist.

Xerostomia can be treated with saliva substitutes. Pilocarpine tablets may help, but cause cholinergic side-effects such as sweating and abdominal cramps. Careful dental hygiene is essential to help prevent premature caries.

Hydroxychloroquine can help the arthritis. Corticosteroids are prescribed for serious complications like vasculitis and neurological problems.

POLYMYOSITIS AND DERMATOMYOSITIS

Definition

Polymyositis (PM) and dermatomyositis (DM) are autoimmune, inflammatory muscle diseases. DM also affects the skin.

Incidence

Both muscle diseases are rare, with a combined incidence of between 2 and 10 cases per million per year. There is a female preponderance of 2 : 1.

Aetiology

The aetiology of PM and DM is unknown. Family studies support a genetic predisposition. Associations with various HLA types have been reported, but are weak.

Pathology

In both conditions, muscle fibres are infiltrated by inflammatory cells and there is subsequent degeneration, necrosis and phagocytosis. The pattern of infiltration and predominant cell type allows PM to be distinguished from DM. Skin biopsy in DM shows the same histological features as in lupus. The autoantibodies commonly associated with inflammatory muscle disease will be discussed later.

Clinical features

Inflammatory muscle disease can affect people of any age, but the peak age of onset is 40–60 years. DM is often seen in children, but PM is unusual in this age group.

Myositis

PM and DM are characterized by symmetrical proximal muscle weakness that develops over weeks to months. Patients find certain tasks increasingly difficult, such as rising from a chair, climbing the stairs or reaching for things above head height.

Involvement of the intercostal muscles and diaphragm can affect ventilation and lead to type 2 respiratory failure. Dysphagia and regurgitation of food result from weakness of the pharyngeal muscles and upper third of the oesophagus. Patients may complain of muscle pain and tenderness. Muscle bulk and tendon reflexes appear normal, except in advanced disease.

Cutaneous manifestations

The skin rashes of DM usually precede the weakness. Typical lesions are:

- *Gottron's papules*—erythematous, scaly papules or plaques over the MCP and PIP joints and also over the extensor surfaces of the knees and elbows.
- A *heliotrope rash* develops on the skin over the eyelids; lilac discoloration is often accompanied by periorbital oedema.
- A *macular erythematous rash* may develop on the face, neck, chest, shoulders and hands.
- *Calcinosis*—this occurs more commonly in juvenile dermatomyositis than in adult disease.
- *Cutaneous vasculitis*—can cause ulceration.
- *Periungual telangiectasia* may be seen and the cuticles are often thickened and irregular.

Some patients develop typical cutaneous features of DM without the muscle disease. They are said to have 'amyopathic DM'.

Extramuscular features of PM and DM

Constitutional features
Fatigue, malaise, weight loss and fever are common.

Skeletal features
Many patients develop polyarthralgia as well as myalgia.

Pulmonary features
Interstitial lung disease occurs in up to 30% of cases. Ventilatory failure can result from weakness of the intercostal muscles and diaphragm. Aspiration pneumonia is a risk in patients with dysphagia.

Cardiovascular features

Myocarditis can present with cardiac failure or arrhythmias, but most cases are asymptomatic. Raynaud's phenomenon and vasculitis can accompany myositis.

GI features

Vasculitis that can result in intestinal haemorrhage or perforation is particularly common in juvenile dermatomyositis.

Malignancy

Approximately 5–15% of adults with inflammatory muscle disease have an underlying malignancy. The association is thought to be much stronger for DM than for PM. Malignancies reported in association with DM include:

- Lung.
- Oesophagus.
- Breast.
- Colon.
- Ovary.

Investigations

Serum levels of muscle enzymes

Serum levels of muscle enzymes are elevated due to myositis. The creatine kinase is measured most commonly and in active disease is at least 10 times the upper limit of normal.

Erythrocyte sedimentation rate

The ESR is usually raised, but does not correlate well with disease activity.

Autoantibodies

Serum autoantibodies to nuclear and/or cytoplasmic antigens are found in more than 80% of patients. The ANA are usually positive. Approximately 30% of patients with PM or DM have myositis-specific antibodies. These can help predict a patient's prognosis and response to treatment. Anti-Jo-1 is an anticytoplasmic antibody and is associated with interstitial lung disease, arthralgia and Raynaud's phenomenon.

Muscle biopsy

This is the most definitive investigation. Histology shows the typical inflammatory cell infiltration of either PM or DM.

Electromyography and nerve conduction studies

Electromyography and nerve conduction studies can show that the weakness is due to a myopathic process, but do not give a specific diagnosis.

Magnetic resonance imaging

MRI can identify areas of muscle inflammation, but again is non-specific.

Management

Corticosteroids are used to control myositis. They are initially prescribed at high doses. Serum creatine kinase is monitored and, as it falls, the corticosteroid dose is gradually reduced. Although the muscle enzymes respond quickly to treatment, the improvement in muscle strength is usually much slower. Many patients with PM or DM require additional immunosuppressive therapy. Methotrexate and azathioprine are commonly used. Cyclophosphamide may be prescribed for patients with severe interstitial lung disease. Physiotherapy plays an extremely important role in the rehabilitation of patients with inflammatory muscle disease. If an underlying malignancy is found, it should be treated appropriately.

Steroid myopathy is a common complication of treatment. It may be difficult to distinguish from active myositis, but should be considered in patients with normal creatine kinase levels whose muscle strength is deteriorating.

Prognosis

The 5-year survival rate of patients with PM and DM has improved and is currently over 80%. However, many patients are left with significant persisting symptoms as a result of their disease or therapy.

SYSTEMIC SCLEROSIS AND RELATED CONDITIONS

Definition

The term 'scleroderma' means hardening of the skin. This is a feature of several disorders (see Fig. 12.11). Localized cutaneous scleroderma is confined to the skin and soft tissues, whereas systemic sclerosis (SSc) involves internal organs as well.

Incidence and prevalence

These are rare conditions. The incidence of scleroderma is 0.6–1.9 per million per year. The UK prevalence is approximately 100 per million. Women are affected four times as often as men.

Aetiology

In most patients, the aetiology is unknown. Specific HLA types are associated with certain subsets of disease, but not with the disease as a whole. Exposure to certain chemicals or drugs has been associated with SSc.

Pathology

The two main pathological processes in SSc are fibrosis and microvascular occlusion. Overactive fibroblasts produce excessive extracellular matrix in the dermis. Perivascular inflammatory infiltration and intimal proliferation lead to narrowing of arteries and arterioles and obliteration of capillaries. There is immune activation and release of cytokines.

Clinical features

Localized cutaneous scleroderma

Localized scleroderma presents with painful, erythematous lesions, which later become fibrotic. The two main types are morphoea and linear scleroderma. Morphoea varies from small, discrete lesions to large, confluent patches that are uncomfortable and disfiguring. Linear scleroderma is commoner in childhood. Bands of sclerosis affect the limbs and lead to growth defects.

Systemic sclerosis

In addition to causing disfiguring skin changes, SSc can have profound effects on many other organs. The disease is divided into limited cutaneous SSc and diffuse cutaneous SSc. Limited disease is twice as common as diffuse and is sometimes referred to as CREST syndrome (CREST = Calcinosis, Raynaud's phenomenon, oEsophageal disease, Sclerodactyly and Telangiectasia). Symptoms develop most commonly in the fifth decade of life.

Skin manifestations

Scleroderma begins with an inflammatory phase. The skin becomes puffy and feels tight and sometimes itchy. These symptoms typically affect the forearms, hands and feet initially. Over several months, skin thickening and induration develop.

Common features found on examination are:

- Sclerodactyly (Fig. 12.12).
- Microstomia (Fig. 12.13).
- Furrowing of skin around the lips (Fig. 12.13).
- Loss of normal skin creases.

Classification of systemic sclerosis and related conditions

Localized cutaneous scleroderma
Morphoea
Linear scleroderma

Systemic sclerosis
Limited cutaneous systemic sclerosis
Diffuse cutaneous systemic sclerosis
Scleroderma *sine* scleroderma

Fig. 12.11 Classification of systemic sclerosis and related conditions.

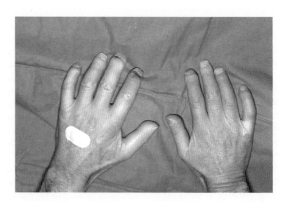

Fig. 12.12 Sclerodactyly.

- Tethering of skin to underlying structures.
- Skin hypo- or hyperpigmentation.
- Flexion contractures of joints.
- In the late stages of scleroderma, the skin becomes thin and atrophic.

The skin changes differ between diffuse and limited cutaneous systemic sclerosis. The main differences are outlined in Figure 12.14.

The effects of systemic sclerosis on other body systems

Involvement of internal organs is more frequent in diffuse than in limited disease.

Cardiovascular manifestations

Raynaud's phenomenon   This occurs in nearly every case of SSc. Severe disease may cause ischaemic

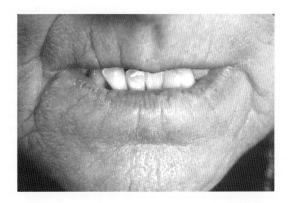

Fig. 12.13 This patient with systemic sclerosis has microstomia and furrowing of the skin around her mouth.

changes in the fingertips and possibly gangrene. The toes, ears, nose and nipples can also be involved.

Cardiac disease   Disease is due to myocardial or pericardial involvement. Myocardial fibrosis can cause cardiac failure and arrhythmias. Pericarditis is often clinically silent.

Pulmonary disease

Pulmonary disease is the most frequent cause of death in SSc.

Fibrosing alveolitis   This affects approximately 25% of patients with limited disease and up to 40% of those with the diffuse cutaneous form.

Pulmonary hypertension   This affects 10–20% of patients. It can be primary (not associated with other lung pathology) or secondary to pulmonary fibrosis. Primary pulmonary hypertension is more common in limited cutaneous SSc, and secondary pulmonary hypertension is more common in diffuse cutaneous SSc.

Renal disease

Scleroderma renal crisis   This implies rapidly progressive renal failure, usually with accelerated hypertension. It tends to occur in patients with diffuse cutaneous disease within 5 years of onset and is often preceded by deterioration of skin disease. Patients present acutely with headaches, visual disturbance and sometimes seizures. Left ventricular failure can occur and

A comparison of skin disease between limited and diffuse cutaneous systemic sclerosis		
	Limited systemic sclerosis	**Diffuse systemic sclerosis**
Distribution of skin fibrosis	Hands* and feet Over the face and neck	Limbs, face, neck and trunk
Skin tethering to underlying structures	Common	Less common
Inflammatory features	Mild	Swelling and pruritus prominent
Telangiectasia	Commonly occur on the face and digits	Less common
Calcinosis	Cutaneous and subcutaneous Calcification common	Less common

*Scleroderma affecting the fingers is often referred to as 'sclerodactyly'

Fig. 12.14 A comparison of skin disease between limited and diffuse systemic sclerosis.

death from renal failure is likely without rapid intervention.

Scleroderma renal crisis is a life-threatening medical emergency that needs urgent treatment.

GI manifestations

Scleroderma can affect any part of the GI tract, but oesophageal problems are particularly common. Reflux oesophagitis and oesophageal dysmotility cause heartburn and dysphagia. Hypomotility can cause bacterial overgrowth in the small bowel and constipation in the large bowel.

Musculoskeletal complications

Most patients suffer with arthralgia and joint stiffness at some time in their disease. Flexion contractures of the interphalangeal joints are common.

Scleroderma *sine* scleroderma

A small minority of patients have the typical vascular or internal organ features of systemic sclerosis without skin sclerosis. They are said to have scleroderma *sine* scleroderma.

Investigations

The diagnosis of scleroderma is clinical. It is important to establish whether patients with SSc have diffuse cutaneous or limited cutaneous disease, as this determines prognosis.

Serological tests

Antinuclear antibodies are found in 95% of patients. The presence or absence of other autoantibodies can help predict complications and prognosis.

For example:

- Anticentromere antibodies are associated with limited disease and a relatively good prognosis. They signify a risk of pulmonary hypertension, but not pulmonary fibrosis.

- Antitopoisomerase-1 (Scl-70) antibodies are associated with diffuse disease and a higher risk of lung fibrosis and renal involvement.

Management

Disease-modifying and antifibrotic therapy

Researchers are still trying to find effective therapies to modify the disease process underlying SSc. Many drugs that affect the immune response have been tested, but none has been very effective. Antifibrotic drugs, such as penicillamine and interferon-α, may help prevent visceral and skin fibrosis if given early.

Screening for complications

This is a very important part in the management of SSc. The blood pressure and renal function should be regularly monitored. Pulmonary function tests and echocardiography will help to detect pulmonary involvement.

Treatment of complications

A lot can be done to treat the organ-related complications. Please see Figure 12.15.

Prognosis

The survival of patients with systemic sclerosis is improving. This probably reflects better management of complications. Estimates of the 5-year survival rate range from 35% to 70%.

THE VASCULITIDES

Definition

Vasculitis is inflammation of blood vessels. It is a feature of many illnesses and can be primary or secondary. The primary vasculitides are uncommon diseases in which vasculitis is the predominant feature. Secondary vasculitis complicates other established diseases such as rheumatoid arthritis (RA), systemic lupus erythematosus (SLE) or HIV infection. Only primary vasculitis will be discussed here.

Fig. 12.15 Treatment of internal organ disease in systemic sclerosis.

Treatment of internal organ disease in systemic sclerosis	
Complication	**Intervention**
Raynaud's phenomenon	Handwarmers Vasodilators • Calcium-channel blockers • ACE inhibitors • Intravenous prostacyclin (iloprost) for severe ischaemia Digital sympathectomy is useful for ischaemia of one or two digits
Pulmonary fibrosis	Prednisolone, with or without cyclophosphamide
Pulmonary hypertension	Anticoagulation Vasodilators • Calcium-channel blockers • Bosentan • Sildenafil • Prostacyclins Diuretics for right ventricular failure, if present
Gastrointestinal problems	Proton pump inhibitor for gastro-oesophageal reflux Antibiotics for small bowel overgrowth Bulk-forming agents for constipation
Renal crisis	Antihypertensives—give immediately • ACE inhibitors • Calcium-channel blockers Temporary dialysis may be required
Cardiac problems	Diuretics and ACE inhibitors for cardiac failure Antiarrhythmics if necessary Corticosteroids for myocarditis

Aetiopathology

Vasculitis is characterized by inflammatory cell infiltration of the blood vessel wall, resulting in fibrinoid necrosis. For this reason, the term 'necrotizing vasculitis' is sometimes used. There is often associated granuloma formation. Vascular inflammation can have severe consequences:

• Aneurysm formation can lead to rupture of vessels and haemorrhage.
• Vessel stenosis or occlusion can lead to distal infarction.

Antineutrophil cytoplasmic antibodies (ANCA) are particularly specific for vasculitis and are helpful for diagnosis and classification. They are antibodies that bind to antigens in the cytoplasm of neutrophils. There are two types of ANCA:

• Cytoplasmic ANCA (c-ANCA) is found in patients with Wegener's granulomatosis and is highly specific.
• Perinuclear staining ANCA (p-ANCA) is found in polyarteritis nodosa, microscopic polyangiitis and Churg–Strauss syndrome.

Classification of primary vasculitis
Large vessel vasculitis Giant cell (temporal) arteritis and polymyalgia rheumatica Takayasu's arteritis
Medium vessel vasculitis Polyarteritis nodosa Kawasaki's disease
Small vessel vasculitis Wegener's granulomatosis* Churg–Strauss syndrome* Microscopic polyangiitis* Henoch–Schönlein purpura Essential cryoglobulinaemic vasculitis
*Vasculitides most commonly associated with ANCA

Fig. 12.16 Classification of primary vasculitis.

Classification of primary vasculitis

The vasculitides are commonly classified on the basis of the size of the vessels they affect (Fig. 12.16).

Clinical features

Many types of primary vasculitis are rare, and detailed knowledge of these individual diseases is beyond the scope of this book. This section will therefore discuss the effects of vasculitis in general, then describe the diseases, allocating the most space to those that occur more frequently.

Vasculitis is potentially life-threatening. The clinical features depend on the size, site and number of blood vessels involved. The most serious problems are due to haemorrhage or infarction of internal organs.

Constitutional features

All primary vasculitic illnesses can cause systemic upset. Features such as fatigue, anorexia, weight loss and fever are common.

Features due to involvement of different body systems

Vasculitis can affect any system of the body (Fig. 12.17). The patient pictured in Figure 12.18 has digital vasculitis.

Giant cell arteritis (GCA) and polymyalgia rheumatica (PMR)

Clinical features

Giant cell arteritis (GCA) is a large vessel vasculitis. It often co-exists with polymyalgia rheumatica (a non-vasculitic illness) which is why they are discussed together here. They have an incidence of approximately 1–5 in 10 000. They both target people over 60 years of age and are twice as common in females than in males. About 50% of patients with GCA have symptoms of PMR and 20–50% of patients with PMR have GCA symptoms.

GCA

Most symptoms are due to inflammation of the carotid artery or its branches, although other large arteries can be involved. The onset of GCA can be insidious or abrupt, with symptoms often appearing overnight. Patients complain of headache, scalp tenderness and sometimes pain on chewing food (jaw claudication). The temporal artery is thickened and tender on examination, sometimes with absent pulsation.

The most feared complication of GCA is blindness. This is due to ischaemic optic neuritis, caused by arteritis of the posterior ciliary artery and branches of the ophthalmic arteries. Patients may experience transient disturbance of vision first. Stroke is another serious potential complication.

PMR

Patients present with symmetrical pain and stiffness in the shoulder and pelvic girdles. Proximal muscles may be tender. Peripheral synovitis affecting medium-sized joints is common.

The effects that vasculitis can have on different body systems	
Body system or organ	**Manifestations of vasculitis**
Skin	Rashes Palpable purpura Ulceration Ischaemia [Fig. 11.18]
Joints	Arthralgia Arthritis
Kidneys	Glomerulonephritis
GI tract	Ischaemia
Nervous system	Neuropathies Stroke
Lungs	Pulmonary haemorrhage

Fig. 12.17 The effects that vasculitis can have on different body systems.

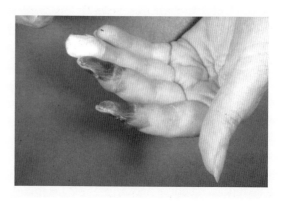

Fig. 12.18 Ischaemic changes in the fingers of a patient with vasculitis.

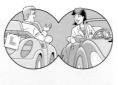

Patients with PMR often complain of muscle weakness. Muscle strength is usually normal in PMR, but patients feel weak because movements are limited by pain.

Most patients with GCA or PMR will be taking corticosteroids for at least 1 year. Prescription of bone-protective drugs for the prevention of osteoporosis should be considered.

Investigations

The diagnosis of PMR is clinical. It is important to exclude malignancy and other connective tissue diseases, which can mimic PMR.

Temporal artery biopsy is the investigation of choice for GCA, but it is not always helpful. The arteritis is patchy and if a 'skip lesion' is biopsied, histology will be normal. Inflammatory cell infiltration, giant cells and granulomata should be seen.

The ESR is usually raised in both conditions, often to at least 70 mm/h. However, a normal ESR does not exclude the diagnoses. Anaemia is common.

Management

Both GCA and PMR should be treated with corticosteroids. Prednisolone at a dose of 10–20 mg is usually prescribed for PMR. Higher doses are required for GCA, particularly in patients with visual symptoms. They should be started promptly to reduce the risk of blindness.

There is usually a dramatic response to corticosteroid therapy with symptoms improving within a few days. Once the disease activity has been suppressed, the corticosteroid dose can be gradually tapered. The slower the dose reduction is, the less likely the patient is to relapse. Azathioprine and methotrexate are sometimes used as steroid-sparing agents if weaning off prednisolone is proving difficult.

Corticosteroids reduce the inflammatory infiltrate within days, so a temporal artery biopsy should be done as soon as possible.

Takayasu's arteritis

This is a rare disease that predominantly affects young women. The arteritis affects the aortic arch and its branches. Symptoms are due to vascular ischaemia and include claudication, dizziness, visual loss and stroke. Immunosuppression may help the acute symptoms. Vascular surgery is often required to bypass obliterated vessels.

Polyarteritis nodosa

Polyarteritis nodosa is a necrotizing arteritis that leads to aneurysm formation. It affects men more frequently than it does women. It is associated with hepatitis B infection. Clinical features include skin ulceration and rashes, peripheral neuropathy, renal disease and gut infarction, which presents with bleeding and abdominal pain. Angiography may show microaneurysms, which are usually found in renal arteries and the coeliac axis. Renal, rectal or sural nerve biopsies can be diagnostic.

Polyarteritis nodosa is treated with corticosteroids and immunosuppressants. Cyclophosphamide is usually used and has improved prognosis.

Kawasaki disease (mucocutaneous lymph node syndrome)

This vasculitis predominantly affects children under the age of 5 years. It was first described in Japan, where most cases occur. It is rare in the western world. Systemic symptoms are prominent. Other features include desquamation of the skin of the hands and feet, conjunctival congestion, cervical lymphadenopathy, arthritis and coronary arteritis, which can lead to acute myocardial infarction.

Fig. 12.19 Clinical features of Wegener's granulomatosis.

Clinical features of Wegener's granulomatosis	
Body system or organ affected	**Clinical features**
Upper and lower respiratory tracts	Subglottic stenosis Lung nodules ± cavitation Pulmonary haemorrhage Pulmonary infiltrates
Kidneys	Glomerulonephritis (often rapidly progressive)
Ear, nose and throat	Sensorineural deafness Nasal discharge, crusting and epistaxis 'Saddling' of the nose due to destruction of the septal cartilage (Fig. 12.20)
Joints	Arthralgia Arthritis
Skin	Rashes Palpable purpura Livedo reticularis
Nervous system	Cranial nerve palsies Peripheral neuropathy Granulomatous meningitis

Wegener's granulomatosis

Wegener's granulomatosis is a granulomatous disorder associated with necrotizing vasculitis. It is strongly linked with the presence of c-ANCA. The peak age of onset is in the fourth and fifth decades. Many systems can be affected (Fig. 12.19), but it is respiratory and renal complications that are the most serious. Survival in Wegener's granulomatosis has improved dramatically since the introduction of cyclophosphamide therapy, which is usually given in conjunction with corticosteroids. Some patients with limited, non-life-threatening Wegener's granulomatosis can be treated less aggressively.

Churg–Strauss syndrome

In Churg–Strauss syndrome, granulomatous, necrotizing vasculitis is found in association with asthma and eosinophilia. Recurrent pneumonia, heart failure, skin lesions, mild renal impairment and peripheral neuropathies can also occur.

Microscopic polyangiitis

Severe renal disease is the main feature of microscopic polyangiitis. Rashes, arthralgia and myalgia are common and lung involvement can present with asthma, pleurisy or haemoptysis.

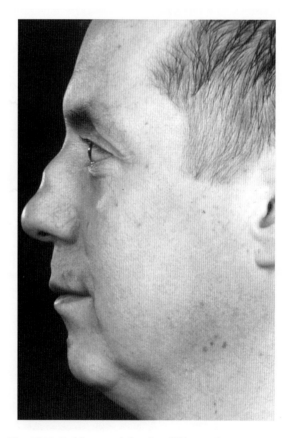

Fig. 12.20 Saddle nose deformity of Wegener's granulomatosis.

Henoch–Schönlein purpura

This vasculitis predominantly affects children. It typically involves the skin, gut, kidneys and joints. Patients can present with a purpuric rash, arthritis, gastrointestinal haemorrhage, abdominal pain and glomerulonephritis.

Essential cryoglobulinaemic vasculitis

This rare vasculitis presents with purpuric skin lesions, arthralgia and renal disease.

Further reading

Ball E, Louis Bridges S Jr 2002 Vasculitis. Oxford University Press, Oxford

Callen J P 2000 Dermatomyositis. *Lancet* **355**: 53–57

Denton C P, Black C M 2000 Scleroderma and related disorders: therapeutic aspects. *Bailliere's Best Pract Res Clin Rheumatol* **14**(1): 17–35

Hazleman B L 2003 Polymyalgia rheumatica and giant cell arteritis. In: Hochberg M C et al (eds) Rheumatology, 3rd edn. Mosby, London, p 1623–1634

Hughes G 1999 Lupus, the facts. Oxford University Press, Oxford

Maddison P Is it a connective tissue disease? In: ABC of Rheumatology, 3rd edn. BMJ Books, London

Metabolic bone disease

Objectives

In this chapter you will learn:

- The risk factors and diseases associated with the development of osteoporosis.
- The common fractures that occur in osteoporotic patients.
- Strategies for fracture prevention in osteoporosis.
- The clinical features and potential complications of Paget's disease.
- The pathways of vitamin D metabolism.
- The differences between rickets and osteomalacia.

OSTEOPOROSIS

Because of the ageing population, fractures resulting from osteoporosis put enormous pressure on hospital services and incur vast costs.

Definition

Osteoporosis is a skeletal disorder characterized by decreased bone mass, leading to increased risk of fracture. Bone mineral density (BMD) is expressed as a T-score. This is the number of standard deviations by which the BMD varies in relation to the mean value for young normal adults. The World Health Organization defines osteoporosis as a T-score of less than −2.5. Osteopenia is defined as a T-score of between −1 and −2.5.

Aetiology and pathology

Peak bone mass is usually attained by the age of 30 and thereafter declines (Fig. 13.1). Bone loss is accelerated in osteoporosis due to an imbalance between the rates of bone resorption and formation, which are governed by activity of osteoclasts and osteoblasts respectively (Fig. 13.2). Risk factors for osteoporosis can be modifiable or non-modifiable (Fig. 13.3).

Osteoporosis is divided into primary (idiopathic or age-related) and secondary (resulting from another disease process). The causes of secondary osteoporosis are shown in Figure 13.4.

Clinical features

Patients either present with pain, deformity or immobility due to fractures, or they are detected by screening measurements of their BMD. Osteoporotic fractures are usually provoked by low-energy injuries. The most common fractures are of the spine, wrist and hip and are discussed below.

Vertebral fractures

Vertebral compression (or wedge) fractures (Fig. 13.5) usually present with thoracic back pain after a minor fall. They are frequently multiple and result in loss of height and a kyphotic deformity. Some patients do not experience pain, but complain that they are shrinking or becoming 'round-shouldered'.

These are stable fractures and treatment is aimed at controlling symptoms with analgesia. Braces are sometimes used, but are poorly tolerated. Newer treatments for controlling pain include vertebro-plasty and kyphoplasty. Both involve the injection of cement into the fractured vertebra.

Wrist

The Colles' fracture results from a fall onto the outstretched hand (FOOSH) resulting in a dinner fork deformity at the wrist. There is dorsal angulation and displacement of the fracture with radial angulation and shortening (Fig. 13.6).

The fracture is usually manipulated under local or regional anaesthesia and placed into a plaster cast. More complex fractures may require surgery, particularly in active patients.

The Smith's fracture is displaced in the opposite direction, i.e. volar or palmar displacement (Fig. 13.6). Such fractures are usually the result of a fall onto a flexed wrist.

Treatment of a Smith's fracture is difficult in a plaster cast alone and most orthopaedic surgeons would now treat a Smith's fracture with internal fixation.

Hip

Of the three common types of osteoporotic fracture, hip fractures place the greatest demand on resources and have the greatest impact on patients in terms of

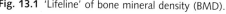

Fig. 13.1 'Lifeline' of bone mineral density (BMD).

Risk factors for osteoporosis	
Non-modifiable	Modifiable
Age	Poor calcium and vitamin D
Race (Caucasian, Asian)	intake
Female sex	Lack of exercise
Early menopause	Smoking
Small size	Alcohol excess
Positive family history	

Fig. 13.3 Risk factors for osteoporosis.

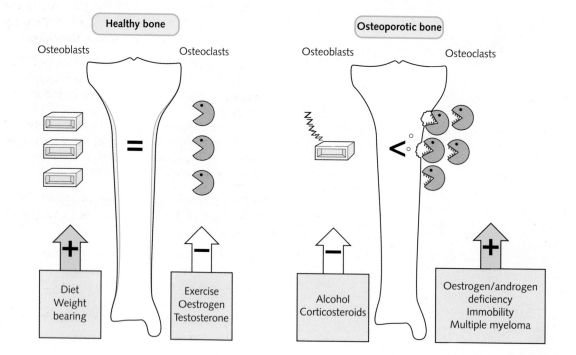

Fig. 13.2 Cell interactions in normal and osteoporotic bone.

Causes of secondary osteoporosis
Hyperthyroidism
Hyperparathyroidism
Hypogonadism
Cushing's syndrome
Rheumatoid arthritis
Inflammatory bowel disease
Coeliac disease
Renal failure
Multiple myeloma
Medications
• Corticosteroids
• Anticonvulsants
• Heparin

Fig. 13.4 Causes of secondary osteoporosis.

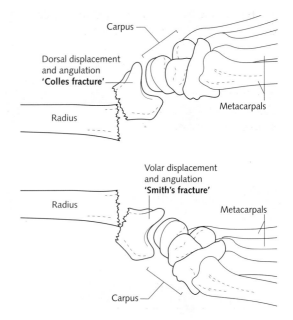

Fig. 13.6 Common osteoporotic distal radial fractures (lateral view).

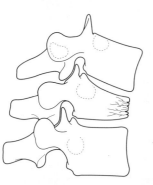

Fig. 13.5 Compression fracture of a thoracic vertebra.

mortality, disability and loss of independence. Approximately one-third of patients with a hip fracture will die within a year of injury.

In the vast majority of cases, femoral neck fractures are treated surgically rather than conservatively. The risk of surgery is balanced against the risks of prolonged bed rest or traction, such as bedsores, deep vein thrombosis and pneumonia. Postoperative patients are mobilized early to minimize these complications. Even when faced with a bed-bound nursing home resident, surgeons still usually operate to provide pain relief.

Hip fractures can be divided into:

- Intracapsular fractures.
- Extracapsular fractures.

The most important distinguishing feature is the blood supply to the femoral head. The blood supply enters the head through the capsule, therefore:

- In an intracapsular fracture (Fig. 13.7A and B), the fracture line is between the blood supply and the head, leading to a risk of avascular necrosis.
- In an extracapsular fracture (Fig. 13.7C), the head is in continuity with its blood supply and therefore the head does not have a risk of avascular necrosis.

This pathophysiology guides the treatment. Intracapsular fractures can be divided into undisplaced and displaced.

- Undisplaced fractures can be treated with internal fixation.
- Displaced fractures (Fig 13.8) are treated with hemiarthroplasty, the femoral head is removed, leaving the artificial head articulating with the normal acetabulum.

Extracapsular fractures are trochanteric or subtrochanteric and are treated with internal fixation with either a dynamic hip screw or an intramedullary nail.

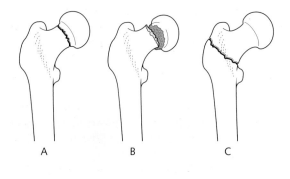

Fig. 13.7 Fractures of the femoral neck: (A) undisplaced intracapsular fracture; (B) displaced intracapsular fracture; (C) extracapsular trochanteric fracture.

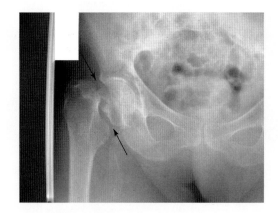

Fig. 13.8 Displaced intracapsular hip fracture.

The subtrochanteric region is a common place for metastatic deposits and care must be taken not to miss these.

Diagnosis and investigation

There are several methods available for measuring BMD. These include dual X-ray absorptiometry (DEXA), quantitative computed tomography and quantitative ultrasound. DEXA is used in most departments to measure BMD at the lumbar spine and hip. BMD cannot be assessed on X-ray, but X-rays are often required to look for fractures.

A full history and examination should be performed when assessing a patient with low BMD. It is important to enquire about risk factors for osteoporosis and to consider the presence of any underlying illnesses, such as those listed in Figure 13.4. Osteoporosis in males and young people is more likely to be due to a secondary cause.

Investigations to exclude a secondary cause will be necessary in some patients. These should include full blood count (FBC), erythrocyte sedimentation rate (ESR), serum calcium, alkaline phosphatase, creatinine, electrophoresis, thyroid stimulating hormone and parathyroid hormone. Serum testosterone should be measured in men.

Management

The aim is to reduce the risk of fractures. This can be achieved by the following methods:

Modification of risk factors for osteoporosis

Patients should change any modifiable risk factors for osteoporosis that they have (see Figure 13.3), for example by stopping smoking and increasing the amount of weight-bearing exercise they do.

Drug therapy to increase bone mass

First line therapy is usually with a bisphosphonate in combination with calcium and vitamin D supplements. Bisphosphonates are anti-resorptive and work by inhibiting osteoclasts. Oestrogen-replacement therapy or raloxifene (a selective oestrogen receptor modulator) can be used in post-menopausal women. Other agents for the treatment of osteoporosis include calcitonin, strontium and parathyroid hormone.

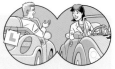

Osteoporosis is often asymptomatic, so the importance of treatment to prevent fractures in the future must be emphasized to patients.

Prevention of falls

The majority of osteoporotic fractures occur as a result of falls. These are more common in the elderly for a number of reasons:

1. Intrinsic factors:
   - Ageing process—leads to slower reaction times (patients unable to stop falling)
   - Poor mobility—patients often have other conditions such as OA
   - Poor eyesight
   - Medical co-morbidity, e.g. syncope/cardiac arrhythmia.
2. Extrinsic factors:
   - Lack of social services
   - Inadequate housing/unsafe local environment.

Falls can be reduced by various interventions such as the avoidance of drugs that have a sedative effect or cause hypotension, the use of walking aids for people with poor mobility and the removal of obstacles in the home.

PAGET'S DISEASE

Definition

Paget's disease is a disorder of bone remodelling.

Incidence

The incidence varies widely across the globe. In the UK, approximately 3% of the population over the age of 40 years are affected by the disease.

Aetiology

The cause of Paget's disease is unknown, but clustering of cases within families has been observed, suggesting a strong genetic contribution. Another hypothesis suggests that it is triggered by a viral infection.

Pathology

There is a dramatic increase in bone resorption, mediated by large multinucleated osteoclasts. Osteoblasts then respond by producing weak, disorganized bone. Repeated cycles of this activity lead to areas of bone becoming abnormally large and deformed with increased vascularity (Fig. 13.9).

Clinical features

Only one-third of patients are symptomatic. They present with bone pain, deformity or fracture. Paget's disease can affect a single part of the skeleton or multiple sites. The commonest sites are the pelvis, lumbar spine, femur, skull and tibia. The affected area may be tender and warm due to increased blood flow.

Paget's disease is usually diagnosed in asymptomatic patients when an X-ray is performed for another reason. For example, pagetic changes may be noticed in the pelvis on an abdominal X-ray.

Figure 13.10 demonstrates some of the possible complications of Paget's disease. Many of these are due to bone overgrowth which can cause localized problems, such as deafness due to auditory nerve entrapment. Osteosarcomas can occur in pagetic bone, but are rare.

Diagnosis and investigation

- Serum alkaline phosphatase levels are elevated and correlate with the extent of skeletal involvement.

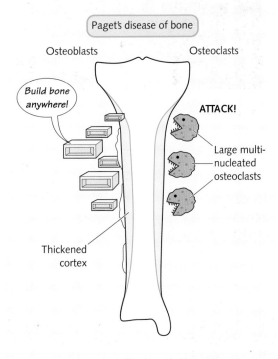

Fig. 13.9 Cell interactions in Paget's disease of bone.

Fig. 13.10 Potential complications of
Paget's disease.

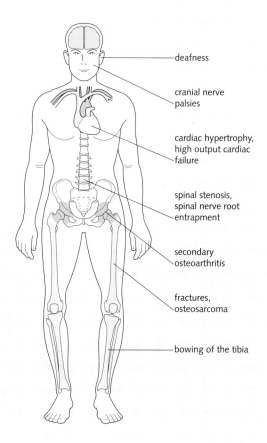

- deafness
- cranial nerve palsies
- cardiac hypertrophy, high output cardiac failure
- spinal stenosis, spinal nerve root entrapment
- secondary osteoarthritis
- fractures, osteosarcoma
- bowing of the tibia

- Plain radiographs show disorganized patterns of affected bone with areas of lysis and sclerosis. The cortex is usually thickened.
- Isotope bone scans will show areas of focal increased uptake.

Treatment

Bisphosphonates are very effective at inhibiting bone resorption and reducing symptoms of Paget's disease. Calcitonin is sometimes used, but is less well tolerated.

Surgical treatment is reserved for complications of:

- Fracture—needs surgical stabilization.

- Deformity—osteotomy is rarely performed.
- Osteosarcoma—these tumours are highly aggressive with a poor prognosis. If the appendicular skeleton is involved, resection or amputation is required followed by chemotherapy.

Pagetic bone is very vascular and bleeds a lot during surgery. Blood should be cross-matched in advance.

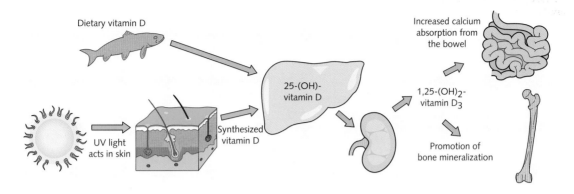

Fig. 13.11 Pathways of vitamin D metabolism.

OSTEOMALACIA AND RICKETS

Both of these conditions are the result of failure of mineralization of bone. Rickets affects the growing skeleton in children and osteomalacia occurs in adults.

Aetiology

Vitamin D deficiency is the commonest cause of both conditions. Hypophosphataemia is a much rarer cause. Figure 13.11 illustrates the pathways of vitamin D metabolism. The causes of vitamin D deficiency are shown in Figure 13.12.

Pathology

Histological examination of bone biopsies in both conditions shows an increased amount of osteoid with deficient mineralization.

Clinical features

The main clinical features of rickets and osteomalacia are:

- Bone pain.
- Skeletal deformity.
- Muscle weakness.

Tetany or convulsions due to hypocalcaemia can occur, but are rare.

Rickets

The growth of children with rickets is impaired. The clinical manifestations depend on the age of the child. Those under 12 months of age may have softening and frontal bossing of the skull. There may be swelling of the epiphyses of the wrists and at the costochondral junctions (the 'rickety rosary'). Older children develop bowing of the long bones and valgus or varus deformities at the knee.

Osteomalacia

Osteomalacia tends to present with vague bone pain, especially in the long bones and pelvis. Severe, localized pain may be due to fracture. The myopathy is usually proximal.

Diagnosis and investigation

The following laboratory abnormalities are usually found:

- Low or low/normal serum calcium.
- Low or low/normal serum phosphate.
- Raised serum alkaline phosphatase.
- Low serum vitamin D.
- Raised parathyroid hormone.
- Low urinary calcium excretion.

Causes of vitamin D deficiency
Low dietary intake plus inadequate sunlight exposure
Intestinal malabsorption (coeliac disease, gastric surgery)
Liver disease
Renal disease
Drugs that affect vitamin D metabolism (anticonvulsants)

Fig. 13.12 Causes of vitamin D deficiency.

The following radiological changes are seen in rickets:

- Delayed opacification of the epiphyses.
- Widened growth plates.
- Thin cortices.

In osteomalacia, the characteristic appearance on X-ray is of 'Looser's zones' which are spontaneous incomplete fractures.

Treatment

Both rickets and osteomalacia can be treated with vitamin D supplementation. The underlying cause of vitamin D deficiency should be addressed.

Further reading

Fitzgerald R H, Kaufer H, Malkani A (eds) 2002 Orthopaedics. Mosby, Philadelphia

Solomon L, Warwick D, Nayagan D (eds) 2001 Apley's system of orthopaedics and fractures, 8th edn. Hodder Arnold, London

Orthoteers website: http://www.orthoteers.co.uk

Crystal arthropathies

GOUT

Definition

Gout is a consequence of hyperuricaemia and uric acid crystal formation. Clinical features include:

- Arthritis.
- Crystal deposition in the soft tissues.
- Renal disease.
- Urolithiasis.

Prevalence

Gout affects between 0.5 and 2.5% of people in the western world. It used to be at least 10 times more common in men than in women. The incidence in women is increasing. There are important links between blood urate and insulin resistance (syndrome X), so musculoskeletal gout may be the tip of a cardiovascular risk 'iceberg'.

Aetiology

Gout is caused by a sustained increase in serum uric acid levels. Uric acid is derived from the breakdown of purine bases, which are components of nucleic acids. It is present in two forms in the body: uric acid and monosodium urate. Synthesis mainly occurs in the liver (Fig. 14.1).

Daily turnover of uric acid is high and approximately two-thirds is renally excreted. Serum levels are related to age, sex, body mass, diet and genetic factors. They are higher in males than in females from puberty until the menopause, when the difference lessens.

Hyperuricaemia is usually due to reduced renal urate excretion, rather than increased production (Fig. 14.2). Diuretic therapy is probably the commonest cause of gout. Hypoxanthine guanine phosphoribosyltransferase (HGPRT) deficiency is a rare inherited disorder that causes gout in childhood. Complete deficiency of HGPRT occurs in the Lesch–Nyhan syndrome.

Some conditions are associated with gout, but do not cause hyperuricaemia. They are shown in Figure 14.3.

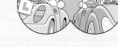

It is important to take a detailed drug and alcohol history from patients presenting with gout. Elderly women presenting with gout are likely to be taking diuretics, whereas younger men often have a history of excessive alcohol consumption.

Pathology

Prolonged hyperuricaemia leads to the formation of urate crystals. These are deposited in the synovium, other connective tissues and the kidney. Joint inflammation occurs when crystals are shed from deposits within the joint and phagocytosed by polymorphonuclear leucocytes. Urate deposition in the kidney can cause interstitial nephritis, renal stones and acute tubular damage.

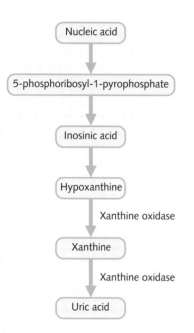

Fig. 14.1 The steps in the synthesis of uric acid.

Causes of hyperuricaemia
Reduced renal excretion
Drugs
• Diuretics
• Low-dose salicylates
• Pyrazinamide
• Ethanol
Renal disease
Hypertension
Increased levels of organic acids
• Lactic acidosis
• Ketoacidosis
• Respiratory acidosis
Hypothyroidism
Hyperparathyroidism
Increased uric acid production
High dietary purine intake (red meat, offal, beer)
Increased turnover of purines
• Lympho- and myeloproliferative disorders
• Polycythaemia
• Haemolytic anaemia
• Severe psoriasis
• Carcinomatosis
Increased purine synthesis
• Hypoxanthine guanine phosphoribosyltransferase (HGPRT) deficiency

Fig. 14.2 Causes of hyperuricaemia.

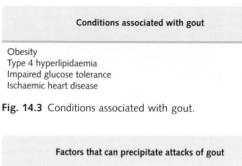

Conditions associated with gout
Obesity
Type 4 hyperlipidaemia
Impaired glucose tolerance
Ischaemic heart disease

Fig. 14.3 Conditions associated with gout.

Factors that can precipitate attacks of gout
Trauma
Intercurrent illness
Surgery
Excess alcohol intake
Starvation
Initiation of drugs that alter urate levels

Fig. 14.4 Factors that can precipitate attacks of gout.

Clinical features

Acute gout

Acute gout is extremely painful. It typically presents as a rapidly accelerating monoarthritis. Symptoms often develop overnight and include severe pain and swelling. The skin overlying the joint is usually shiny, warm and red and the joint is extremely tender. Attacks subside spontaneously within a few days to a couple of weeks.

The first metatarsophalangeal (MTP) joint is the commonest to be affected, but the ankle, knee, elbow, wrist and hand joints can also be involved. A polyarticular presentation, mimicking rheumatoid arthritis (RA) is rare. Acute gout can also affect bursae and is a common cause of olecranon bursitis. Several factors can provoke an acute attack of gout. These are shown in Figure 14.4.

Initially, acute attacks resolve, leaving the patient free of symptoms. Some people have no further problems, but most will have a further attack within a few years. Without treatment, the acute attacks can become more frequent, sometimes merging into each other.

The majority of people with hyperuricaemia never develop gout. Asymptomatic hyperuricaemia is much more common.

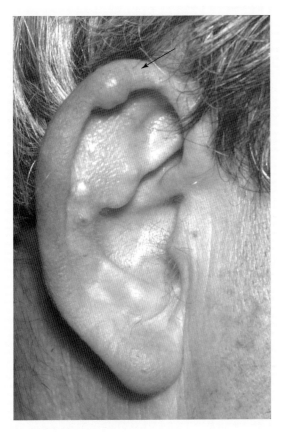

Fig. 14.5 Tophus formation in the pinna.

Chronic gout

Musculoskeletal features

Chronic gout occurs in patients with uncontrolled hyperuricaemia, who have had recurrent attacks of acute gout for years. It is characterized by tophus formation and joint destruction. Tophi are soft tissue deposits of urate. They commonly develop in the digits, helix of the ear (Fig. 14.5), bursae and tendon sheaths. They can interfere with function and sometimes ulcerate, discharging chalky white material. Cartilage destruction and bony erosion in chronic gout can lead to deformities.

Renal disease

Urate deposition in the renal interstitium and collecting tubules can cause a nephropathy. Uric acid stones can also form in the urinary tract.

Investigations

Synovial fluid analysis

This is the single most important test in the diagnosis of suspected gout. Synovial fluid should be obtained by needle-aspiration of symptomatic joints and examined with a microscope under polarized light. Monosodium urate crystals are needle-shaped and show strong negative birefringence. This means that crystals parallel to the plane of light appear yellow, whereas those at right angles are blue. Aspirated material from tophi can be examined in a similar way. Synovial fluid Gram stain and culture should be performed to exclude infection.

Synovial fluid should be examined soon after aspiration to increase the chance of seeing crystals.

Blood tests

Serum uric acid should be measured, but the discovery of hyperuricaemia is not diagnostic of gout. The erythrocyte sedimentation rate (ESR) and C-reactive protein (CRP) are usually raised in acute gout and a full blood count may reveal a polymorphonuclear leucocytosis.

Radiology

Radiological changes do not usually appear until years of recurrent gouty attacks have elapsed. Radiographs show soft tissue swelling and opacities due to tophi. Erosions may be seen. They typically have overhanging edges and, unlike in RA, the surrounding bone is sclerotic.

Management

Management of acute gout

Acute gout should be treated promptly with one of the following drugs:

- Non-steroidal anti-inflammatory drugs (NSAIDs) are used most commonly, and should be continued until the pain and inflammation subside.

Indications for prophylactic treatment of gout
Recurrent attacks
Tophi
Polyarticular disease
Renal disease

Fig. 14.6 Indications for prophylactic treatment of gout.

Metabolic diseases predisposing to CPPD deposition
Hypothyroidism
Hyperparathyroidism
Haemochromatosis
Acromegaly
Gout

Fig. 14.7 Metabolic diseases predisposing to CPPD deposition.

- Colchicine should be used at a dose of 500 μg twice or thrice daily as higher doses often cause gastrointestinal side-effects.
- Corticosteroids are a useful therapy for patients who are unable to tolerate NSAIDs or colchicine. They should not be used for long-term treatment.

Prophylactic therapy

Drugs that lower serum urate can be used to prevent attacks of gout: indications for prophylactic treatment are listed in Figure 14.6. Allopurinol is the most popular drug. It reduces uric acid synthesis by inhibiting the enzyme xanthine oxidase. Other drugs work by increasing renal urate excretion.

Changes in the serum urate can precipitate episodes of gout. Urate-lowering therapy should not be commenced until an acute attack has settled completely and NSAIDs or colchicine should be co-prescribed for the first few months.

Correction of risk factors

Attempts should be made to identify each patient's risk factors for gout. The factors listed in Figure 14.4 that are known to precipitate acute attacks should be avoided if possible.

CALCIUM PYROPHOSPHATE DIHYDRATE (CPPD) DISEASE

Definition

CPPD disease is an arthropathy associated with the deposition of calcium pyrophosphate dihydrate crystals. It can present as an acute synovitis, often referred to as 'pseudogout', or as a chronic arthritis.

Prevalence

CPPD disease is less common than gout, but estimates of prevalence vary greatly. It is predominantly a disease of the elderly and has a slight female preponderance.

Aetiology

The cause of CPPD deposition is unknown. Associations with osteoarthritis (OA) and various metabolic diseases are recognized (Fig. 14.7), but not well understood.

Pathology

CPPD crystals are deposited mainly in cartilage, but also in the synovium, joint capsule and tendons.

Clinical features

The two main clinical presentations of CPPD disease are:

- Acute synovitis (pseudogout).
- Chronic arthritis (pyrophosphate arthropathy).

Pseudogout

This is the commonest cause of acute monoarthritis in the elderly. Patients present with an acute onset of joint pain, stiffness and swelling, sometimes accompanied by fever. The knee is the commonest site, but the ankle, wrist, elbow and shoulder are also targets. Attacks rarely affect more than one joint at a time. As with gout, examination reveals a swollen, erythematous and tender joint. Attacks usually resolve within a few weeks.

Chronic pyrophosphate arthropathy

This has many similarities to OA. Onset is gradual and symptoms include pain, stiffness and loss of function. Commonly affected joints are knees, hips, shoulders, elbows, wrists and metacarpophalangeals (MCPs; particularly the 2nd and 3rd). Some patients develop acute attacks of synovitis. Examination reveals signs of OA, at times with synovitis. Pyrophosphate arthropathy can be distinguished from OA by the involvement of wrists, elbows and ankles and the episodes of synovitis.

Investigations

Synovial fluid examination

Synovial fluid examination with polarized light microscopy is the key to the diagnosis. The CPPD crystals are either rhomboid or rod-shaped and show weak positive birefringence. Gram stain and culture of synovial fluid should be performed to exclude infection.

Radiology

CPPD causes the following radiographic signs:

* Chondrocalcinosis.
* OA-like changes.

Calcification of cartilage (chondrocalcinosis) is often seen in the menisci of the knee, triangular cartilage of the wrist (Fig 14.8) and the symphysis pubis. The cartilage loss, sclerosis, cysts and osteophytes seen in OA all occur in pyrophosphate arthropathy.

Other investigations

CPPD deposition in younger patients is unusual and should be investigated by screening for the underlying associated metabolic disorders (see Fig. 14.7).

Management

Attacks of pseudogout should be treated with analgesics. Joint aspiration and corticosteroid injection often produce rapid relief of symptoms, and colchicine can also be effective. Unlike gout, there is no specific treatment for chronic pyrophosphate arthropathy. It should be managed in a similar way to OA, with emphasis on weight

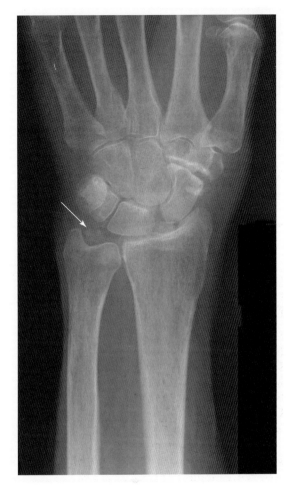

Fig. 14.8 X-ray of the wrist showing calcification of the triangular cartilage.

reduction, physiotherapy, pain control and, when necessary, joint replacement. Episodes of synovitis can be improved by intra-articular corticosteroid injection.

Further reading

Agudelo C A, Wise C M 2001 Gout: diagnosis, pathogenesis and clinical manifestations. *Curr Op Rheumatol* **13**: 234–239

Doherty M 2003 Calcium pyrophosphate dihydrate crystal-associated arthropathy. In: Hochberg M C et al (eds) Rheumatology, 3rd edn. Mosby, London, p 1937–1950

Objective

You should be able to:

- Describe normal variations of gait and joints commonly referred to paediatric clinics.
- Recognize the clincal features of developmental dysplasia of the hip (DDH) and know how to investigate and treat it.
- Recognize and describe features of Perthes disease and a slipped upper femoral epiphysis (SUFE).
- Describe the different ages that the three childhood hip conditions usually present and know how to treat these conditions.
- Recognize the clinical features of clubfoot.
- Describe features and management of osteogenesis imperfecta.
- Understand the common causes of knee pain in children including Osgood–Schlatter disease and osteochondritis dissecans.
- Define and describe the features of juvenile idiopathic arthritis and understand the management principles.
- Know the orthopaedic problems associated with cerebral palsy.

Of all the joint disorders affecting children the most important to the orthopaedic surgeon are those affecting the hip. Many of these children will require hip replacement surgery in adult life with the most severely affected having such surgery in their 20s or 30s.

NORMAL VARIANTS

The majority of referrals to paediatric orthopaedic surgeons are for normal variations in growth of a healthy child brought in by anxious parents. The single most reassuring feature is the symmetrical appearance of the limb. If the child has only one side affected then the condition is much more likely to be pathological.

Examples of normal conditions commonly referred are:

Flat feet

This condition is usually physiological, painless and may be associated with laxity of ligaments. Simple advice only is required as even the use of insoles is questionable and most children develop normally regardless. Pain or fixed deformity suggests an underlying pathological condition.

Toe walkers

Often a child who is beginning to walk does so on tiptoes. Usually the child 'grows out' of this but examination is required to exclude a tight Achilles tendon or an underlying condition such as cerebral palsy.

In-toeing gait

Causes of in-toeing are at three levels: the hip, the tibia and the foot.

Persistent femoral torsion leaves the patient with an excessive internal rotation and the child often sits in a W position rather than cross-legged (Fig. 15.1).

The natural history of this condition is of spontaneous resolution as the child grows, but a small number require femoral osteotomy.

Internal tibial torsion also results in in-toeing but almost always resolves with no treatment.

In the foot, metatarsus adductus (inwardly pointing forefoot) is the cause of in-toeing and again this usually resolves over time.

Bow legs (genu varum)

It is normal for toddlers to have bow legs and they almost always grow out of this over time. Very rarely,

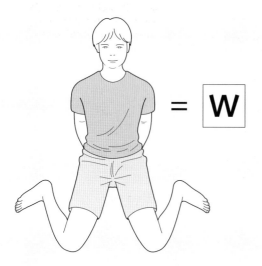

Fig. 15.1 Child sitting in the 'W' position in excessive femoral anteversion.

pathological conditions such as <u>rickets</u> can cause bowing but the child is usually <u>older and</u> the disease on <u>one side only.</u>

Knock knees (genu valgum)

Older children <u>3–8 years </u>old gradually become more <u>valgus</u> as they <u>grow normally,</u> and again the majority <u>straighten spontaneously.</u> Pathological genu valgum is <u>rare,</u> usually <u>asymmetrical,</u> severe and <u>progressive. </u>

PAEDIATRIC HIP DISORDERS

Developmental dysplasia of the hip <u>(DDH)</u>

Introduction

Previously called CDH (congenital dislocation of the hip) this disorder is due to <u>failure of normal development of the acetabulum</u> resulting in abnormal <u>hip anatomy.</u> This disorder encompasses the spectrum of disease from a <u>frankly dislocated hip</u> to <u>acetabular dysplasia</u> (in which the slope of the acetabulum is too steep).

Incidence

The incidence is approximately 2 per 1000, although at birth 5–20 per 1000 hips will be unstable. The majority of these settle, stabilize and develop normally without treatment.

Aetiology and pathology

The condition is seven times more common in <u>females.</u> It is also more common in certain races (northern Italy and North American indigenous population).

DDH is associated with:

- <u>Breech</u> presentation.
- <u>Family history.</u>
- <u> Other congenital deformities.</u>

The <u>left side</u> is more commonly affected but the condition is <u>bilateral in 20%.</u>

The acetabulum relies on the presence of the femoral head for normal development. In DDH there is <u>excessive laxity of the joint</u> with a <u>shallow acetabulum</u> (socket) (Fig. 15.2). This allows the femoral head to develop out of the socket, in severe cases forming a <u>false acetabulum</u> (located above the normal one).

Clinical features

The majority are picked up on <u>routine baby</u> check and referred appropriately.

Late-presenting DDH can occur as the child <u>begins to walk.</u> The child will have a <u>limp</u> and <u>shortness of one leg</u> (if unilateral).

The clinical findings of DDH include:

- <u>Loss of abduction.</u>
- <u>Leg length discrepancy.</u>
- <u>Asymmetrical posterior skin crease.</u>

The special tests for dislocated hips are called <u>Barlow's</u> and <u>Ortolani's</u> tests.

Barlow's test

This is an attempt to <u>dislocate a reduced hip.</u>

The examiner's hand is placed so that the child's knee is flexed to 90° and the examiner's thumb is on the medial aspect of the thigh with the middle finger on the trochanter (Fig. 15.3). The child's hip is flexed to 90° and slightly adducted with a slightly downward force applied to try to dislocate the hip. A clunk is felt if positive.

Ortolani's test

This is an attempt to reduce a dislocated hip.

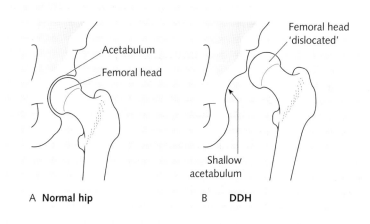

Fig. 15.2 Anatomy of the hip showing (A) normal and (B) pathological hip development.

A **Normal hip**   B   **DDH**

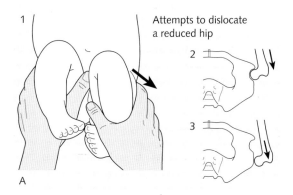

Fig. 15.3 Barlow's test: attempts to dislocate a reduced hip.

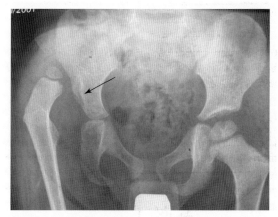

Fig. 15.4 X-ray showing developmental dysplasia of the hip.

Both hips are examined together. The hand is placed in a similar position and the hip is flexed to 90° and then gently abducted. The test is positive if the hip reduces with a clunk.

Diagnosis and investigation

All babies are screened clinically by examination at birth but unfortunately this is unreliable. At-risk babies with the factors listed above are screened with ultrasound. If there is doubt this investigation can be repeated.

An older child should be investigated with X-rays, which once the femoral head has ossified should clearly show if there is a dislocation (Fig. 15.4).

Management

This depends on whether the hip is dislocated and, if so, whether the hip is easily reducible.

Conservative
A Pavlik harness abducts the leg, keeping the hip in joint.

Surgical
If the hip is not reduced, closed or open, reduction is performed.

A variety of surgical osteotomies to the pelvis or femur can be used to maintain reduction and 'normalize anatomy'.

Prognosis

The outcome depends upon the degree of dysplasia and whether or not complications such as osteonecrosis develop. Secondary osteoarthritis is common in this group of patients.

Perthes disease

Introduction

This is a rare disease in which there is segmental avascular necrosis of the femoral head of unknown aetiology.

Incidence

Approximately 1 in 800 are affected.

Aetiology and pathology

Perthes disease is four times more common in boys and is bilateral in 15%. It usually presents between the ages of 4 and 10.

The condition is associated with:

- Family history.
- Lower socioeconomic groups.
- Low-birthweight children.
- Delayed bone age.

Following bone death the femoral head changes, initially showing collapse and fragmentation followed by repair and eventual remodelling, which may take many years.

Variable amounts of the head are involved and this has an effect on outcome. Sometimes the head migrates out of the joint (subluxation).

Clinical features

The child (usually a boy) presents with a gradual history of hip or knee pain associated with a limp. Clinical features will show loss of hip motion, particularly abduction, and there may be fixed deformity. Complete loss of abduction is a worrying sign and may signify subluxation of the hip.

Diagnosis and investigation

Perthes disease in an acutely presenting child could be confused with septic arthritis and therefore blood tests including white cell count (WCC) and inflammatory markers should be performed (all normal in Perthes disease).

A plain X-ray (Fig. 15.5) is the mainstay of diagnosis. The features of Perthes on X-ray are:

- Loss of epiphyseal height.
- Increased density.
- Subchondral fracture, partial collapse and fragmentation of the head.

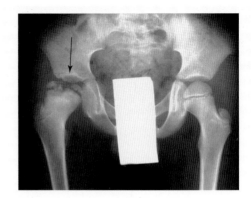

Fig. 15.5 X-ray of Perthes disease.

- Abnormal shape and size of femoral head.
- Subluxation.

Treatment

This depends upon the age of the patient and the extent of the disease.

Conservative

75% of children require no treatment and will have a good long-term outcome. Young patients with less than 50% involvement of the femoral head have a good prognosis.

Surgical

Older patients (8 years) with greater than 50% involvement have a poor prognosis, and significant early osteoarthritis is likely. These children may require containment of the femoral head with surgery, e.g. a pelvic or femoral osteotomy.

Slipped upper femoral epiphysis (SUFE)

This condition is a disorder in which there is structural failure through the growth plate of an immature hip.

Incidence

Approximately 3 per 100 000 children are affected.

It is more common in boys than in girls, usually occurring during the early adolescence growth spurt between 11 and 14 years of age.

Aetiology and pathology

Classically the boy is overweight and has delayed puberty.

The exact cause is not known but may relate to failure of the epiphyseal cartilage to mature as the child grows. Some hormonal conditions are associated.

The slip results in the epiphysis lying posterior and inferior to the femoral neck.

Approximately 60% are bilateral.

Clinical features

The child presents with groin or knee pain (or both) and a limp. The history can be acute or gradual.

Examination findings reveal an external rotation deformity with limitation of most movements. There may be a slight leg length discrepancy. Check for evidence of hypogonadism, hypopituitarism and hypothyroidism.

Diagnosis and investigation

Diagnosis is based on X-ray changes. An anteroposterior (AP) X-ray is taken, but it is the frog lateral which most clearly demonstrates the pathology (Fig. 15.6).

Management

Surgical
All slips should be urgently fixed in situ to prevent further displacement.

Attempts to reduce severe slips are associated with avascular necrosis.

Prognosis

There is a high incidence of secondary degenerative osteoarthritis.

> The age of the child at presentation gives the biggest clue to the diagnosis. DDH is diagnosed at birth. Septic arthritis usually occurs between the ages of 0 and 5 years. Perthes disease presents between the ages of 4 and 10 years. SUFE usually presents in overweight adolescent boys approximately 11–14 years old.

CONGENITAL TALIPES EQUINOVARUS (CLUBFOOT)

Congenital talipes equinovarus (CTEV) encompasses a deformity of the lower limb with calf wasting and the classical inwardly pointing foot.

Incidence

The incidence is approximately 1 per 1000 live births. Males are affected twice as often as females.

Aetiology and pathology

The exact aetiology is not known but arrest of normal limb bud development in utero may be the cause. Genetic factors play a role, with family history being important.

The basic pathology is at the level of the subtalar joint with a cavus deformity (high arch) and metatarsus adductus (Fig. 15.7). The Achilles tendon is also tight, resulting in an equinus deformity.

Associated soft tissue contractures occur on the medial side.

Clinical features

The condition is easily noted at birth as a fixed varus and equinus deformity of the foot. The calf is underdeveloped when compared with the normal side.

The baby should be examined for associated syndromes or conditions (such as DDH).

Diagnosis and investigation

The diagnosis is a clinical one and X-rays are usually taken after initial treatment or surgery.

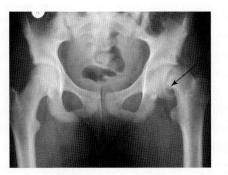

Fig. 15.6 X-ray of SUFE.

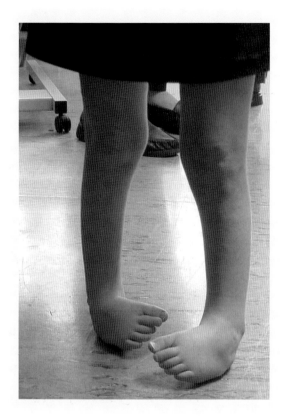

Fig. 15.7 Untreated talipes.

Management

Conservative

Initial treatment is with serial casting changed weekly for up to 3 months.

Surgical

Surgery is reserved for those that fail to correct fully or for later recurrence.

Prognosis

The foot and limb will never be normal in terms of appearance but most patients lead a normal life.

OSTEOGENESIS IMPERFECTA

Also known as brittle bone disease, this disorder predisposes to multiple fractures.

Incidence

The condition is rare.

Aetiology and pathology

Osteogenesis imperfecta (OI) is usually inherited as an autosomal dominant condition, although sporadic and recessive cases can occur.

There are four different types of OI.

The primary abnormality is a defect in the synthesis of type 1 collagen.

Clinical features

The child may present with a low-energy fracture and the diagnosis is made subsequently, following examination and investigation.

Blue sclera are pathognomonic but not always present. Children are usually small with bony deformities (including scoliosis) and joint abnormalities. Associated features include deafness and joint laxity.

Diagnosis and investigation

X-rays may show:

- Multiple fractures.
- Deformity.
- Thin-looking cortex.

Treatment

Conservative

Gentle handling is needed to prevent fractures.

Bisphosphonates such as pamidronate can be given intravenously to try to improve bone strength.

Surgical

Sheffield intramedullary telescoping rods are the mainstay of treatment for prevention of deformity and further fracture.

Established deformity is treated with osteotomy.

Prognosis

The outcome depends on the type of OI; some are incompatible with life.

CEREBRAL PALSY (CP)

Definition

This is a non-progressive neuromuscular disorder that results from injury to an immature brain.

Incidence

2 per 1000 births.

Aetiology and pathology

The cause is often unknown, but can include prematurity, perinatal anoxia, perinatal infection including meningitis, and kernicterus.

Clinical features

There is a mixture of muscle weakness and spasticity. This leads to characteristic joint deformities (see Fig. 15.8). There may be athetosis and ataxia. This can be associated with varying degrees of cognitive impairment and emotional disturbance. Children may also develop seizures.

Diagnosis and investigation

CP is a clinical diagnosis which is based on a thorough birth and developmental history and is normally apparent within the first 2 years of life. MRI of the brain may show periventricular leukomalacia.

Management

Conservative

Depending upon the severity of the disease, children will benefit from physiotherapy, occupational therapy, speech and language therapy and other forms of special needs care.

Surgical

In children who have not developed fixed contractures, intramuscular botulinum injections can temporarily reduce spasticity. For fixed deformity, soft tissue release or tendon lengthening is required to improve function. Severe muscle imbalance can result in bone deformity, sometimes requiring corrective osteotomy.

Characteristic joint deformities associated with cerebral palsy

Flexion at elbows and wrists with clasped fingers
Adductor spasticity of the hips resulting in a 'scissors stance'
Flexion at the hips and knees
Equinus deformity of the feet

Fig. 15.8 Characteristic joint deformities associated with cerebral palsy.

NON-ACCIDENTAL INJURY

Non-accidental injury (NAI) is becoming increasingly recognized and is often diagnosed late but it is important as the child may die.

Clinical features

The history is often vague, inappropriate or changes each time it is told. In young children (<2 years) it is rare for accidental fractures to occur, particularly in long bones. Late presentation is often a feature of NAI.

The child may have external features of abuse such as bruising in other areas of the body away from the fracture. The child may be withdrawn, particularly when the parents are present.

Diagnosis and investigation

In suspected cases a skeletal survey or bone scan is performed to look for occult fractures. Certain fractures such as of the rib or tibial metaphysis are typical of NAI.

Conditions such as osteogenesis imperfecta can be confused with NAI.

Management

The child should be admitted for protection if NAI is strongly suspected and the fracture should be treated in the usual way.

Paediatricians and social workers are involved.

Prognosis

A child left in an abusing environment has a 5% risk of death.

PAEDIATRIC KNEE CONDITIONS

Osgood–Schlatter disease

Definition

Osgood–Schlatter disease is traction apophysitis of the tibial tuberosity.

Incidence

The condition is common, usually in adolescent boys.

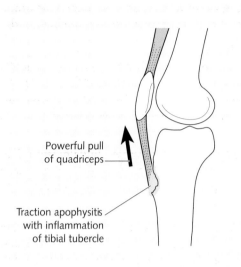

Powerful pull
of quadriceps

Traction apophysitis
with inflammation
of tibial tubercle

Fig. 15.9 Osgood–Schlatter disease.

Aetiology and pathology

It occurs during a period of rapid growth and is related to the pulling force of the patellar ligament on the tibial tuberosity (Fig. 15.9).

It is more common in athletic individuals.

Clinical features

The patient complains of localized pain over the tubercle. The pain is usually made worse by activity and relieved by rest.

Clinically a tender swollen tuberosity is found.

Diagnosis and investigation

Fragmentation and sclerosis of the tibial tuberosity is present.

Sometimes a visible ossicle remains.

Management

Conservative

Treatment is with rest if the knee is very inflamed, with simple analgesia and modification of activities.

Parents are usually very worried and need reassurance.

The child may choose to 'put up' with the pain and continue sporting activities but this has no detrimental effect and will not prolong the natural history of the disease process.

Surgical

Surgery is used only for a painful ossicle.

Prognosis

The natural history is complete resolution of symptoms after 2 years.

Osteochondritis dissecans

Definition

Osteochondritis dissecans is a small area of avascular bone on an articular surface, usually of the knee.

Incidence

The incidence is 4 per 1000.

Presentation is between 10 and 20 years of age and is more common in boys.

Aetiology and pathology

The condition is most common in the knee (medial femoral condyle) but can affect other joints.

It is thought to be due to repeated trauma in a susceptible patient.

Clinical features

The patient has intermittent ache, swelling and 'catching' in the knee. The patient may complain of the knee giving way owing to acute sharp episodes of pain.

Diagnosis and investigation

X-rays show a variably sized lesion on the medial femoral condyle, which is fragmented in the child but in mature adults the lesion shows as a clear, demarcated sclerotic zone. The lesion can be attached or be a loose body.

CT scan further defines the lesion, although MRI has superseded this. An isotope bone scan confirms the presence of activity and hence healing potential.

Management

Conservative

Activity modification with avoidance of sporting activity is adequate to allow small well-fixed lesions to heal.

Surgical

Lesions that become detached or give significant persistent symptoms require surgical stabilization. If the fragment becomes a loose body, removal may be the only option.

JUVENILE IDIOPATHIC ARTHRITIS

Definition

Juvenile idiopathic arthritis (JIA) is persistent inflammatory arthritis occurring in childhood. It does not include 'specific' diseases such as systemic lupus erythematosus (SLE), or the arthritis of inflammatory bowel disease.

JIA has been classified into seven subtypes (see Fig. 15.10). This classification is based partly on the number of joints involved 3 months into the disease process. It is useful as it gives a guide to prognosis.

Clinical features

Joint disease

Children develop symptoms and signs of joint inflammation similar to those in adults, including joint pain, stiffness and swelling. Presentation depends on the joints affected and the age of the child. A 12-year-old with knee synovitis will complain of pain, whereas a 2-year-old may just be irritable and reluctant to mobilize.

Eye disease

Some forms of JIA can be associated with anterior uveitis. Acute anterior uveitis presents with pain and redness of the eye. Chronic anterior uveitis, however, is more insidious and can cause significant visual loss.

Constitutional symptoms

Fatigue, malaise and other systemic symptoms affect JIA patients, in particular those with systemic onset

---

The subtypes of JIA
Oligoarticular disease
Extended oligoarticular disease
Polyarticular disease—rheumatoid factor negative
Polyarticular disease—rheumatoid factor positive
Systemic onset disease
Enthesitis-related arthritis
Psoriatic arthritis

Fig. 15.10 The subtypes of JIA.

---

disease. Growth retardation is an important consequence of prolonged inflammation in childhood.

JIA subtypes

Oligoarticular disease   Between one and four joints are affected, commonly in the lower limb. The prognosis is good; many children 'grow out of it'. This group of patients has the greatest risk of developing chronic anterior uveitis.

Extended oligoarticular disease   Initially fewer than four joints are involved, but these patients gradually develop a polyarthritis after the first 3 months. The outcome is often poor.

Polyarticular disease   More than four joints are affected from an early stage. There are two types. Rheumatoid factor negative arthritis targets small and large joints and tends to persist into adult life. Rheumatoid factor positive arthritis is the equivalent of adult RA. It is seen mainly in teenage girls and frequently has a poor outcome.

Systemic onset disease   This arthritis is characterized by prominent systemic symptoms. It was previously known as Still's disease. Patients present with a swinging fever, plus any of the following features:

- Evanescent rash.
- Hepatomegaly.
- Splenomegaly.
- Anaemia.
- Lymphadenopathy.
- Serositis, especially pericarditis.

The differential diagnosis includes infection and malignancy. Joint involvement may be mild or absent initially.

Enthesitis-related arthritis   Inflammation of entheses, e.g. Achilles tendonitis, is a prominent feature. Enthesitis-related arthritis encompasses juvenile ankylosing spondylitis (AS). A positive family history of AS or related diseases is common and patients are often HLA-B27 positive.

Psoriatic arthritis   This is usually oligoarticular and often involves weight-bearing joints. A personal or family history of psoriasis is common.

Investigations

The diagnosis of JIA is essentially clinical. X-rays are helpful in excluding other causes of joint pain, such as malignancy, but are usually normal in early JIA.

Blood tests are useful, but not diagnostic. Full blood count may reveal anaemia or thrombocytosis and the erythrocyte sedimentation rate (ESR) and C-reactive protein (CRP) are usually elevated. Serum rheumatoid factor should be measured. It is also important to know if the patient has positive anti-nuclear antibodies (ANA), as they are associated with an increased risk of uveitis.

Management

All children with JIA should be seen by a specialist.

Physiotherapy
This is vital to maintain mobility and function. Hydrotherapy is commonly used and is popular with children. Splinting is sometimes required to prevent deformity.

Drug treatment
Initial treatment is with non-steroidal anti-inflammatory drugs. Disease-modifying therapy with drugs such as methotrexate is used when symptoms persist. Corticosteroids may be necessary in severe or systemic onset disease. Biological agents, such as the anti-tumour necrosis factor-α drugs, are indicated for seriously ill children with persistent major synovitis or systemic features.

Eye screening
Children should have their eyes examined regularly by an ophthalmologist.

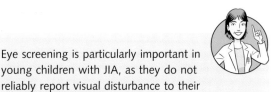

Eye screening is particularly important in young children with JIA, as they do not reliably report visual disturbance to their parents.

Further reading

Cassidy J T, Petty R E 2001 Textbook of pediatric rheumatology. Saunders, Philadelphia

Solomon L, Warwick D, Nayagan D (eds) 2001 Apley's system of orthopaedics and fractures, 8th edn. Hodder Arnold, London

Orthoteers website: http://www.orthoteers.co.uk

Objectives

You should be able to:

- Understand the terms 'fracture' and 'pathological fracture'.
- Classify and describe fractures.
- Recognize the clinical features of a broken bone and know how to investigate this.
- Understand the basic principles of fracture management.
- Describe some of the common methods of surgical fixation of fractures.
- Describe the complications of fractures.

In this chapter we will discuss the basic principles of managing fractures.

Advanced trauma life support and the management of a multiply injured patient is covered in Chapter 17.

Incidence

Fractures are very common and most of us will have at least one during a lifetime. They occur in peaks during childhood, young adult life and again in the elderly when osteoporosis has weakened bony structure (see Ch. 13).

Definition

A fracture is a break in the continuity of the cortex of the bone.

Pathology and aetiology

Fractures can occur through normal bone if the force applied is large enough, or be pathological and occur through abnormal or diseased bone. Figure 16.1 shows the causes of pathological fractures.

In children the fracture may occur through the growth plate (physis), and these injuries are classified as shown in Figure 16.2.

The mechanism of injury dictates the fracture pattern. A twisting injury produces a spiral fracture and a direct blow from the side a transverse or oblique fracture. See Figure 16.3.

As the force applied increases so does the severity of injury; a patient falling 50 feet will have more serious injuries than one twisting an ankle. A bone fails because the load exceeds its strength.

Fractures can be open (associated with a wound; see Fig. 16.4 and Ch. 17) or closed (skin intact). Open fractures allow contamination of the bone ends, predisposing to deep bony infection (see Ch. 18).

Injuries may also involve the joint surface (intra-articular) or the bone may be in lots of pieces (comminuted).

A segmental fracture occurs in the diaphysis (shaft) at two levels, leaving a 'floating segment'.

When concentrating on the bone it is easy to forget the soft tissues surrounding the bone. It is the soft tissues that will eventually provide a healing environment via blood vessel attachment to the injured bone.

Clinical features

The patient almost always gives a clear history of an injury such as falling off a slide, playing football or a simple trip. Difficulty can arise if the patient cannot give a history (e.g. because of dementia), in which case the history may be obtained from the carer or a relative but sometimes there is no history of a fall.

Patients will complain of severe pain and they may have noticed a deformity (e.g. 'my ankle pointed the wrong way, doctor').

Underlying causes in pathological fractures
Underlying causes in pathological fractures
Osteoporosis

Tumours
• Benign
• Malignant
   —Metastasis (most common by far)
   —Primary

Paget's disease
Metabolic bone disease • Osteomalacia/rickets • Hyperparathyroidism • Osteogenesis imperfecta
Other malignancy • Lymphoma • Myeloma
Rheumatoid arthritis
Infection

Fig. 16.1 Underlying causes in pathological fractures.

The whole patient should be examined for associated injuries and then the injured limb.

The affected limb will be swollen and bruised with significant tenderness to palpation. Fracture crepitus can be felt and heard on movement but this is cruel and unnecessary (plus moving the fracture excessively may further damage soft tissues).

It is very important to note:

- Skin condition (i.e. open or closed, but also note blisters and abrasions).
- Peripheral nerve function—any weakness or numbness of the hand or foot.
- Distal vascular status—assess peripheral pulse and capillary refill.

Compare the abnormal with the normal limb.

The patient may also have a clinical deformity associated with a particular fracture, such as a dinner fork deformity in Colles' fracture.

Patients with suspected spinal injuries need to be log-rolled for examination and a full peripheral nervous system examination performed.

Diagnosis and investigation

X-rays should be taken in two planes at 90° to each other (anteroposterior (AP) and lateral) to give accurate information on the suspected fractured bone (Fig. 16.5). If there may be an associated joint injury, X-rays of the joint are needed. Special views are taken for certain fractures (e.g. scaphoid views).

Type I
Fracture through epiphysis only

Physis

Type II (most common)
Fracture travels through physis but part of metaphysis is involved

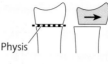

Type III
Epiphyseal segment separated (intra-articular fracture)

Type IV
Fracture crosses physis and involves joint interface
Requires accurate reduction to prevent growth problems leading to deformity

Type V
Crush injury
Difficult to initially diagnose becomes obvious later when growth arrest occurs

Fig. 16.2 The Salter–Harris classification of fractures of the growth plate (physeal fractures).

Computed tomography (CT) scans are helpful to plan surgery in very severe multi-fragmentary intra-articular fractures.

Magnetic resonance imaging (MRI) or isotope bone scans are occasionally used to diagnose a fracture where doubt exists. MRI is also useful in the follow-up of certain fractures to look for avascular necrosis.

Describing fractures

This is something all medical students are very bad at!

Fig. 16.3 Fracture patterns.

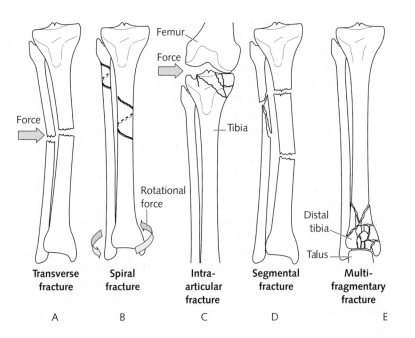

Transverse fracture	Spiral fracture	Intra-articular fracture	Segmental fracture	Multi-fragmentary fracture
A	B	C	D	E

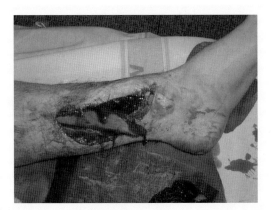

Fig. 16.4 An open tibial fracture.

- Where in the bone, i.e. metaphysis/diaphysis/epiphysis.
- Fracture pattern; transverse, oblique, spiral, segmental, multi-fragmentary.
- Deformity (Fig. 16.6):
  —Displacement
  —Angulation
  —Shortening
  —Rotation (can be difficult to appreciate unless the joints above and below are seen).
- Joint: intra-articular, dislocation.
- **C** is for soft tissues: look for air (may indicate an open fracture), swelling or joint fluid.

Follow the steps outlined below:

- Name and age of patient, and date of X-ray.
- Remember **ABC.**
- **A** is for Adequacy and Alignment (Is the film rotated? Of acceptable quality, i.e. too light or too dark?).
- **B** is for Bone.
  - State which bone, e.g. tibia.

Remember to add important clinical features when describing the fracture:
- General condition of patient
- Skin (open or closed)
- Neurovascular status.

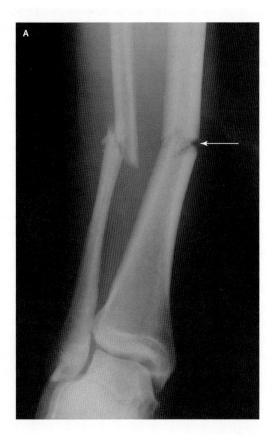
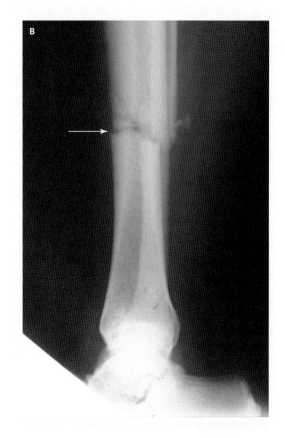

Fig. 16.5 Fracture of the tibia: (A) AP view showing angulation; (B) lateral view.

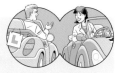

Often the decision about whether or not to operate on a patient's wrist fracture is difficult. If non-operative treatment is chosen it is important to warn the patient if a deformity is likely once they come out of plaster. Most patients function very well without pain despite having a "crooked looking wrist" and are happy to accept this if it is explained clearly.

Management

The basic principles for the treatment of any fracture are:

- Reduction of any deformity (displacement, angulation, rotation), i.e. put the bones back into the correct place.

- Stabilization (maintain reduction until healing occurs).
- Rehabilitation (rehabilitate the limb and the person back to normality).

Reduction

Reduction can be performed open or closed.

- Closed reduction is performed by manipulating the fracture into position. A Colles' fracture is a good example of a fracture treated with closed reduction.
- Open reduction is performed in the operating theatre and involves a surgical procedure to open up the fracture site and accurately reduce the bones under direct vision.

Intra-articular fractures are treated with open reduction so that the joint can be accurately reduced, minimizing the risk of secondary osteoarthritis.

Fig. 16.6 Deformity associated with fractures.

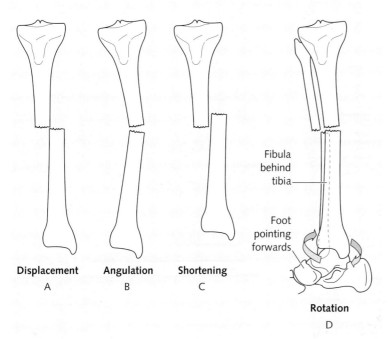

Displacement
A

Angulation
B

Shortening
C

Fibula behind tibia

Foot pointing forwards

Rotation
D

Stabilization

The fracture can be stabilized by conservative or operative treatment. The choice of treatment depends on the bone and fracture characteristics.

Internal fixation allows early mobilization and prevents displacement but there are risks of surgery.

Plaster casts avoid the risk of surgery but there is a chance the fracture will re-displace, and deformity may result if malunion occurs.

Conservative

A plaster of Paris cast is the most common form of conservative treatment used.

The cast should immobilize the joint above and below the fracture and be moulded into position in order to minimize the position 'slipping' in a cast.

Traction used to be widespread on orthopaedic wards but is rarely used nowadays. Traction uses weight to pull fracture fragments into alignment and maintain reduction. The disadvantage of traction is the prolonged treatment with risks of bedsores, deep vein thrombosis (DVT) and chest complications.

Operative

Operative treatment is always required for open fractures and displaced intra-articular fractures. Other fractures may be treated in this way, particularly if they are unstable.

There are several different methods of surgical stabilization (Fig. 16.7):

1. Percutaneous wiring: commonly performed at the wrist. Wires are passed across the fracture site to hold the bone reduced. They are removed at 4–6 weeks.
2. Internal fixation: a plate and screws hold the fracture rigidly.
3. Intramedullary nail: a nail is passed in the medullary cavity and locked at both ends. This is commonly used in the tibia and femur.
4. External fixation: pins or wires inserted into the bone are held by a 'frame' externally.

Rehabilitation

Following healing, or if the fracture is stable, the limb can be mobilized and range of movement exercises begun. The physiotherapist may need to

Fig. 16.7 Methods of surgical stabilization of fractures.

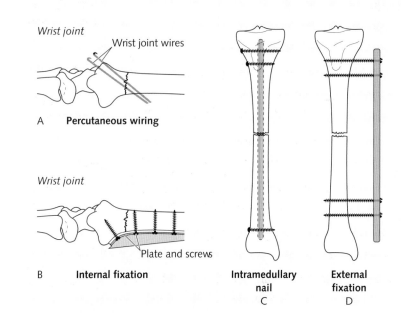

Wrist joint — Wrist joint wires

A **Percutaneous wiring**

Wrist joint

Plate and screws

B **Internal fixation**

Intramedullary nail
C

External fixation
D

instruct the patient in the use of crutches for restricted weight bearing.

Rehabilitation of the limb may often take as much time as the fracture took to heal.

Following a hip fracture elderly patients require intensive input from physiotherapy, occupational therapy and social workers in order to become self-caring and safe prior to discharge.

Complications of fractures

Any complication can be local or general, and immediate, early or late.

Immediate

Local

Initial displacement can cause the skin to tear, resulting in an open fracture. Fracture fragments may press on nerves, producing a nerve palsy (common in the humerus, resulting in radial nerve palsy) or blood vessels, producing ischaemia (e.g. femur—popliteal vessels). See Figure 16.8.

Very occasionally nerves and blood vessels are torn completely and repair is needed.

General

Haemorrhage from fractures can be excessive, especially from femoral, pelvis, open or multiple fractures. Hypovolaemic shock may result.

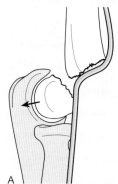

A
Supracondylar fracture of humerus pressing on the brachial artery

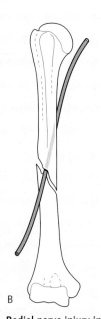

B

Radial nerve injury in humeral fracture

Fig. 16.8 Neurovascular complications of fractures.

Early

Local

Compartment syndrome This is an important complication and results from excessive pressure developing in closed fascial muscle compartments. Following a fracture, swelling can cause the blood supply to the muscle to be impaired. This occurs at the level of small vessels, and peripheral pulses are usually still present. The patient will complain of excessive pain (more than normal) and pain on passive movement of the digits is demonstrated. Paraesthesia develops early as a result of ischaemia of the nerves. The diagnosis is clinical (sometimes confirmed with pressure monitoring), and if present requires urgent surgical fasciotomy (release of compartments).

Infection This can occur early or late following operative stabilization or open fracture. See Chapter 18.

Complex regional pain syndrome (CRPS) This unusual condition can occur after any injury or operation. The exact cause is not known but is thought to relate to the sympathetic nervous system.

Usually the upper limb is affected. The patient has red, swollen shiny fingers with excessive joint stiffness. Atypical pain is also a feature. Physiotherapy is the mainstay of this difficult condition.

General

Deep vein thrombosis DVT can occur after any lower limb injury. Prevention in the form of mechanical (foot pumps, graduated compression stockings) or chemical (heparin, aspirin) agents is routinely used.

Diagnosis is often difficult as the limb will be swollen and may be painful because of the injury. If in doubt obtain a duplex scan or venogram. Some at-risk patients are treated prophylactically with warfarin.

Fat embolus This important condition is common after long bone fractures (particularly of the femur) and occurs due to fat entering the circulation and embolizing to the lungs. The condition occurs because the medullary canal of long bones contains fat. Early stabilization of fractures reduces the risk.

The patient presents with shortness of breath, petechial haemorrhages and sometimes confusion from low circulating Po_2 usually 2–3 days after injury.

This condition is potentially very serious and may lead on to acute adult respiratory failure (ARDS), which can be fatal.

Treatment is supportive with oxygen and fluids. Transfer to a high-dependency unit is advised.

Late

Delayed union/non-union

Some fractures are slow to unite or fail to do so despite adequate treatment. Certain fractures (e.g. of the tibia) are more prone to this and it is more likely if the initial injury was high energy or complicated by compartment syndrome. Further surgery may be required to encourage the bone to heal.

Malunion

The fracture heals but in an abnormal position. This is usually due to inadequate stabilization of the fracture. The resulting deformity may reduce movement in an associated joint and predisposes to late arthritis.

Osteoarthritis

Osteoarthritis, which is discussed in Chapter 9, is more common after intra-articular fractures.

Stiffness

Prolonged immobilization can result in severe joint stiffness.

Contracture

Untreated compartment syndrome or vascular complication can result in contracture. Volkmann's ischaemic contracture is an example.

Growth disturbance

Fractures occurring through the growth plate can cause deformity if the growth arrest is partial (i.e. one side of the limb grows, the other does not) or shortness of the limb if complete. Treatment of such problems is complex.

Further reading

Charnley J 1999 The closed treatment of common fractures, new Golden Jubilee edn. Colt Books, Cambridge (*gives an excellent practical account of plaster and traction techniques*)
Orthoteers website: http://www.orthoteers.co.uk

Objectives

You should be able to:

- Understand the principles of Advanced Trauma Life Support (ATLS).
- Define and understand the management of open fractures.
- Understand basic spine anatomy and recognize structures that can be injured.
- Understand the signs and consequences of pelvic trauma.

When taking a history from a multiply injured patient, the assessment should be rapid to avoid delays in diagnosis of life threatening conditions. Specifically ask about significant past medical history or illnesses, allergies, and drug history. Seek a collateral history from others such as paramedics or people at the scene for clues about the mechanism (e.g. damage to the car) and to gain an idea of the patient's initial condition.

Definition

Trauma can refer to any bodily injury but in the context of surgery normally refers to a patient with major isolated or multiple injuries.

Incidence

Trauma is the leading cause of death in the first four decades of life, the majority from road traffic accidents.

Clinical features

The Advanced Trauma Life Support (ATLS) program and the Golden Hour

This system prioritizes interventions so that life threatening injuries are treated first. This can be remembered simply as 'ABCDE' and is summarized in Figure 17.1. The *golden hour* is the first hour after injury and it is during this period a number of treatable complications of trauma manifest clinically.

Airway

Lack of oxygenated blood delivered to the brain and other major organs causes rapid death in the injured patient. A protected, unobstructed airway is a priority in order to avoid hypoxia. A patient's airway can be compromised with:

- A decreased level of consciousness (head injury, hypoxia, hypovolaemia, drugs).
- Facial trauma.
- Neck trauma.
- Aspiration of vomit or teeth.
- Swelling of subcutaneous tissues associated with burns or smoke inhalation.

Assessment of airway patency should be rapid (see Fig. 17.2). All trauma patients should receive oxygen initially.

C spine control

All trauma patients should be assumed to have unstable neck injuries until proven otherwise, especially in those with an altered conscious level or with injuries above the level of the clavicle. The cervical spine can be immobilized manually or with an appropriately sized hard collar, sandbags and tape across the patient's forehead.

Breathing

Adequate ventilation is required in order to oxygenate blood and therefore major organs such as the brain. Causes of ventilatory compromise include:

- Central nervous system depression (head injury, alcohol, drugs, cervical spine injury).
- Tension pneumothorax (needs immediate decompression **before** a chest X-ray!).
- Open pneumothorax.

Priorities for ATLS	
A	Airway with cervical spine control
B	Breathing
C	Circulation with haemorrhage control
D	Disability/Neurological status
E	Exposure and Environment

Fig. 17.1 Priorities for ATLS.

Neurological assessment using AVPU	
A	Alert
V	Responds to Verbal Stimuli
P	Responds to Pain
U	Unresponsive

Fig. 17.3 Neurological assessment using AVPU.

Signs and symptoms of airway and breathing compromise		
Signs	Airway compromise	Inadequate ventilation
Look	Poor respiratory effort Agitation (hypoxia) Cyanosis Decreased consciousness (unable to protect airway) Tongue, loose teeth, vomit or blood	Asymmetrical rise of chest wall (flail chest, pneumothorax) Laboured breathing Increased respiratory rate Visible penetrating wounds Low oxygen saturations
Listen	Stridor (upper airway obstruction causing inspiratory noise) Hoarse voice (burns)	Unequal air entry (haemopneumothorax) Wheeze
Feel	Remove visible obstructions	Trachea pushed to one side (tension pneumothorax) Tenderness or crepitus (rib fractures) Unequal chest expansion Percussion (hyperresonant = pneumothorax, dull = haemothorax)

Fig. 17.2 Signs and symptoms of airway and breathing compromise.

- Rib fractures.
- Haemothorax.
- Flail chest.

Fig 17.2 shows some signs of airway and ventilatory compromise.

Circulation

Shock is defined as inadequate organ perfusion and tissue oxygenation. The most common cause of this in the trauma patient is hypovolaemia secondary to haemorrhage.

It is important to recognize hypovolaemic shock so that treatment is not delayed. The patient should have capillary refill, pulse rate, blood pressure, urinary output and conscious level closely monitored. Clinical findings allow the doctor to estimate the circulating blood volume (approximately 5L in adults). Blood pressure can be normal with up to 30% blood loss, but as the patient decompensates, there is tachycardia, hypotension and confusion.

There are five areas to look at for potential blood loss—chest, abdomen, pelvis, long bones . . . and on the floor (e.g. arterial bleeding).

Conscious level

This is based on the Glasgow Coma Scale (GCS) and ranges from 3 to 15. This should be monitored regularly to observe for deterioration in the patient's condition. A simpler method to determine conscious level is AVPU (see Fig. 17.3).

Exposure and secondary survey

Look from head to toe for other injuries.

This includes log-rolling the patient (with C spine control) to assess for trauma to the back and spine.

Investigations

A trauma series of X-rays (performed in the resuscitation area) should include at least chest and pelvis films, and if indicated C spine films. Blood tests include full blood count, urea and creatinine, clotting and blood should be grouped and saved in case the patient needs a blood transfusion.

Treatment

Treat life threatening conditions first, in the order of ABCDE. It is then important to identify all other injuries through the secondary survey so that they can be managed by the relevant surgical specialties.

OPEN FRACTURES

Definition

This is when there is an external wound leading to the fracture site potentially allowing contamination with bacteria (see Fig. 16.4).

Incidence

Approximately 23 per 100 000 patients per year.

Aetiology and pathology

Most open fractures are high energy injuries, and are associated with significant damage to soft tissues. They can also occur when the fracture is grossly angulated or displaced, and the sharp fracture end exits through the skin. The greatest risk to the bone is infection and the development of chronic osteomyelitis.

Clinical features

Check ABCDE. Assess the fractured limb for deformity and neurovascular status. Any wound around the fracture site should be assumed to communicate with the bone. Also assess for evidence of compartment syndrome (still possible in open fractures).

Management

Photograph and then dress the wound with a betadine soaked swab. Splint the limb and start intravenous antibiotics as soon as possible. Give tetanus prophylaxis if immunizations are not up to date. The wound should be aggressively debrided in theatre within 6 hours to avoid bacterial infection of the fracture. The fracture can then be stabilized with a suitable method of internal or external fixation.

SPINAL INJURIES

Definition

Includes fractures and subluxations/dislocations of vertebrae. Also includes damage to the spinal cord even in absence of a fracture.

Incidence

Common injury in the trauma patient. 10–20% of patients with a spinal fracture will have a second spinal fracture at another level.

Aetiology and pathology

Most often occur after road traffic accidents (RTA). Other examples include neck injuries from diving into a shallow pool, thoracic injuries from hyper-

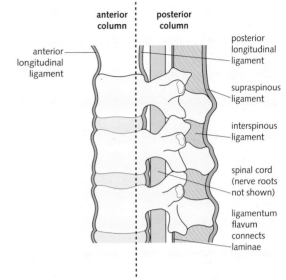

Fig. 17.4 Anatomy of the spine divided into anterior and posterior columns.

flexion and lumbar injuries which commonly occur from falls from a height. Thoracolumbar injuries classically occurred as a result of wearing a lap belt in an RTA. In elderly patients with osteoporosis, low energy trauma can result in simple wedge fractures (Fig. 13.5).

The stability of the spine depends on the bony structures and the integrity of strong ligaments. It can be thought of as two columns (Fig. 17.4). Fractures involving one column only such as anterior wedge fractures are stable (Fig. 13.5) and can be treated conservatively. Fractures involving both columns such as a high energy burst fracture (Fig. 17.5) are often unstable. Injuries may involve the bony structures only, both ligaments and bones or purely ligaments. This means even if the X-ray is normal you cannot assume the spine is stable as **all** the ligaments may be torn!

Be careful with spinal injuries. It is very distressing for the patient and staff if fractures are missed. To exclude injury you need good X-rays (and/or CT) and an awake patient who has not just had morphine to allow proper examination. If in doubt get senior help.

Clinical features

The conscious patient will complain of pain at the level of injury (beware in patients with decreased conscious level). **Patients with facial or head injuries should be presumed to have a significant neck injury until proven otherwise.**

Clinical examination may reveal tenderness, a boggy swelling, bony step, or a gibbus. The patient should be log-rolled with C spine control in order to examine the thoracic and lumbar spine. Check limbs for abnormal neurology. A full neurological examination should include a rectal examination for anal tone and sensation (sacral nerves). Knowledge of dermatomes and myotomes will guide the doctor to the level of spinal cord injury if present.

Remember that spinal injury may cause bradycardia and hypotension (spinal shock). These patients should receive intravenous fluids cautiously.

Diagnosis and investigation

Neck—AP, lateral (to at least T1) and odontoid peg views.

Thoracic and lumbar spine AP and lateral views if indicated.

X-rays can be normal, even with spinal cord trauma.

Further imaging includes CT for fractures and MRI to look for ligament and spinal cord damage.

Treatment

This depends on the stability of the fracture.

Stable fractures can be mobilized.

Unstable fractures require immobilization (e.g. halo vest), bracing or possibly internal fixation.

Prognosis

The patients with spinal cord damage have the worst prognosis and often require extensive rehabilitation on a spinal unit.

PELVIC FRACTURES

These are high energy injuries commonly associated with massive bleeding, urethral, bladder and abdominal injuries.

Incidence

Rare injuries but careful assessment of the polytraumatized patient is necessary to avoid missing such injuries. Most deaths in polytrauma patients occur as a result of pelvic fractures.

Aetiology

The pelvis can be thought of as a stable ring formed from the sacrum, ilium and pubis bones held together by strong ligaments. The basic mechanisms of injury are anteroposterior compression (blow from the front; Fig. 17.6), lateral compression (side

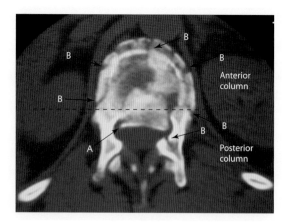

Fig. 17.5 Axial CT scan showing an unstable two-column burst fracture (arrows 'B') with retropulsion of a bone fragment (arrow 'A') into the spinal canal.

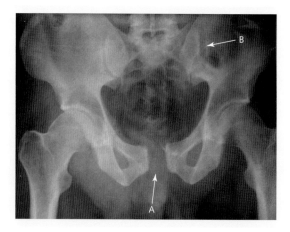

Fig. 17.6 X-ray of an open book pelvic fracture. There is widening at the symphysis pubis (arrow 'A') and the left sacroiliac joint (arrow 'B').

impact), vertical shear forces (usually fall from height) or a combination of all three.

Clinical features

The patient will have pain and may be shocked due to blood loss.

Clinical examination may reveal blood at the urethral meatus (urethral tear) and bruising in the scrotal region. Rectal examination may reveal blood or a boggy, high riding prostate (urethral tear). Bone fragments may be palpable. **Do not** assess pelvic stability by bi-manual compression of the iliac wings ('springing' the pelvis) as this may displace a clot and cause re-bleeding.

Diagnosis and investigation

An AP X-ray of the pelvis should be checked for fractures, symmetry and normal contours. Once stable a CT scan more accurately defines the fracture.

Emergency treatment

The patient should be managed according to ATLS protocol and resuscitated with intravenous fluids. Those patients who either transiently respond or do not respond are likely to have ongoing bleeding. There is haemorrhage from bones, the pelvic venous plexus and rarely, arteries.

Bleeding can be reduced by stabilizing the pelvis. This can be done immediately by tying a bed sheet around the pelvis to close the pelvic ring. Emergency external fixation can then be applied. If this fails, angiography and embolization of bleeding vessels is performed.

Stable fractures require pain relief and mobilization.

Unstable fracture patterns require surgical fixation.

Prognosis

Mortality can be high, especially when the patient has associated head, chest or abdominal injuries. Complications such as urethral tears, sciatic nerve damage or persistent sacroiliac pain can affect quality of life in the long term.

Further reading

Committee on Trauma, American College of Surgeons. Advanced Trauma Life Support® for Doctors. Chicago, IL: American College of Surgeons, 2004
Orthoteers website: http://www.orthoteers.co.uk

Infection of bones and joints

Introduction

Bone and joint infection has become much less common in western society over the last century. This is explained by increasing use of antibiotics and the general improvement in nutrition and health of the population as a whole.

Infection does still occur and needs to be recognized and treated promptly to avoid potentially serious complications.

In this chapter we will talk about osteomyelitis (infection in bone) and septic arthritis (infection in a joint).

Blood supply to bone is from the endosteum and periosteum.

OSTEOMYELITIS

Infection of bone can be caused by direct inoculation (exogenous) or blood-borne bacteria (haematogenous).

In childhood or adolescence osteomyelitis is usually caused by haematogenous spread of bacteria. In adults the source is more likely to be exogenous, most commonly due to infection developing after surgery or after injury (particularly in the case of an open fracture).

Incidence

Osteomyelitis is now uncommon.

Aetiology and pathology

In children there is often a history of preceding trauma, which may predispose the limb to infection. The most common infecting organism overall is *Staphylococcus aureus*, but streptococcal (neonates particularly) and Gram-negative infections can also occur. If unusual organisms are present, consider specific predisposing factors as listed in Figure 18.2, for example patients with AIDS can get fungal infections.

The three most common causes of osteomyelitis are:

- Post-trauma osteomyelitis.
- Post-surgery osteomyelitis.
- Acute haematogenous osteomyelitis.

Post-trauma osteomyelitis

An open fracture means the skin is broken allowing bacteria direct access to the bony surfaces. Large dirty wounds associated with high-energy injuries are more likely to result in post-trauma osteomyelitis. Urgent surgical debridement and lavage are required in order to remove contaminated material and dead bone. Inadequate or delayed surgery often leads to osteomyelitis due to bacteria being harboured within dead bone. In these circumstances the fracture will often fail to heal.

Post-surgery osteomyelitis

Many surgical procedures in orthopaedics involve using implants such as hip replacements or plates

Fig. 18.1 Sequence of events in osteomyelitis. The primary focus of infection (A) has spread through bone, causing the death of cortical bone and formation of a subperiosteal abscess (B). Infection can spread into the joint (C) causing septic arthritis. Death of a segment of bone (sequestrum) occurs (D), and the area is surrounded by new subperiosteal bone (involucrum).

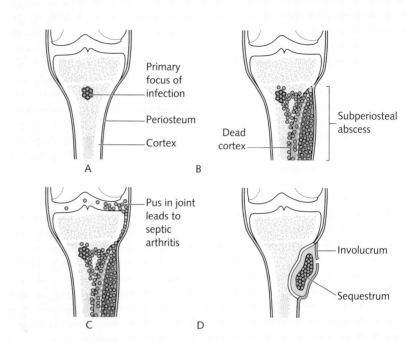

and screws. These 'foreign bodies' can harbour infection if at the time of surgery bacteria are introduced. For this reason orthopaedic surgeons are strict about aseptic techniques in the operating theatre and use antibiotics as prophylaxis. Despite this, infection does still occur and may spread around the implant, devitalizing bone.

Acute haematogenous osteomyelitis

This form of osteomyelitis is usually seen in children and may develop spontaneously.

The pathogenesis of acute haematogenous osteomyelitis is as follows (Fig. 18.1):

1. Trauma to affected limb.
2. A bacteraemia that settles in the metaphysis of a long bone.
3. The metaphysis has a good blood supply but is thought to have very few phagocytic cells capable of fighting infection, therefore allowing the infection to develop.
4. Inflammation and pus formation within the bone.
5. Pus escapes through small holes in bone (harversian canals) to form a subperiosteal abscess.

6. Pus is now present on both sides of the bone, causing this part of the bone to die.
7. Dead bone, now called the sequestrum, harbours infection.
8. Periosteal new bone called involucrum forms as the body tries to fight the infection.
9. In older children the physis (growth plate) acts as a barrier, preventing further spread of infection.
10. In neonates and infants spread can occur across the physis via the epiphyseal artery.
11. In some joints the capsule extends down to the metaphysis. If pus escapes here, then septic arthritis will result.

Acute osteomyelitis can easily become chronic if the sequestrum is neglected or not completely excised at surgery.

Other conditions associated with osteomyelitis

The above three causes of osteomyelitis are the most common but it also occurs in the other conditions listed in Figure 18.2.

Sadly we are now seeing more and more cases of bone and joint infection in intravenous drug users.

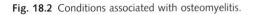

Conditions associated with osteomyelitis	
Congenital	**Acquired**
Sickle cell disease	Diabetes
Haemophilia	Renal failure
	Intravenous drug use
	Malnutrition
	Immunosuppression
	HIV/AIDS

Fig. 18.2 Conditions associated with osteomyelitis.

When you consider that these patients are often malnourished, immunosuppressed (possibly HIV positive), frequently inject themselves deeply with dirty needles and often neglect small abscesses it is not difficult to understand why.

Clinical features

Acute osteomyelitis causes pain, fever and loss of funtion (often a limp if the lower limb is involved).

It is more common in the tibia and femur. The limb will be tender to palpate, erythematous and possibly swollen.

At the extremes of age (neonate, infant or elderly) the symptoms and signs are often non-specific (such as general malaise). These patients can be seriously ill and it can be extremely difficult to pinpoint the exact site of the problem.

Occasionally a patient presents with multiple sites affected or there may be another focus of infection which has then spread from or to bone, for example infective endocarditis. This is called seeding of infection.

In post-surgery and post-trauma osteomyelitis the wound will be painful, red and inflamed. Normally, once postoperative pain has settled, patients are comfortable and can mobilize without pain. If pain persists or increases, infection is a possible cause. Eventually wounds will break down and discharge. If left untreated a sinus will result.

A limb with chronic osteomyelitis will be swollen and have thickened 'woody' skin. Here the focus of infection remains within the bone as a sequestrum and the infection remains quiet for a period of time (can be many years) and then flares up unexpectedly, often producing an abscess. A chronic discharging sinus can result.

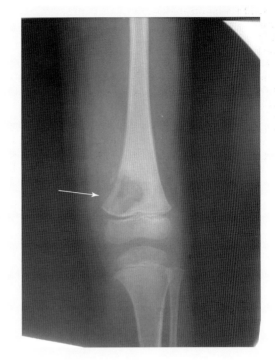

Fig. 18.3 Brodie's abscess.

Diagnosis and investigation

The diagnosis may be obvious on clinical features, particularly if the history reveals a clear predisposing factor.

A raised white cell count (WCC), erythrocyte sedimentation rate (ESR) and C-reactive protein (CRP) will be present on blood tests.

Initially X-rays will be normal, but after 10 days, features of lysis, periosteal elevation and new bone formation are seen. Later the sequestrum may be seen as a sclerotic area. A Brodie's abscess may be seen in the distal femur (Fig. 18.3).

Early osteomyelitis can be detected before X-ray changes, using bone scanning (shows increased uptake) or magnetic resonance imaging (MRI).

It is very important to send microbiology specimens such as blood cultures prior to starting antibiotics.

Management

Conservative

The patient needs adequate analgesia, splintage of the affected limb and appropriate antibiotics. Consultation with the microbiologist is advisable.

As the majority of infections are with *Staph. aureus*, flucloxacillin and fusidic acid are usually the first-line antibiotics, given initially intravenously for 6 weeks.

Antibiotic-resistant strains such as MRSA are becoming more prevalent and if suspected then vancomycin is usually the antibiotic of choice (consult a microbiologist).

Provided the patient does not have an abscess or dead bone present, then antibiotics will suffice.

Surgical

If an abscess is present this should be drained surgically. Dead bone, the sequestrum, needs to be removed.

In a chronic case if the patient and surgeon decide to attempt to cure the infection, extensive surgery is required to remove the implant and all infected bone. Techniques for doing this vary depending on the extent of involvement and the site.

It is possible to simply treat the 'flare-ups' and suppress the infection with antibiotics when required.

Complications

Complications occur if:

- Osteomyelitis persists.
- The physis is damaged, leading to growth disturbance and deformity.
- The infection spreads to the joint, causing septic arthritis.

Prognosis

For acute osteomyelitis the outcome is good and the majority make a full recovery provided none of the above complications occur. In chronic cases following surgery or trauma many surgical procedures are often required and amputation is not an uncommon outcome.

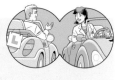

Chronic osteomyelitis is very difficult to treat. It may remain dormant for many years and then flare up intermittently causing pain and loss of function. These flare-ups are often managed simply with antibiotics. Some people cannot tolerate long-term loss of function of the limb in which case amputation may be indicated.

SEPTIC ARTHRITIS

Septic arthritis is infection within a synovial joint.

Incidence

The condition is uncommon, but is seen more often in children, young adults and the elderly. It is more common in the developing world and in patients with a predisposing factor. In children, it is less common than osteomyelitis.

Aetiology and pathology

Infection reaches a joint via the haematogenous route, direct spread from the metaphysis or penetrating trauma/surgery. Associated conditions are similar to those for acute osteomyelitis (see Fig. 18.2) with the addition of rheumatoid arthritis and crystal arthropathy.

Certain organisms are more common at different ages. *Haemophilus influenzae* used to be the most common infecting organism in infants prior to the introduction of the vaccination programme. In young sexually active adults the most likely infecting organism is *Neisseria gonorrhoeae*.

In haematogenous septic arthritis the bacterium settles in the synovium, which may be inflamed due to trauma or disease. Proliferation of bacteria causes an inflammatory response by the host with numerous leucocytes migrating into the joint. The variety of enzymes and breakdown products produced damages the delicate articular cartilage very quickly (within hours) and if left unchecked permanent damage will ensue (Fig. 18.4).

Clinical features

The patient will have an acutely hot swollen joint with a fever and be systemically unwell. An infant or young child will be distressed, unwell and difficult to assess. There may be a history of recent infection such as otitis media.

Septic arthritis is more common in the hip and knee but can present in the shoulder, elbow and wrist.

Any movement at all causes intense pain, and weight bearing will not be tolerated. If the joint is superficial an effusion is palpable.

In neonates and infants the diagnosis may be less obvious, particularly if the joint is deeply

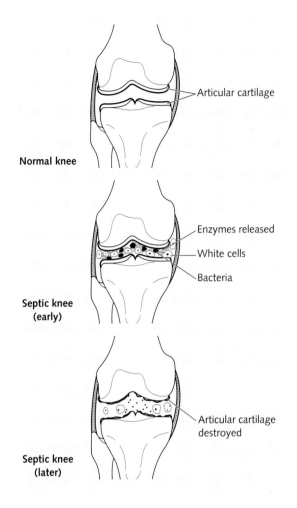

Normal knee

Articular cartilage

Enzymes released

White cells

Bacteria

Septic knee (early)

Articular cartilage destroyed

Septic knee (later)

Fig. 18.4 Sequence of events in septic arthritis.

situated such as the hip. These patients may be seriously ill.

Patients with an infected joint will not let you put the joint through a passive range of movement. It is too painful!

Diagnosis and investigation

- WCC, CRP and ESR will be raised.
- X-rays will be normal initially and show joint destruction late.

- If available, ultrasound scanning is useful to see if there is a joint effusion where the hip is the suspicious joint.
- If the joint aspirate is cloudy, it is sent for urgent Gram stain, culture and examination for crystals.

Management

Conservative

Relieve pain by giving analgesia and splinting the limb. Give appropriate antibiotics as directed by the microbiologist, depending on the age of the patient and any predisposing illness.

Surgical

Unlike in osteomyelitis, the treatment of septic arthritis is always surgical drainage. This should be done as an emergency to limit the damage to the joint cartilage.

Complications

- Seeding of infection can occur to the spine or other organs.
- Recurrence of infection.
- Joint destruction with long-term arthritis or even anklyosis (bony fusion across the joint).
- Avascular necrosis (particularly in the hip).

Prognosis

If treated promptly, prognosis is good, but if joint destruction occurs it is very poor.

TUBERCULOSIS

Incidence

Tuberculosis (TB) is common in global terms and causes significant morbidity and mortality in Africa and Asia.

TB is making a 'comeback' in the UK with over 10 000 cases per year, most of which are in the Asian community.

Aetiology and pathology

TB is due to *Mycobacterium tuberculosis* or *Mycobacterium bovis* infection.

137

Histologically the classical appearance is of caseating necrosis.

Musculoskeletal tuberculosis results when primary TB (lung) becomes widespread or when later reactivation or reinfection occurs (immunosuppressed patients).

Clinical features

Patients have general symptoms of ill-health such as malaise, weight loss, cough and loss of appetite. The most common musculoskeletal sites affected by TB are the spine, hip and knee.

Unlike other orthopaedic infections, TB presents with gradual symptoms of pain and may be initially diagnosed as osteoarthritis or inflammatory arthritis.

Diagnosis and investigation

The two commonest tests are the Mantoux and Heaf tests, which are skin hypersensitivity tests.

For confirmation, large samples of bone or synovial fluid are required which need to be cultured for a prolonged period (6 weeks).

If mycobacterial infection is suspected, samples should be submitted to a Ziehl–Neelsen stain and the mycobacteria appear as red acid–alcohol-fast organisms.

X-rays show variable amounts of joint destruction with periarticular osteopenia.

In the spine, vertebra plana may be found with almost complete collapse of the vertebral body (see Fig 23.9).

Treatment

Drugs commonly used are rifampicin, isoniazid and ethambutol.

A spinal abscess may need drainage with stabilization of the spine.

Ankylosed joints from old treated TB can be replaced (usually the hip).

Further reading

Solomon L, Warwick D, Nayagan D (eds) 2001 Apley's system of orthopaedics and fractures, 8th edn. Hodder Arnold, London

Orthoteers website: http://www.orthoteers.co.uk

Objectives

You should be able to:

- Recognize the common symptoms of fibromyalgia.
- Understand the strategies employed in the management of patients with fibromyalgia.

Definition

Rheumatologists meet many patients suffering from chronic widespread pain that cannot be explained by an inflammatory or articular problem. There are often associated symptoms such as depression, fatigue and sleep disturbance. Fibromyalgia is a diagnosis used to describe this collection of clinical features, particularly when they are accompanied by the finding of soft tissue tenderness on examination. However, the existence of fibromyalgia as a disease is a matter of debate. Many physicians recognize the clinical features above, but feel that giving patients a label may reinforce their illness behaviour.

Prevalence

Fibromyalgia is common. The prevalence is estimated to be between 2 and 5%.

Aetiology

The aetiology of fibromyalgia is unknown, but several risk factors for the condition are recognized. These include:

- Female sex.
- Middle age.
- Stress.

There is some overlap between the features of fibromyalgia and other syndromes that have a functional component (Fig. 19.1).

Pathogenesis

The roles of various neurotransmitters, hormones and peptides have been examined in fibromyalgia; in spite of much research, the pathogenesis has not been explained.

Clinical features

Fibromyalgia predominantly affects women between the ages of 30 and 60 years. Patients usually report a long history of widespread pain which responds poorly to analgesia. Other common symptoms are shown in Figure 19.2.

Fatigue is often severe and follows minimal exertion. Sleep disruption is common and patients frequently complain that they wake feeling unrefreshed. Psychiatric problems, such as anxiety and depression, are thought to affect as many as 20% of fibromyalgia sufferers.

The only significant finding on musculoskeletal examination is the presence of soft tissue tenderness, usually at multiple sites. Common sites of tenderness are shown in Figure 19.3.

Investigations

Fibromyalgia is a clinical diagnosis based on recognition of symptoms and tender points. The only role of investigations is in the exclusion of other conditions. Certain diseases can mimic fibromyalgia, including systemic lupus erythematosus (SLE), hypothyroidism, osteomalacia and polymyalgia rheumatica.

Management

There is no specific treatment for fibromyalgia. Quality of life for most patients remains poor. The following treatment strategies may help.

Education

- Informs patients about the condition.
- Reassures them that they do not have a destructive arthritis.

- Emphasizes that they will not harm their joints by exercising.

Physiotherapy

A graded aerobic exercise regime can improve fitness and reduce pain and fatigue.

Cognitive behavioural therapy

This encourages patients to develop mechanisms to cope with their symptoms.

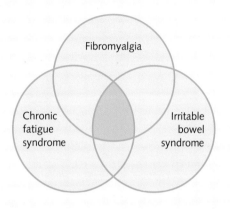

Fig. 19.1 Overlap between fibromyalgia and other syndromes.

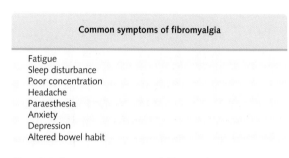

Common symptoms of fibromyalgia
Fatigue
Sleep disturbance
Poor concentration
Headache
Paraesthesia
Anxiety
Depression
Altered bowel habit

Fig. 19.2 Common symptoms of fibromyalgia.

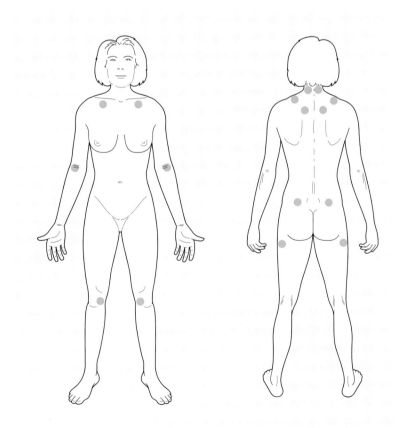

Fig. 19.3 The 'tender points' of fibromyalgia.

Drug therapy

Low-dose amitriptyline can help improve sleep, fatigue and pain.

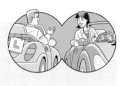

It is important to give patients with fibromyalgia information about the condition when you make the diagnosis. Many patients are told that the news is good, they don't have arthritis and can 'get on with their lives'. They often leave clinic thinking that the doctor hasn't taken them seriously and thinks the pain is 'in their head'. It is helpful to explain that the pain is real, but is arising from the tendons, ligaments and muscles rather than the joints. Although certain activities will be painful, gentle exercise will not harm them and, if continued, can lead to an improvement in symptoms.

Further reading

Arthritis Research Campaign patient information leaflet
Goldenberg D L 2003 Fibromyalgia and related syndromes. In: Hochberg M C et al (eds) Rheumatology, 3rd edn. Mosby, London, p 701–712
Ryan S Fibromyalgia. In: ABC of Rheumatology, 3rd edn. BMJ Books, London

You should be able to:

- Describe how to reduce the risk of infection in orthopaedics.
- Understand the basic priciples of joint surgery for osteo- and rheumatoid arthritis.
- Understand the term 'osteotomy' and give an example of its use.
- Understand what is meant by arthroscopy and on which joints this is most commonly performed.
- Understand the term arthroplasty and know the main indication for this type of surgery.
- Describe which joints are commonly fused and why.

Orthopaedic operations are very common and this chapter outlines the principles of surgery.

STERILITY

Infection is the major concern in elective orthopaedic surgery. Deep infection in joint replacement surgery is disastrous when it occurs as simple measures such as antibiotics and abscess drainage will not eradicate the infection. The patient may be worse off than before surgery and require lengthy hospital stays with extensive further surgery and significant risks.

The risk of infection is minimized by the following preoperative, perioperative and postoperative factors.

Preoperative factors

- Cleaning the skin.
- Avoidance of concurrent infection (e.g. urinary tract infection).
- Preoperative antibiotics on induction of anaesthesia.
- A healthy, well-nourished patient.

Perioperative factors

- Clean laminar airflow theatre (air is specially filtered).
- Adequate skin preparation and impervious exclusion drapes.

- Exhaust suits (enclosed clothing with air evacuation to prevent skin contaminants falling onto the wound).
- Sterile instruments and prostheses.
- Careful surgical technique (including haemostasis).
- The use of antibiotic loaded cement in joint arthroplasty

Postoperative factors

- Wound dressing.
- Prophylactic antibiotics for possible bacteraemia (e.g. during catheterization).
- Postoperative antibiotics.

OPERATIONS

There are several things a surgeon can do for a painful joint.

Joint debridement

A diseased joint can be debrided surgically in an attempt to improve range of movement or to reduce symptoms such as pain and swelling.

Debridement means removing diseased tissue. Osteophytes are often removed in osteoarthritis but debriding a joint does not cure or stop the progression of the disease process.

Examples of joints where debridement is performed include the first metatarsophalangeal (MTP) joint in hallux rigidus. See Figure 20.1.

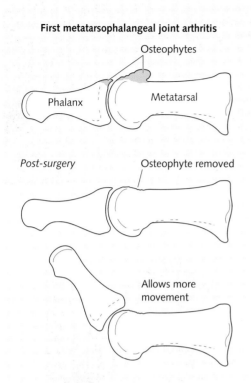

First metatarsophalangeal joint arthritis

Osteophytes

Phalanx Metatarsal

Post-surgery Osteophyte removed

Allows more movement

Fig. 20.1 Joint debridement.

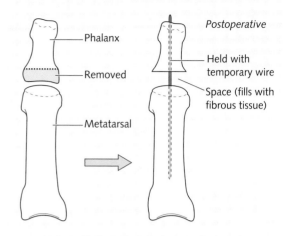

Phalanx

Removed

Metatarsal

Postoperative

Held with temporary wire

Space (fills with fibrous tissue)

Fig. 20.2 Excision of a joint.

The operation leaves the joint unstable and it may still be painful.

Joint arthrodesis

Arthrodesis or fusion is performed to make the bones 'heal' together across a joint. Movement is obviously lost but if the fusion is sound then the joint will be pain-free.

Bones are most commonly fused around the foot and ankle or hand and wrist, usually in patients with rheumatoid arthritis. Examples include ankle fusion, subtalar fusion and wrist fusion.

Fusion can be achieved by different means, such as:

- Internal fixation (screws, staples, plates) (Fig. 20.3, top).
- Intramedullary nail (Fig. 20.3, bottom).
- External fixation.

A bone graft may be used.

Joint arthroplasty

Almost any joint can now be replaced. The primary reason to replace a joint is pain.

The advantage of replacement over fusion is that movement is maintained and therefore function can return to near normality.

Implants are usually a combination of a metal and high-density polyethylene bearing to keep frictional forces to a minimum. The joint surfaces are also highly polished for low friction.

Arthroscopy

'Keyhole surgery' techniques have become routine in recent years.

In the past, arthroscopy was seen as a diagnostic procedure but now a number of operations are possible by purely arthroscopic means. Examples are stabilization or rotator cuff repair in the shoulder, and meniscal repair or anterior cruciate ligament reconstruction in the knee.

It is now commonplace for many joints to be arthroscoped, including the shoulder, ankle, hip and wrist.

Joint excision (excision arthroplasty)

This operation has been mostly superseded by joint replacement. It is still occasionally performed for severe arthritis of the first MTP joint (Keller's procedure) and also in the hip (Girdlestone's procedure) if the patient has had an infected joint. See Figure 20.2.

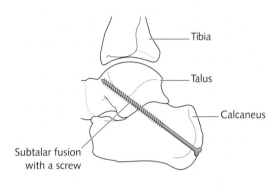

Tibia

Talus

Calcaneus

Subtalar fusion
with a screw

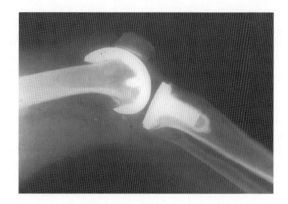

Fig. 20.4 Total knee replacement.

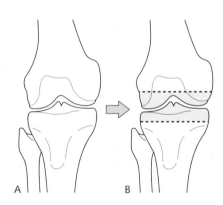

A   B

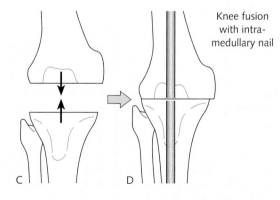

Knee fusion
with intra-
medullary nail

C   D

Fig. 20.3 Joint fusion.

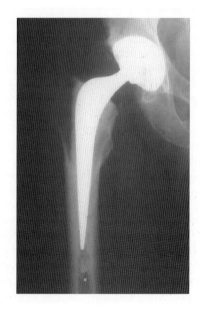

Fig. 20.5 Total hip replacement.

The joint components are either cemented in place or uncemented (press fit).

Joint replacements are available for almost any joint although the most reliable are:

- Knee (Fig. 20.4).
- Hip (Fig. 20.5).
- Shoulder.
- Elbow.

The vast majority of replacements should last over 10 years but this is partly dependent on the patient. A young patient is more likely to wear out a prosthesis.

The most common reasons for failure of an implant are loosening, infection and fracture (Fig. 20.6).

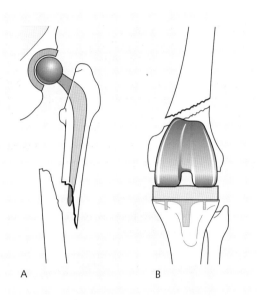

A   B

Fig. 20.6 Periprosthetic fracture of the femur: (A) at the hip; (B) at the knee.

Osteotomy/deformity correction

An osteotomy is an operation to break a bone and realign the joint or deformity.

As described in Chapter 9, the most common place for this to occur is at the knee to offload the medial compartment, which may be arthritic.

Deformity can occur for other reasons (see Ch. 5) and correction of such deformity is an important part of orthopaedic surgery. The two most common reasons for deformity needing correction are mal-union of fractures (tibia and femur) and congenital deformity (e.g. clubfoot). This is an expanding area of orthopaedics with a lot of interest in correction of complex multiple deformities.

It is also possible to lengthen bones gradually with external fixation usually in the form of circular frames with a variety of hinges and movable rods. See Figure 20.7.

Operations for rheumatoid arthritis

In Chapter 10 there is a lot of information about the diagnosis and medical treatment of rheumatoid arthritis but the majority of patients with rheumatoid disease will have surgery at some stage and

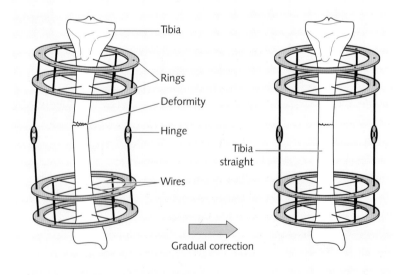

Tibia

Rings

Deformity

Hinge

Wires

Tibia straight

Gradual correction

Fig. 20.7 Deformity correction with frames. (A) The use of an external fixator 'frame' to achieve gradual correction of a deformity over several weeks. Note that the frame is also bent but straightens out as the bone is corrected.

A

some have multiple operations (you may come across a patient with shoulders, elbows, hips and knees replaced, and both wrists and ankles fused!).

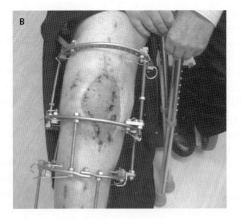

Fig. 20.7 (*Continued*) (B) Ilizarov frame on a fractured tibia.

Synovectomy

The aim of this operation is to remove the synovial lining of the diseased joint or the tenosynovium around tendons. The procedure needs to be performed early and has three possible beneficial effects:

1. Reduction of swelling.
2. Slowing of disease progression.
3. Prevention of tendon rupture.

Unfortunately it is impossible to remove the whole synovium with synovectomy, and symptoms often return. This procedure is usually performed around the wrist.

Operations commonly performed on rheumatoid patients are shown in Figure 20.8.

Further reading

Canale S T 2006 Campbell's operative orthopaedics, 11th edn. Mosby, St Louis, vols 1–4

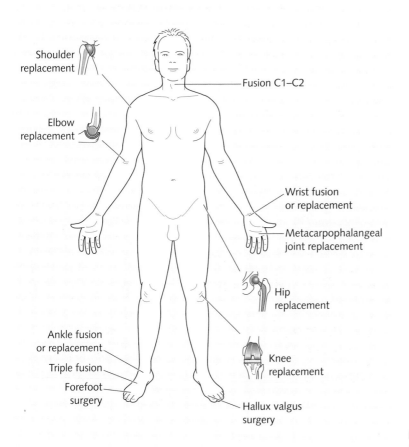

Fig. 20.8 Common operations for rheumatoid patients.

Pre- and postoperative care

Objectives

You should be able to:

- List ways to prevent complications from orthopaedic surgery.
- Understand the purpose of preoperative assessment and think of examples of important conditions that may be discovered at this stage.
- Classify complications of surgery.
- List the local and general complications of surgery.
- Outline basic postoperative care.
- Treat low blood pressure and low urine output postoperatively.
- Define shock and know the five major causes.

Orthopaedics is a surgical speciality and one of the tasks of a junior doctor is to assess patients prior to surgery and look after them postoperatively.

Any surgical procedure has risks and complications, and knowledge of these helps minimize and prevent them.

Patients now need to be made aware of these important complications before informed consent is obtained.

Complications are divided into:

- Local (specific to that operation), and
- General (common to any operation).

We further subdivide complication on the basis of the time that has elapsed after surgery, into:

- Immediate (within 24 hours).
- Early (days/weeks).
- Late (months/years).

PREOPERATIVE ASSESSMENT

Complications can be minimized by careful preoperative preparation. Any concurrent medical problems need to be stabilized and new conditions identified, investigated and treated appropriately.

Elective patients are seen a few weeks before surgery in the preoperative assessment clinic. The following should be recorded.

General

- Observations (BP, pulse, temperature): the patient may have undiagnosed atrial fibrillation (AF) or hypertension.
- History including past medical history and drug history: the patient may be on warfarin and will need this to be stopped prior to surgery and may need admission for intravenous heparin.
- Detailed systemic enquiry: the patient may have shortness of breath on exertion and chest pain (angina). Such a patient following investigation may even go on to have coronary bypass surgery prior to the orthopaedic operation.
- Examination: e.g. the patient may have a heart murmur.
- Blood tests (unnecessary in young, fit patients for simple surgery): full blood count (FBC), glucose, urea and electrolytes (U&E), liver function tests (LFTs) and clotting screen. Sickle cell test for patients of Afro-Caribbean origin. Arterial blood gases may be required if the patient has chest disease.
- Blood can be grouped and saved and cross-matched if significant blood loss is expected.
- Urinalysis for diabetes mellitus or urinary tract infection (UTI). If a patient has an UTI, it should be treated prior to any orthopaedic operation.
- Electrocardiogram (ECG) and chest X-ray (if indicated).

- Further investigations should be ordered if required, e.g. cardiac echo in aortic stenosis.

Informed consent should be taken by a surgeon capable of performing the operation so that particular risks and expectations can be explained to the patient. This means the pre-registration House Officer is not the best person for the job!

Local

The patient should be asked if the limb is still painful because the surgery may be unnecessary.

The limb is examined.

Note skin condition (there may be a rash or skin breakdown over the operation site), pulses, range of movement and look for any distal infection. For example, a knee replacement procedure should not be carried out in a patient with an infected ingrowing toenail.

IMMEDIATE PREOPERATIVE CARE

Additional monitoring such as an arterial line and central venous line can be inserted in the anaesthetic room for patients expected to have a complicated anaesthetic.

A urinary catheter is important to assess fluid balance in patients who may lose significant amounts of blood.

Intravenous antibiotics and deep vein thrombosis (DVT) prophylaxis are also given if necessary.

BASIC POSTOPERATIVE CARE

General

Patients are taken to recovery until fully awake, then transferred to a high-dependency unit (HDU) or the ward.

Regular recordings are made of BP, pulse and oxygen saturation.

Adequate pain relief is very important.

Check sensation, perfusion, pulses and function of digits distal to the operative field.

After major surgery requiring an inpatient stay, patients will need:

- FBC and U&E checked the day after surgery.
- X-rays of the joint operated upon.

Once patients are well, every effort is made to mobilize them and encourage early safe discharge. DVT prophylaxis is continued until patients are mobile.

A multidisciplinary approach is needed to achieve this, with physiotherapy, occupational therapy, social workers, nursing staff and sometimes physicians having input.

Home modifications are required for patients having a joint arthroplasty.

Local

Elevation in a Bradford sling (for an arm) or on a Braun's frame (Fig. 21.1) is very important to reduce swelling.

Distal neurovascular observations are performed to check the perfusion and function of the limb distal to the operation.

As soon as possible, physiotherapy is encouraged, to mobilize the limb.

COMPLICATIONS

General

Respiratory

Chest infections

Complications affecting the respiratory system are very common postoperatively.

A chest infection typically presents early with fever and shortness of breath. Elderly patients may be confused.

There may be signs of consolidation on examination and a low Po_2.

Treatment is with physiotherapy, nebulizers and antibiotics.

Pulmonary embolus

Immobile orthopaedic patients with traumatized limbs are very susceptible to deep vein thrombosis. Risk is reduced by mechanical (foot pumps, graduated compression stockings) and chemical agents (heparin, clexane, aspirin, warfarin) and early mobilization.

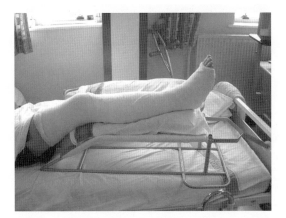

Fig. 21.1 Braun's frame used to elevate a lower limb.

If the clot propagates and then breaks off it travels to the lungs (a pulmonary embolus), which can be fatal. The patient becomes acutely short of breath and has pleuritic chest pain with signs of tachycardia, tachypnoea and a low PO_2. An ECG may show a sinus tachycardia, arrythmias or the classical but rare S1Q3T3.

Treatment should be started immediately in the form of low molecular weight subcutaneous heparin if suspected and diagnosis is proven with a computed tomographic pulmonary angiogram (CTPA)

Cardiac

Myocardial infarction (MI)
MI is a relatively common postoperative complication, particularly in the elderly or those with preexisting heart disease. Patients do not always have typical central crushing chest pain radiating to the left arm associated with sweating and nausea and the cardiac event may be silent or occur during anaesthesia. This should be suspected in any patient with unexplained hypotension.

Diagnosis is made based on raised troponin cardiac enzymes and electrocardiograms (ECGs).

Treatment includes oxygen and aspirin. Further agents may be used based on an opinion from the physicians (it is usually impossible to give thrombolytic drugs to postoperative patients owing to the risk of bleeding).

Left ventricular failure
This can result from a cardiac event or from aggressive fluid management over the perioperative period.

It is important not to give too much fluid, particularly to elderly patients with little physiological reserve.

These patients present with shortness of breath, and signs include a raised jugular venous pressure (JVP) and bibasal crackles. Simple measures such as sitting the patient up and giving oxygen can dramatically improve the patient's condition. Further treatment includes diuretics and nitrates.

Blood loss and blood transfusion

Most patients do not require a blood transfusion postoperatively, even after a total hip or knee replacement. Blood transfusions are expensive (£400 per unit) and are associated with transfusion reactions, transmission of infections (hepatitis, HIV, vCJD) and immunosuppression. Therefore blood should be prescribed sparingly. Most patients can tolerate a Hb of 8 g/dL even if they have pre-existing ischaemic heart disease.

Gastrointestinal

Bleeding
The most important complication of the gastrointestinal (GI) system is bleeding, and the most common reason for this on the orthopaedic wards is non-steroidal anti-inflammatory drug (NSAID) therapy.

Patients with haematemesis or melaena have a suspected upper GI bleed until proven otherwise. Diagnosis is confirmed with upper GI endoscopies performed as soon as possible. Supportive measures including starting a proton pump inhibitor (PPI), cross-matching of blood, fluid resuscitation, careful observations and oxygen are required.

Referral to a gastroenterologist or surgeon is needed.

Paralytic ileus
This is a less serious complication presenting with abdominal distension and nausea. Operations or trauma to the spine predispose to ileus, which usually spontaneously corrects after a few days on intravenous fluids and a nasogastric tube.

Renal

Renal failure
Pre-existing renal impairment is common in orthopaedic patients and the additional insult of a

fracture or surgery with the associated blood loss can tip the balance, causing renal failure.

Factors influencing the development of renal failure include drugs (diuretics, NSAIDs) and hypovolaemia. It is very important to keep patients well hydrated with enough fluid to prevent prerenal failure.

Careful monitoring of fluid input with hourly urine output and daily urea and electrolyte measurement are important when assessing such a patient.

Low urinary output postoperatively is almost always due to hypovolaemia and patients require fluid. It is very important to carefully assess fluid balance, so that diuretics are not given to such patients just to increase the output. This may precipitate renal failure!

Urinary tract infection

Urinary tract infections postoperatively are very common. Diagnosis is made on urinalysis and a midstream urine (MSU) sample is sent to microbiology. Antibiotics are started until culture and sensitivity results are known.

Local

Figure 21.2 lists local complications, their timing, causes, signs and symptoms, and management.

SHOCK

Shock is defined as an inability to maintain adequate tissue perfusion and oxygenation.

Every doctor should be able to recognize shock.

On the orthopaedic wards the most likely causes are hypovolaemic, septic and cardiogenic shock, although neurogenic shock can occur after spinal cord injury. Anaphylactic shock is less common, but possible if patients are allergic to drugs or latex.

Hypovolaemic

Haemorrhage is the most likely cause of hypovolaemic shock, which is due to inadequate circulatory volume. These patients require intravenous fluids and sometimes blood to restore blood pressure.

Cardiogenic

The heart is unable to maintain adequate cardiac output, usually because of infarction. Intravenous fluids may further overload the heart and positive inotropes such as noradrenaline may be required.

Neurogenic/spinal

This is due to peripheral vasodilatation secondary to spinal cord injury.

It is important not to overload such a patient with fluid in an attempt to raise the blood pressure (the BP remains low because of loss of peripheral resistance). A sytolic blood pressure of 100 mmMg is normally acceptable in these patients.

Septic

Peripheral vasodilatation is due to bacterial endotoxins in severe infection.

Anaphylactic shock

This occurs in patients already sensitized to an allergen. There is an aggressive immune response resulting in massive histamine release from basophils. The patient may rapidly deteriorate, and develop a generalized urticaria, with stridor (upper airway narrowing), wheeze and shortness of breath. There is massive vasodilatation and a tachycardia associated with hypotension. Treatment should be rapid including emergency airway procedures, oxygen, nebulizers, intravenous hydrocortisone, antihistamines (chlorphenamine) and intramuscular or intravenous adrenaline and fluid resuscitation.

Treatment

Basic treatment of shock should be instituted immediately and includes oxygen therapy and

		Local complications of orthopaedic surgery		
Postoperative timing	**Complication**	**Cause**	**Signs/symptoms**	**Management**
Immediate—first 24 hours	Tight cast	Swelling Dressing/cast too tight	Pain, tingling in toes/fingers Poor distal perfusion Numbness Ischaemia of limb	Elevation Split cast
	Compartment syndrome	Swelling in a closed fascial compartment (usually post fracture)	PAIN, pain on passive stretch, tense compartments Altered sensation	Fasciotomy
	Primary haemorrhage	Technical problem at surgical site, e.g. bleeding vessel Other risk factors include: major surgery, e.g. total hip replacement; drugs, e.g. warfarin; obesity	Haemodynamic instability Anxiety Slow capillary refill Tachycardia Hypotension Low urine output Confusion	Replace losses—fluids +/− blood Reverse cause, e.g. warfarin Pressure dressing Clamp drains If heavy bleeding reexplore wound
	Nerve injury	Usually retractor, e.g. sciatic nerve in hip replacement	Pain, weakness, paraesthesia	Wait and see. Usually recovers
Early—first 4 weeks	Secondary haemorrhage	Occurs at 5–10 days usually secondary to infection	Bleeding with signs of infection	Treat infection. Wound debridement and washout
	Infection (see Chapter 18)	Infection at time of surgery. Can occur later with haematogenous seeding	Early: red, hot, swollen, discharging, temperature Late: persistent pain, loosening of prosthesis	Early: debridement and washout Late: removal of implant and debridement Reimplantation at second stage once infection treated
	Wound dehiscence (breakdown)	Within first week: usually due to poor surgical technique Later: invariably infection and poor healing	Wound gapes open Other features in keeping with infection may be present	Early: clean wounds are taken back to theatre for primary closure Later: treat infection as above
Late (in theory these can occur at any time)	Dislocation of total hip replacement	Patient: inappropriate patient activity, poor stem or cup position Excessive wear Infection	Severe pain, shortening External rotation (anterior) Internal rotation (posterior)	Reduce hip Abduction brace for 6 weeks if early Revision surgery if there is a problem with position of implant
	Periprosthetic fracture	Intraoperative: if a prosthesis is too big for the bone when inserted Late: loosening of the prosthesis, infection or trauma	Increased pain, deformity, unable to weight bear	Intraoperative: fixation of fracture Late: revision of prosthesis
	Heterotopic ossification	Abnormal bone formation in soft tissues: more common in head injured patients and with hip surgery or trauma	Stiffness	Surgical excision and immediate NSAIDs or radiotherapy postoperatively
	Aseptic loosening	Loosening of prosthesis occurs because particle wear of the implant triggers macrophages. These cause osteolysis around the prosthesis	Pain, instability	Revision of the prosthesis

Fig. 21.2 Local complications of orthopaedic surgery.

fluid resuscitation, with catheterization to monitor urine output and regular observation. Admission to a high dependency unit (HDU) should be considered if the patient is unstable or requires intensive input.

Further reading

Sweetland H, Conway K 2004 Crash course in surgery. Mosby, Edinburgh

Bone tumours/malignancy

Objectives

You should be able to:

- Classify bone tumours and know which types are most common.
- List which tumours most commonly metastasize to bone.
- Describe symptoms associated with bone metastasis.
- Describe typical X-ray features of primary and secondary bone tumours.
- Outline available treatments for primary and secondary bone tumours.
- Define different benign and malignant bone tumours including chondromas and sarcomas.
- Give examples of haemopoietic disease which can present with bone destruction.
- Give a prognosis for individual malignant tumours.

This chapter concerns bone tumours (primary and secondary) and other malignant conditions presenting as a musculoskeletal disorder.

You will notice that we have listed secondary bone tumours before primary. This is because metastatic disease of bone is far more common than primary malignancy.

- Secondary bone tumours—metastasis from:
  —Lung
  —Breast
  —Prostate
  —Kidney
  —Thyroid
  —Bowel.
- Primary bone tumours:
  —Osteosarcoma
  —Ewing's sarcoma
  —Chondrosarcoma.
- Soft tissue sarcomas.
- Haemopoietic diseases:
  —Myeloma
  —Leukaemia
  —Lymphoma.

SECONDARY BONE TUMOURS

Incidence

Secondary bone tumours are the most common bone-destroying lesions in the older patient.

Aetiology and pathology

The tumours most likely to metastasize to bone are listed above. Metastatic lesions are most commonly found in the spine, pelvis, ribs and proximal long bones.

The mechanism of metastasis is shown in Figure 22.1.

Bone is destroyed by metastatic disease and weakened, predisposing to fracture. The majority of metastases appear osteolytic but those from prostate cancer appear sclerotic.

Clinical features

Patient with a known primary

The patient has a clear history of previous malignancy, which in the case of breast carcinoma may have been many years previously. Unrelenting bone pain in the axial skeleton then makes the patient seek medical help. Night pain is often a feature that does not respond to simple analgesia. There may be constitutional symptoms such as weight loss and malaise.

Patient with no known primary

The patient presents with bone pain as described above but with no history of previous malignancy. In this case it is important to ask about symptoms suggestive of malignancy such as cough and haemoptysis (lung), urinary symptoms (prostate) or

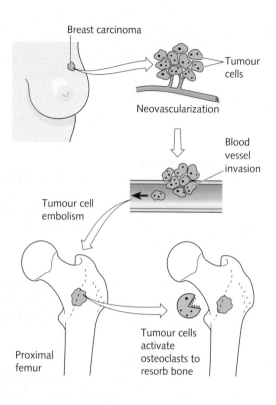

Fig. 22.1 Mechanism of long bone metastasis.

change in bowel habit (bowel). Patients often do not have any symptoms of the primary. Clinical examination should concentrate on likely sources of primary tumours; therefore examine:

- Breast.
- Chest.
- Prostate (per rectum).
- Thyroid.
- Abdomen (kidney and bowel).

Fracture

Usually the patient has a history of bone pain preceding the event (usually minor trauma) that caused the fracture. The patient is then either admitted or seen in a fracture clinic.

Patients who present with significant fractures after a very minor injury (e.g. after lifting a suitcase) may have a malignancy.

Spinal cord compression

Patients with maligancy can present 'off their legs' with weakness and a demonstrable spinal level (change in sensation corresponding to the vertebral level affected). There may be a history of preceding spinal bony pain and then weakness, numbness and then loss of bladder and bowel control. Urgent radiotherapy may shrink the tumour and preserve spinal cord function.

It can be a very difficult decision whether or not to operate on a patient with spinal cord compression in the presence of malignancy. There are significant risks of surgery but most spinal surgeons will try to stabilize the spine if at all possible to preserve the patient's mobility and dignity. The patient will know they are terminally ill but will not want to spend the last few months of life immobile and incontinent.

Spinal bony pain in patients with known metastatic disease needs investigation and treatment before spinal cord compression results.

Diagnosis and investigation

Any bone-destroying lesion could be due to infection or malignancy. Therefore:

- Check the white cell count (WCC) and inflammatory markers—C-reactive protein (CRP) and erythrocyte sedimentation rate (ESR). These are raised in infection but may also be raised in malignancy (myeloma).
- Further blood tests may identify the primary such as carcinoembryonic antigen (CEA) or prostate-specific antigen (PSA).
- Plain X-rays will usually show an osteolytic lesion; however, significant bone loss (>50%) is needed before it is apparent on X-ray examination.
- If strong clinical suspicion exists then an MRI scan is more sensitive.

- Cortical thinning suggests impending fracture.
- A bone scan will be hot and is useful to exclude further lesions.
- In an unknown primary, further investigation to find the primary is warranted (see Algorithm for the investigation of sinister back pain, Fig. 1.5).

Treatment

Treatment depends on the primary and on the life expectancy of the patient. A multidisciplinary approach is required involving oncologists.

Conservative

- Adequate analgesia and splintage.
- Radiotherapy is used frequently for bony metastatic pain.
- Chemotherapy may have a role in certain tumours.
- Hormonal therapy is useful in breast disease.
- Intravenous bisphosphonates are now being used to inhibit osteoclastic resorption of bone.

Surgical

- Intramedullary fixation of long bones is performed for fracture or impending fracture.
- Joint arthroplasty is sometimes used around the hip and shoulder.
- Spinal decompression and stabilization for acute cord compression.

Prognosis

The prognosis depends on the primary.

Patients with renal tumours and a solitary metastasis may be cured by resection of both.

PRIMARY BONE TUMOURS

Primary tumours of bone can be benign or malignant.

Benign bone tumours

Enchondroma

An enchondroma is a benign bone lesion of cartilaginous origin.

Incidence

They are quite common, occurring usually in adulthood.

Aetiology and pathology

Enchondromas develop from aberrant cartilage ('chondroma') left within bone ('en'). They are usually found in the metaphysis of long bones (femur or humerus) but are also common in the hand. See Figure 22.2.

Clinical features

An enchondroma is usually asymptomatic and may be found incidentally. Large lesions causing cortical erosion can be painful and the patient may notice a swelling, particularly in the hand.

Diagnosis and investigation

Typical features on X-ray show a well-demarcated calcifying lesion in the metaphysis of the bone. Serial X-rays may be obtained to make sure the lesion is not growing rapidly.

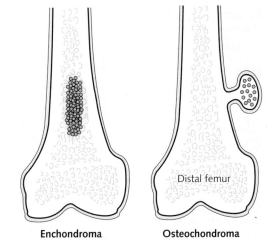

Enchondroma   Osteochondroma

Fig. 22.2 Benign cartilage tumours.

Treatment

Usually no treatment is required, but if the lesion is significantly painful or associated with fracture, excision or curettage may be performed.

Osteochondroma

Incidence

This is the most common benign bone lesion, presenting from childhood through to adult life.

Aetiology and pathology

The lesion develops from aberrant cartilage remaining on the surface of the cortex. It is usually found around the knee, most commonly on the distal femur.

The pathological appearance is of a bone lesion continuous with the cortex of the bone, capped with hyaline cartilage. It can be sessile or pedunculated.

Clinical features

The majority are asymptomatic, presenting incidentally or as a swelling. Rarely, pain or pressure effects on nerves or vessels occur.

Diagnosis and investigation

The typical appearance of a pedunculated lesion in continuity with the cortex clinches the diagnosis. If there is doubt, computed tomography (CT) or magnetic resonance imaging (MRI) may reassure.

Treatment

Usually no treatment is needed; rarely, excision is carried out, if symptomatic.

Prognosis

It is extremely rare for either osteochondroma or enchondroma to undergo malignant change.

Osteoid osteoma

Osteoid osteoma is a painful self-limiting benign bone lesion.

Incidence

The lesion is uncommon, usually presenting between 5 and 30 years of age.

Aetiology and pathology

It is caused by a nidus of osteoblasts located in the cortex of bone, and is usually found in the tibia, spine or femur.

Clinical features

Patients have intense pain, particularly at night. Tenderness over the lesion is usual. In the spine a scoliosis may be present.

Diagnosis and investigation

X-ray features show a radiolucent nidus surrounded by a dense area of reactive bone.

CT scans confirm and accurately locate the lesion (Fig. 22.3).

Treatment

Pain is typically relieved by aspirin.

CT-guided ablation is now preferred over surgical excision.

Prognosis

The tumour is eventually self-limiting.

Fibrous dysplasia

This is not strictly speaking a bone tumour.

Incidence

Fibrous dysplasia is relatively common, usually presenting in the first three decades.

Aetiology and pathology

It is most commonly found in the tibia, femur and ribs, and is caused by developmental abnormality of bone with numerous fibrous proliferations.

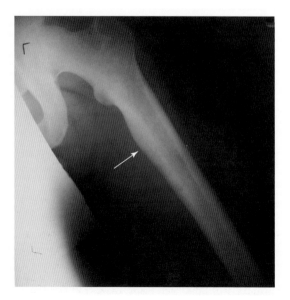

Fig. 22.3 X-ray showing an osteoid osteoma.

Clinical features

The condition is usually asymptomatic, discovered as an incidental finding, but can present with pain, swelling, deformity or fracture.

Diagnosis and investigation

A typical ground glass appearance is diagnostic.

Treatment

No treatment is usually required, but if significant, curettage and bone grafting can be performed.

Malignant primary bone tumours

Primary malignant bone tumours are very rare indeed. We will discuss two of those most likely to be encountered.

Osteosarcoma

Incidence

There are approximately 1–2 cases per million of population. Presentation is in adolescence and young adulthood or in the elderly where they develop in Pagetic bones.

Aetiology and pathology

Paget's disease or radiation can predispose, but most cases occur sporadically. The tumour is highly malignant and secretes osteoid. Local spread occurs quickly, destroying the cortex, but it may also metastasize.

The most common location is around the knee; other sites include the proximal humerus and femur.

Clinical features

The patient presents with pain and sometimes also swelling. Clinically there is usually warmth over the affected area and there may be a palpable mass.

Diagnosis and investigation

X-rays (Fig. 22.4) may show:

- An ill-defined lesion with an indistinct zone of transition.
- Sclerotic or lytic areas within the lesion.
- Cortical destruction.
- Codman's triangle (elevation of periosteum).
- 'Sunray spicules' (calcification within the tumour but out of the bone).

Biopsy may be necessary to confirm the diagnosis. Further investigations such as CT and MRI are required to stage the lesion.

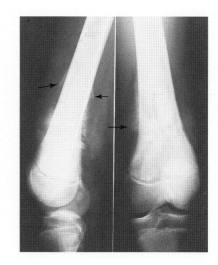

Fig. 22.4 X-ray of osteosarcoma (from Klippel J H, Dieppe P A (eds) 1998 Rheumatology, 2nd edn. Mosby, London).

Treatment

A combined multidisciplinary team approach is adopted.

Preoperative chemotherapy followed by limb salvage surgery is performed if possible. Occasionally amputation is required.

Prognosis

5-year survival is 60%.

Ewing's sarcoma

Incidence

Ewing's sarcoma is extremely rare (less common than osteosarcoma), occurring between 5 and 25 years of age.

Aetiology and pathology

Histologically this is a small cell sarcoma. It occurs as frequently in flat bones as in long bones, being most common in the femur or tibia (long bone), pelvis or vertebra (flat bones).

These tumours are highly malignant and often large at presentation.

Clinical features

Patients present with pain and may be unwell with a fever. Clinically the area is warm and swelling may be present.

Diagnosis and investigation

Diagnosis is usually made on X-ray appearance (Fig. 22.5), which is classically a lytic lesion with a laminated periosteal reaction (onion skinning).

Fig. 22.5 Pathology specimen in advanced Ewing's sarcoma (from Hochberg M C, Silman A J, Smolen J S et al 2003 Rheumatology, 3rd edn. Mosby, Edinburgh).

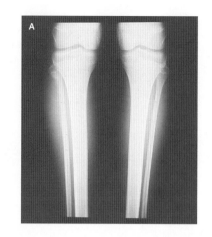
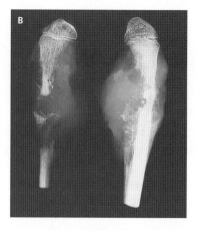

CT and MRI help to stage the lesion. Biopsy may be necessary.

Treatment

A combined multidisciplinary team approach is adopted.

Preoperative chemotherapy and radiotherapy followed by limb salvage surgery is performed if possible.

Prognosis

5-year survival is 60%.

HAEMOPOIETIC DISEASES

Lymphoma and myeloma can present with bone destruction.

Lymphoma

Incidence

Lymphoma is rare but can occur at any age.

Aetiology and pathology

It is a small cell bone tumour arising from the marrow, which can occur in any bone, most commonly around the knee.

Diagnosis and investigation

- X-rays show a long lesion with mottled bony destruction.
- Isotope bone scanning excludes further lesions.
- Biopsy confirms the diagnosis.

Treatment

Chemotherapy and irradiation are commonly used in conjunction.

Myeloma

Incidence

This is a rare tumour occurring between 50 and 80 years of age.

Aetiology and pathology

Lesions are due to a plasma cell malignancy, and are found usually in the spine, ribs or clavicle.

Clinical features

Bony pain is common and there may be a pathological fracture. Systemic symptoms of fatigue and fever are very common.

Diagnosis and investigation

Patients will have a high erythrocyte sedimentation rate (ESR) and may have hypercalcaemia. Serum electrophoresis and urinary analysis for Bence Jones proteins confirm the diagnosis.

X-rays show classic punched-out lytic lesions.

Treatment

Chemotherapy is the mainstay with surgical stabilization or radiotherapy for impending fracture.

Prognosis

Overall prognosis is poor, with survival averaging 2 years.

LEUKAEMIA

The last malignancy to mention is leukaemia—a malignancy of white blood cells.

Leukaemia is the most common malignancy of childhood and about one-third of patients have bone pain. Leukaemia can also present with an acutely hot, swollen joint very similar to septic arthritis.

Further reading

Canale S T 2006 Campbell's operative orthopaedics, 11th edn. Mosby, St Louis, vols 1–4

Solomon L, Warwick D, Nayagan D (eds) 2001 Apley's system of orthopaedics and fractures, 8th edn. Hodder Arnold, London

Orthoteers website: http://www.orthoteers.co.uk

Disorders of the spine

Objectives

You should be able to:

- Discuss the likely causes of back pain.
- Know 'red flag' signs associated with sinister causes of back pain.
- Outline the presentation and treatment of musculoskeletal back pain.
- Know how and when to investigate back pain.
- Recognize the difference between spinal stenosis and a prolapsed intervertebral disc.
- Know the difference between spinal claudication and vascular claudication.
- Define spondylolysis and spondylolisthesis.
- Outline the diagnosis and treatment of discitis and vertebral osteomyelitis.

MUSCULOSKELETAL BACK PAIN

Back pain is extremely common and causes a significant burden on the resources of westernized societies in terms of lost working days.

Definition

Musculoskeletal back pain is not a single specific disease entity but rather a collection of ill-defined conditions presenting with low back pain. This diagnosis should only be made after other pathological conditions have been excluded.

Incidence

60–80% of the population will have back pain at some stage in their lives.

Aetiology and pathology

As back pain is so common it is difficult to define clear aetiological factors for its occurrence.

It is known, however, that patients with chronic back pain are more likely to smoke, have a medicolegal claim pending and be over 30 at presentation.

There is much controversy about the exact pathology. One problem is that a lot of the pathological changes seen will also be present in the healthy 'normal' population with no symptoms.

Implicated structures are listed in Figure 23.1.

- Facet joint arthritis shows the typical features of osteoarthritis (OA) with joint space destruction and osteophyte formation.
- Degenerative disc disease occurs with ageing and is related to decreased water content in the nucleus pulposus. The disc space narrows and the segment is said to become more mobile. It is this abnormal movement, together with an inability to distribute load, that causes pain.

An interesting point is that patients rarely present after the age of 60 and as the patient enters old age usually the symptoms subside. This is said to be due to stiffening of a mobile spine.

Clinical features

There are two typical clinical scenarios.

An acutely presenting patient with a history of back pain over days or weeks

Pain is usually solely located to the back, possibly following a precipitating incident.

Pain is severe and the patient may have difficulty getting into a comfortable position. Sometimes the patient has pain referred down the back of the leg but this differs from true sciatica (radicular pain) in that back pain is still the predominant feature and the pain does not radiate to the foot.

Possible causes of musculoskeletal back pain

Bone/periosteum
Paraspinous muscles spasm/sprain
Facet joint arthritis
Disc/degenerative disc disease
Posterior longitudinal ligament

Fig. 23.1 Possible causes of musculoskeletal back pain.

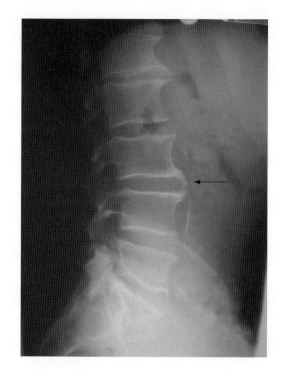

Fig. 23.2 Osteoarthritis of the spine.

The pain is mechanical (i.e. worse on movement).

Clinical examination will show muscle spasm with loss of lumbar lordosis. The patient may find it difficult to walk and spinal movements will be minimal.

Sciatic stretch testing and peripheral nerve examination will be negative.

The chronic patient who has unrelenting back pain for many years

The patient will be unable to work, may be overweight and depressed. Usually the patient has seen numerous doctors, physiotherapists and other allied health workers including alternative medical practitioners.

The back pain is usually unrelenting and does not have any relieving factors. Leg pain may or may not be present.

Clinical examination rarely shows any significant features other than reduced movements. Inappropriate signs (Waddell's signs) may be present (e.g. increased pain on applying mild downward pressure to the head).

Diagnosis and investigation

The majority of patients with a short history (less than 6 weeks) and mechanical symptoms need no further investigation.

Prolonged symptoms need investigation to exclude sinister causes of back pain.

Blood tests including full blood count (FBC), liver function tests (LFTs), calcium, myeloma screen, erythrocyte sedimentation rate (ESR) and C-reactive protein (CRP) should all be normal in mechanical back pain.

X-rays may show:

- Normal appearances.

- Minor disc narrowing.
- Facet joint arthritis (Fig. 23.2).

Magnetic resonance imaging (MRI) or computed tomography (CT) scanning are rarely helpful and may be misleading if they highlight an abnormality that may not be significant.

Treatment

Conservative

Analgesia, non-steroidal anti-inflammatory drugs (NSAIDs) and physiotherapy are used for acute low back pain. Prolonged bed rest should be avoided.

Chronic patients are very difficult to treat and need a multidisciplinary approach to try to break the pain cycle. Psychological input may be required, as may the 'pain team'. Occasionally facet joint injections for localized disease can relieve symptoms.

Surgical

This is controversial but some advocate spinal fusion in a few very selected patients with degenerative disc disease.

Prognosis

Most acute back pain episodes settle spontaneously and the patient returns to normal.

Once chronic, the condition becomes extremely difficult to treat.

PROLAPSED INTERVERTEBRAL DISC

Definition

A disc prolapse occurs when part of the nucleus pulposus herniates through the annulus fibrosus and presses on a spinal nerve root.

Incidence

Disc prolapse is common—up to 3% of men and 1% of women will suffer with sciatica related to a prolapsed intervertebral disc. Usual presentation is between 35 and 55 years of age.

Aetiology and pathology

There is good evidence that manual workers involved in heavy lifting have increased incidence of disc prolapse. Regular automobile use is also said to be a risk factor.

The herniation of disc material tends to occur posterolaterally where the annulus is thinner. Central disc prolapse can occur and press on the combined nerve roots, including those supplying the bladder and bowel (cauda equina syndrome). Prolapse can occur without spinal root involvement in which case the patient will have symptoms of back pain but not true sciatica.

Disc prolapse most commonly occurs at L4–L5 or L5–S1 level but can occur at any level (including cervical and rarely thoracic). The nerve root crosses its space before exiting the spine beneath the pedicle (L4–L5 disc presses on L5 nerve root). See Figure 23.3.

Clinical features

Sciatica is a symptom of nerve root irritation. The patient complains of severe pain radiating down the leg into the toes. There may be numbness and tingling in the foot and weakness of the foot. Patients find it very uncomfortable to sit, and either stand or lie down. Coughing and sneezing worsen the pain.

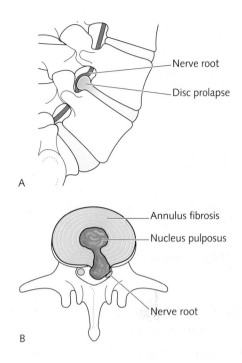

A

B

Fig. 23.3 Prolapsed intervertebral disc.

In cauda equina syndrome there is bladder and bowel dysfunction with possibly urinary retention and saddle anaesthesia.

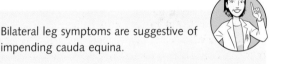

Bilateral leg symptoms are suggestive of impending cauda equina.

Clinically a patient will have an abnormal posture, stooping to the affected side and standing with the knee flexed to relieve pressure on the dura (Fig. 23.4).

Nerve root tension signs such as straight leg raising will be positive.

The crossover sign may be positive (elevation of the opposite or normal leg gives pain shooting down the affected leg).

Numbness in a dermatomal distribution and weakness with loss of reflexes may be present.

In cauda equina there is loss of anal tone and reduced perianal sensation.

Check for any sinister features (see Ch. 1, p. 4, Fig. 1.2).

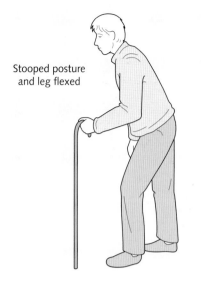

Stooped posture
and leg flexed

Fig. 23.4 Posture in prolapsed intervertebral disc.

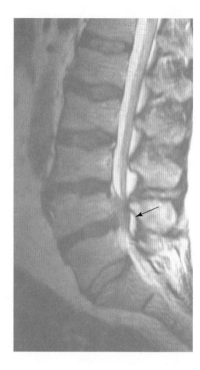

Fig. 23.5 MRI scan of prolapsed intervertebral disc at L4–L5 level.

Diagnosis and investigation

In older patients blood tests described above should be performed to exclude any sinister causes.

X-rays are usually normal and are performed to exclude bony pathology such as spondylolisthesis.

MRI scanning is now the investigation of choice in patients with persistent symptoms (Fig. 23.5).

Treatment

Conservative

A short period of bed rest followed by gentle physiotherapy with adequate analgesia (including NSAIDs) is the initial treatment for most discs.

Surgical

The only indications for urgent surgical discectomy are cauda equina syndrome and progressively worsening neurological deficit.

If patients have prolonged symptoms (>6 weeks) then surgery is considered.

Prognosis

70% of acute disc prolapses settle spontaneously with conservative treatment.

SPONDYLOLISTHESIS

Definition

This means slipping of one vertebral body on another.

It is easy to get confused with the terminology. A spondylolysis is a defect in the pars interarticularis which may allow the vertebra to slip forward causing a spondylolisthesis (forward slippage of one vertebra on another).

Incidence

The condition is common (approximately 5% of the population) but most are asymptomatic. It is more common in Caucasian males.

Aetiology and pathology

Certain sports predispose to spondylolysis (gymnasts and fast bowlers in cricket).

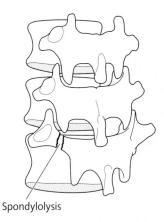

Spondylolysis

Fig. 23.6 Classic 'Scottie dog' appearance of spondylolisthesis.

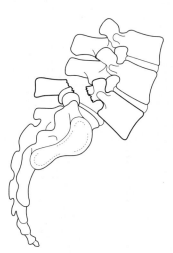

Fig. 23.7 An L5–S1 spondylolisthesis with a pars defect.

Spondylolisthesis can be caused by differing pathology.

The slip usually occurs at the L5–S1 level. The degree of slip is normally assessed as a percentage and graded 1–4. There can be an associated kyphosis or scoliosis.

Clinical features

This condition is the most common cause of persistent back pain in children.

Initially back pain is the sole presentation but if the slip becomes severe then nerve root irritation will occur, causing sciatica. Radicular symptoms are more common in the adult patient.

There is tenderness over the spine but sometimes well-preserved movements (except in the arthritic type of spondylolisthesis); classically hyperextension is painful.

Diagnosis and investigation

Oblique X-rays may show the classic 'collar on Scottie dog' appearance (Fig. 23.6), and the lateral X-ray will show the degree of slippage (Fig. 23.7).

CT scans clearly demonstrate the lesion.

MRI should be performed if nerve root irritation is suspected.

Treatment

Conservative

Initial rest and restriction of activities may allow a spondylolysis to heal before a slip occurs.

In adult patients a trial of conservative treatment is advised with physiotherapy, analgesia and activity modification.

Surgical

Persistent pain, radiculopathy and significant deformity are indications for surgery.

Fusion with metalwork and bone graft is commonly performed.

Prognosis

The outcome is variable, depending on the type and degree of slip.

SPINAL STENOSIS

Definition

Spinal stenosis is caused by degenerative changes narrowing the spinal canal and causing compression of the nerve roots.

Incidence

This is a common disorder mainly affecting men over 50 years of age.

Aetiology and pathology

Spinal stenosis is more common in heavy manual labourers.

It is usually secondary to degenerative changes. Thickening of soft tissues, osteophytes and posterior disc bulge encroach into the spinal canal (Fig. 23.8).

It is thought that ischaemia of the spinal nerves during exercise produces the classic symptoms.

Clinical features

Typically patients present with discomfort when walking, with pain referred to the buttock, calves and feet. Back pain is usually present. Pain is worse on extension and relieved by rest or flexion of the spine.

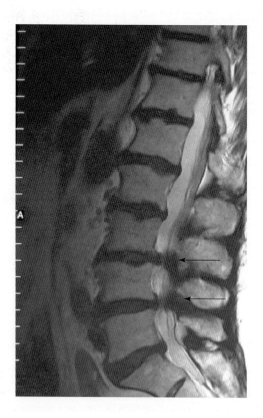

Fig. 23.8 MRI scan of spinal stenosis.

Examination will reveal stiffening of the spine but sciatic stretch testing may be normal.

It is important to examine the peripheral vascular system in such patients as vascular claudication presents in a similar way.

Diagnosis and investigation

X-rays will usually show degenerative changes.

MRI shows the degree of stenosis and nerve root involvement.

If suspected, exclude peripheral vascular insufficiency with Doppler scans.

Treatment

Conservative

Weight loss, physiotherapy, activity modification and NSAIDs may relieve symptoms enough to avoid surgery.

Surgical

Severe symptoms not responding to conservative measures require surgical decompression.

Prognosis

The condition tends to be progressive.

DISCITIS/VERTEBRAL OSTEOMYELITIS

Definition

Discitis is infection of the disc space, and vertebral osteomyelitis infection of a vertebral body.

Incidence

They are becoming more common, although still rare.

Presentation can be at any age.

Aetiology and pathology

Conditions associated with other bone and joint infection (see Ch. 18), particularly intravenous drug use and immunocompromised patients, predispose to spinal infection. Patients with recent sepsis from pneumonia or urinary tract infection (UTI) can subsequently develop discitis by seeding of infection.

Common infecting organisms are *Staphylococcus aureus* and streptococci but tuberculosis should be considered.

Clinical features

Patients are unwell with a pyrexia and complain of severe unrelenting back pain.

Clinical examination may reveal a swelling and in severe cases a gibbus. There is pain on palpation, reduced movement and possible abnormal neurology.

Discitis commonly presents late, the patient often having 6–12 weeks of symptoms before the correct diagnosis is made.

Diagnosis and investigation

The white cell count (WCC), ESR and CRP are elevated.

X-rays show narrowed disc space (discitis) and bony destruction (osteomyelitis) (Fig. 23.9).

An isotope bone scan will be hot in the affected area.

MRI scanning should be performed to detect any epidural abscess.

CT guided biopsy should be obtained for culture and sensitivity.

Treatment

Conservative

Intravenous antibiotics are given for 6 weeks.

Surgical

Any abscess should be drained and an unstable spine with significant deformity needs stabilization.

Prognosis

Prognosis is variable: childhood cases respond well and should return to normality; severe adult infections can be life-threatening and surgery carries significant risk.

SCOLIOSIS

Definition

This is a lateral deviation and rotational abnormality of the spine.

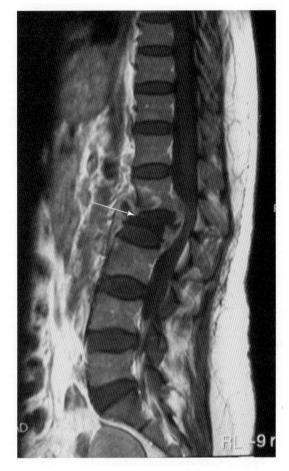

Fig. 23.9 MRI showing TB of the spine. There is complete collapse of the vertebra (arrowed) with resultant kyphosis.

Incidence

Up to 2.5% of the population are affected by idiopathic scoliosis.

Aetiology and pathology

Causes of scoliosis are listed in Figure 23.10.

In idiopathic scoliosis the exact cause is not known.

Curves are thoracolumbar (Fig. 23.11).

Clinical features

Pain is not usually a feature; rather the patient or relatives complain of deformity, in the form of an asymmetrical rib hump, spinal curve and limb length inequality. For clinical examination, the rib hump is more prominent on forward flexion (Fig. 23.12).

169

Fig. 23.10 Causes of scoliosis.

Causes of scoliosis		
Type	**Pathology**	**Example**
Congenital	Abnormal development of spine	Hemivertebra
Idiopathic	Unknown	Adolescent idiopathic scoliosis
Neuromuscular	Abnormal muscle forces acting on the spine	Cerebral palsy
Secondary	Curve develops secondary to another process	Leg length discrepancy

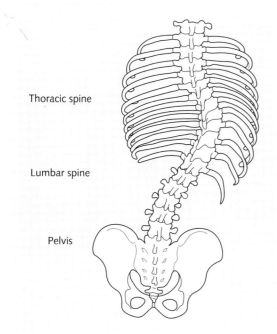

Thoracic spine

Lumbar spine

Pelvis

Fig. 23.11 Thoracolumbar curve in scoliosis.

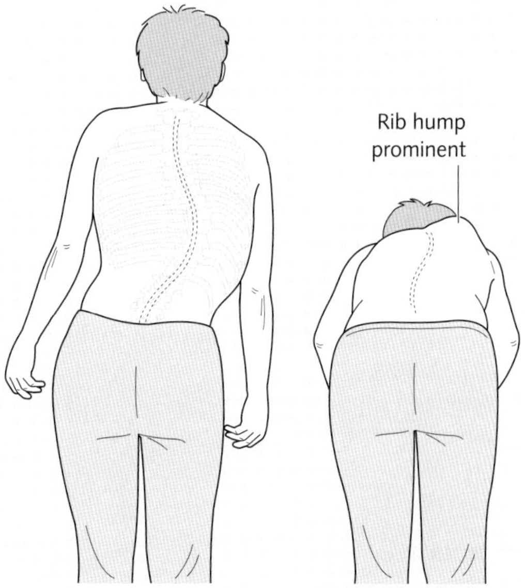

Rib hump prominent

Examined from behind   **On forward flexion**

Fig. 23.12 Examination of a patient with scoliosis.

Very severe deformity reduces chest expansion which can be life-threatening.

Diagnosis and investigation

Standing X-rays show the curve, and serial films are important to monitor the progress of the curve.

A significant increase in the severity of the curve is often an indication for surgical stabilization.

MRI scans are performed to exclude any associated spinal cord abnormality.

Treatment

Conservative

The treatment depends on the angle of the curve measured on the X-rays. In idiopathic scoliosis the initial treatment is bracing for mild to moderate curves.

Surgical

All congenital, most neuromuscular and severe or progressive idiopathic curves will require surgical stabilization, fusion and correction.

170

Prognosis

The majority of curves are minor and require little treatment.

Very severe neuromuscular curves can lead to death due to cardiorespiratory compromise.

Further reading

Solomon L, Warwick D, Nayagan D (eds) 2001 Apley's system of orthopaedics and fractures, 8th edn. Hodder Arnold, London
Orthoteers website: http://www.orthoteers.co.uk

Objectives

You should be able to:

- Define what is meant by a 'locked knee' and give causes.
- Outline how to treat meniscal tears and describe which tears should be repaired.
- Describe the classical history of an anterior cruciate ligament rupture and how this differs from a meniscal tear.
- Understand the mechanism of collateral ligament injuries and how these should be managed.
- Describe why the patella does not normally dislocate and describe which two groups of people suffer patella dislocations.
- Describe shoulder anatomy and explain why this is the joint most prone to dislocation.
- Classify shoulder dislocations and know how to manage them.
- Outline the surgical indications for treatment of ACL and PCL ruptures and also shoulder and patellar dislocation.
- Diagnose and manage ankle sprains.

KNEE INJURIES

Introduction

The knee is commonly injured in sport—particularly soccer, rugby and skiing.

We will discuss injuries to the menisci, ligamentous injuries of the knee and patellar dislocation.

Meniscal injuries

The menisci are two semicircular fibrocartilage structures that lie between the femoral and tibial articular surfaces (Fig. 24.1). They act as 'shock absorbers' and are prone to injuries caused by the large forces crossing the knee.

Incidence

Meniscal injuries are common, usually occurring in young adult patients who participate in sports.

Pathology and aetiology

The medial meniscus is more commonly injured because it is fixed in comparison to the more mobile lateral meniscus.

Meniscal tears can be traumatic or degenerative:

- Traumatic tears. The meniscus is normal and injury usually occurs after landing or twisting with the knee flexed. This can be associated with a ligamentous injury such as an anterior cruciate ligament (ACL) tear. A chronically unstable knee is prone to further tears.
- Degenerative tears. These occur in an older population through abnormal cartilage. They may occur with little or no injury.

Types of meniscal tears (Fig. 24.2)

1. Bucket handle. The tear extends over a distance, remaining attached at the anterior and posterior horns. It can be displaced (in which case the cartilage flips over) or undisplaced (the cartilage remains in its normal position). A locked knee results when a large bucket handle tear flips over and becomes trapped in the joint, resulting in loss of complete extension.
2. Radial.
3. Horizontal cleavage.
4. Flap/parrot beak.

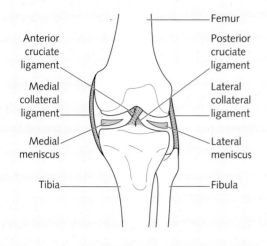

Fig. 24.1 Basic anatomy of the knee.

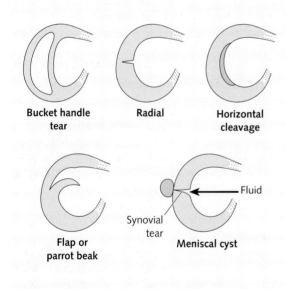

Fig. 24.2 Meniscal lesions.

Of clinical importance is how peripheral the tear is. Very peripheral tears occur through vascular tissue and are amenable to repair, as these tears can heal. Meniscal tears further away from the blood supply (i.e. further into the knee) cannot heal.

Meniscal cysts result from synovial fluid being pumped into the meniscal tear. A valve effect means the fluid in the cyst cannot drain back into the knee. See Figure 24.2.

Clinical features

Patients usually give a history of injury while playing sport, the incident occurring during a tackle or when twisting or changing direction.

A patient may present immediately after injury with a painful locked knee, or with a gradual chronic nagging pain over months or years following minor injury. This variation reflects how the different types and positions of tears manifest clinical symptoms.

Mechanical symptoms such as locking and catching suggest meniscal pathology. A 'clicking joint' does not necessarily mean there is pathology.

A more major injury with acute swelling and instability suggests associated ligamentous injury.

Examination may reveal:

- A locked knee.
- An effusion:
  —A large acute effusion suggests a very peripheral tear (which bleeds) or an associated injury
  —A small chronic effusion is common.
- Joint line tenderness; this is an important part of the examination and is usually positive in a patient with a torn meniscus.
- A meniscal cyst, which may be palpable over the lateral joint line.

A variety of special tests are described for meniscal tears and none is very reliable.

Diagnosis and investigation

In most cases the diagnosis is made solely on the basis of history and examination.

X-rays are usually normal and are performed to exclude osteoarthritis or other rare causes of knee pain.

Magnetic resonance imaging (MRI) is very useful to confirm the presence of torn menisci, particularly in patients with a dubious history.

The most accurate way to confirm the diagnosis is with arthroscopy of the knee.

Management

Conservative

Initially RICE (rest, ice, compression, elevation) is used for an acutely swollen knee. Early physiotherapy is essential to encourage movement.

Surgical

Surgery is now performed using arthroscopic techniques.

For peripheral bucket handle tears, meniscal repair has the advantage of retaining the meniscus.

For tears not amenable to repair, meniscal resection is commonly performed. Partial meniscectomy removes the damaged portion only, leaving a stable rim and reducing the risk of osteoarthritis in the future.

Prognosis

Removal of the meniscus leads to osteoarthritic changes developing in the knee because of increased load on the articular surface.

Meniscal repair is successful in 70% of cases.

Ligamentous injuries of the knee

Anterior cruciate ligament (ACL)

Incidence

1 per 3000 of the population per year are affected.

Aetiology and pathology

The ACL is the primary restraint to anterior tibial translation. The mechanism of injury is usually a twisting or valgus strain pattern of injury commonly occurring in soccer or skiing (Fig. 24.3).

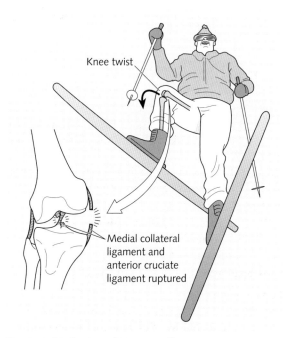

Fig. 24.3 Mechanism of injury in ACL rupture.

The knee is usually extended or slightly flexed with the foot fixed. Associated injuries to the medial collateral ligament and either meniscus are common.

ACL-deficient knees are liable to further meniscal tears.

Clinical features

With an acute ACL rupture, the patient will be unable to play on and may have to be carried from the field. Many patients present a long time after injury with symptoms of instability.

The patient often hears a 'pop' or feels 'something go' inside the knee.

Swelling typically occurs within a few hours unlike meniscal tears which swell over 24 hours, because the ACL is more vascular than the menisci.

Once initial symptoms have settled, the patient may complain of giving way of the knee. This occurs when the patient tries to turn rapidly. Classically the patient will report being able to run in a straight line but not being able to 'twist and turn'.

Clinically, patients have a tense effusion after an acute injury.

The anterior drawer, Lachmann's and pivot shift tests are positive (see Ch. 29).

Diagnosis and investigation

The majority can be diagnosed clinically.

In some patients it is difficult to elicit positive examination findings and in those patients an MRI scan or examination under anaesthetic (EUA) is useful to confirm the diagnosis.

X-rays will usually be normal.

Management

Conservative Initial treatment is with RICE and physiotherapy. A proportion of patients can modify their activities and manage with a hamstring rehabilitation programme only.

Surgical ACL reconstruction is indicated for functional instability of the knee. With modern techniques this is now performed arthroscopically using a hamstring tendon graft. Meniscal tears can also be addressed at the time of surgery.

Prognosis

Chronic instability associated with meniscal pathology leads to early osteoarthritis (OA). Early ACL reconstruction can protect the knee from further meniscal injury.

Fig. 24.4 Mechanism of injury in
PCL injuries.

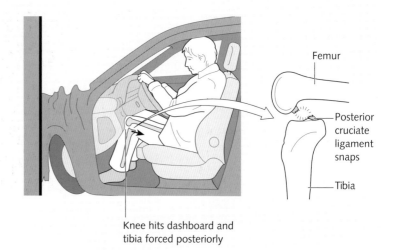

Femur

Posterior
cruciate
ligament
snaps

Tibia

Knee hits dashboard and
tibia forced posteriorly

Posterior cruciate ligament (PCL)

The PCL is the primary restraint to posterior movement of the tibia on the femur.

Incidence
PCL injuries are rare.

Aetiology and pathology
PCL injuries occur either in sporting activities or from road traffic accidents (dashboard injury) (Fig. 24.4).

Classically it is a goalkeeper's injury in soccer, the mechanism of injury being the knee combining with an onrushing attacking player forcing the tibia backwards. The PCL can also rupture when the knee is forcibly hyperextended.

The majority of PCL tears occur in combination with other ligamentous injuries.

Clinical features
The patient will have a substantial injury to the knee and will usually be unable to bear weight. Swelling is usually less obvious than with an ACL injury.

Patients complain less of instability than with ACL injuries.

Clinically, patients will have a posterior sag and positive posterior drawer test.

Careful assessment is needed to look for associated injuries such as lateral collateral injuries.

Treatment
Conservative Almost all isolated PCL injuries can be treated with rehabilitation alone.

Surgical Patients with combined injuries or symptomatic instability require reconstruction.

Prognosis
In the short term PCL injuries often follow a benign course and are often asymptomatic in certain sports players (a professional rugby league team will have several players who are PCL deficient).

Osteoarthritis develops in the long term (25 years).

Lateral collateral injuries

Incidence
These are rare injuries.

Aetiology and pathology
Isolated lateral collateral ligament (LCL) injuries occur when a varus strain is placed on the knee (i.e. a hit from the medial side; Fig. 24.5).

Associated injuries to the PCL or ACL can occur.

Clinical features
The patient will complain of pain and possibly instability.

In the normal knee the LCL is easily palpable as a cord-like structure. When the LCL is ruptured, the area is tender and indistinct.

Opening up of the joint on the lateral side will be present on collateral testing.

Management
Almost all isolated injuries heal well with conservative treatment.

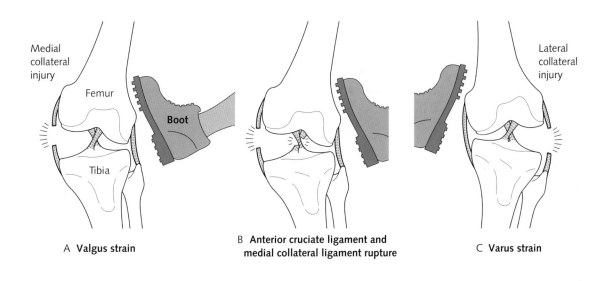

Fig. 24.5 Mechanism of injury in collateral ligament tears.

Medial collateral injuries

Incidence
These are common injuries in isolation or combined with ACL injury.

Aetiology and pathology
There is a valgus strain pattern of injury. The injury can be complete or partial, and can be associated with ACL injury.

Clinical features
This is usually a sporting injury; the patient may feel 'something go' but an effusion is not a feature of an isolated medial collateral ligament (MCL) tear (it is an extra-articular structure).

Tenderness over the broad attachment of the MCL and opening up of the joint on collateral stressing are examination features.

Management
Treatment is with physiotherapy and bracing for 6 weeks. Minor tears heal well without bracing.

Surgical advancement is sometimes required for chronic unstable injuries.

Prognosis
The knee usually returns to normal after a period of rehabilitation.

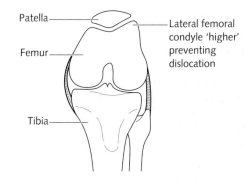

Fig. 24.6 Anatomical features that prevent lateral dislocation of the patella.

Patellar dislocation

Introduction
The patella is prevented from dislocation by anatomical features such as a large lateral femoral condyle and the insertion of vastus medialis oblique (VMO) (Fig. 24.6).

Incidence

Patellar dislocation is quite common.

Aetiology and pathology

Patellar dislocation can be habitual or traumatic.

Habitual dislocators are often young women with ligamentous laxity and a hypoplastic femoral condyle. This group get recurrent dislocations after minor injuries, often without trauma, and are difficult to treat.

Traumatic dislocations occur during sports, usually with the knee slightly flexed with side impact. The dislocation occurs laterally and damage may occur to the joint surface. Structures along the medial border of the patella are torn.

Clinical features

A first-time dislocation is extremely painful and the patient arrives in casualty with the patella laterally placed.

Often there is tenderness over the medial side of the knee and an effusion.

Later when the acute injury has settled the patient may have patella apprehension and a J-sign (see Ch. 29). Habitual dislocators may show evidence of generalized laxity in other joints such as fingers, thumbs, elbows and knees.

Diagnosis and investigation

X-rays should be taken after reduction, including a tunnel and skyline view looking for any osteochondral defects.

Management

Conservative

Initial reduction is required, usually under sedation in the accident and emergency (A&E) department.

Physiotherapy is required once pain and swelling allows improvement of range of movement and quadriceps strength.

Surgical

Large osteochondral defects should be repaired or removed arthroscopically.

Recurrent dislocations may require surgical realignment. Repair or reconstruction of the medial patello-femoral ligament is gaining in popularity.

SHOULDER DISLOCATION

Incidence

The shoulder is the most commonly dislocated large joint in the body.

Aetiology and pathology

The shoulder is at risk of dislocation because the joint has very little inherent bony stability, with reliance instead on capsule, ligaments and rotator cuff muscles. The joint has 'sacrificed' stability for movement.

The dislocation can be anterior or posterior. Anterior dislocation (Fig. 24.7) accounts for 98% and usually occurs when the arm is forced back in a 'ball throwing' position of external rotation and abduction.

Posterior dislocations occur with epileptic seizures and electrocutions.

In anterior dislocation the capsule is damaged antero-inferiorly, leaving a so-called Bankart lesion predisposing to further dislocations. Recurrent dislocations cause a Hill–Sachs lesion due to impaction of the glenoid on the posterior part of the humeral head.

In older patients the rotator cuff is torn rather than a Bankart lesion developing.

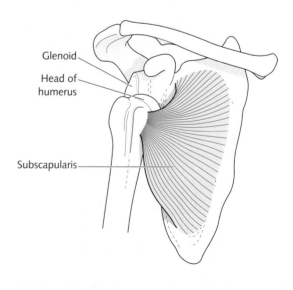

Fig. 24.7 Anterior dislocation of the humerus.

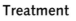

Clinical features

The patient is often a sports player—typically rugby—and has an acute injury to the shoulder as described above. The injury is intensely painful and the shoulder is held supported by the other arm (Fig. 24.8).

Examination findings include:

- Loss of normal contour.
- Palpable glenoid.
- Complete loss of movement.

Diagnosis and investigation

Anterior dislocation is usually obvious and confirmed with X-rays (also performed to exclude a fracture).

Posterior dislocation is often missed as the initial anteroposterior (AP) X-ray looks normal to the untrained eye. This should be suspected in any patient who has fixed internal rotation of the shoulder.

The 'light bulb sign' (Fig. 24.9A) should raise suspicion but the diagnosis is made on axillary view (Fig. 24.9B) or CT scan.

Treatment

Conservative

The dislocation needs to be promptly reduced in the A&E department under sedation.

Posterior dislocation often requires a general anaesthetic and may need open reduction.

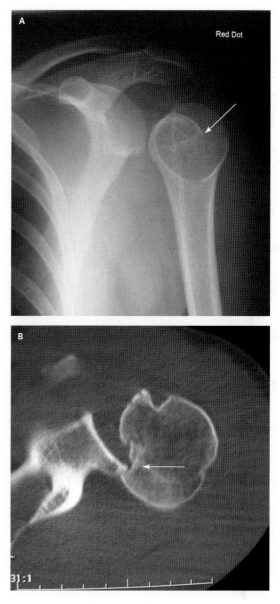

Fig. 24.9 Posterior dislocation of the shoulder: (A) AP X-ray showing the 'light bulb' sign; (B) CT scan showing axillary view. There is posterior subluxation of the head with impaction of the head from the glenoid rim (arrowed).

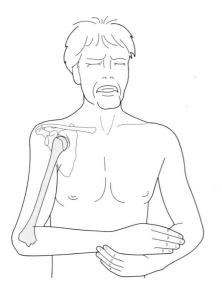

Fig. 24.8 Abnormal shoulder contour in anterior dislocation of the humerus.

Once the dislocation is reduced, the joint is rested in a collar and cuff and once the pain has settled, supervised early rehabilitation with the physiotherapist can commence.

Surgical

Surgery is reserved for the recurrent dislocations to repair bone or labral defects.

Prognosis

A young male sportsman has an 80% chance of recurrent dislocation following anterior dislocation of the shoulder.

In the more elderly population shoulder stiffness is more of a problem than recurrence.

Your current textbook may advise 6 weeks' immobilization for patellar and shoulder dislocations to allow the 'soft tissues to heal'. This is old-fashioned thinking and a short period of rest (3–5 days) is now followed by early rehabilitation.

ANKLE SPRAIN

Incidence

This is a very common injury.

Aetiology and pathology

The injury is commonly found on the sports field but anyone can have an ankle sprain. The mechanism of injury is inversion with damage to the lateral ligament complex.

As the talus tilts in the ankle mortice, the anterior talofibular and calcaneofibular ligaments are torn (Fig. 24.10).

Clinical features

The patient experiences pain and may feel 'something go'; swelling occurs rapidly.

Chronic ankle instability leads to giving way of the joint.

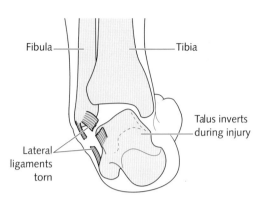

Fig. 24.10 Ankle ligament rupture.

Clinically the patient has a variable amount of swelling and tenderness over the lateral ligament complex.

Patients may have instability of the ankle joint with a positive anterior drawer test and opening of the lateral side.

Diagnosis and investigation

X-rays are performed only if there is bony tenderness or inability to weight bear (Ottowa ankle rules).

Management

Conservative

All sprains are treated conservatively initially with analgesia, RICE and physiotherapy.

Surgical

Arthroscopy of the ankle is sometimes performed for associated osteochondral injuries.

Rarely, ligament reconstruction is required for a chronically unstable ankle.

Further reading

Solomon L, Warwick D, Nayagan D (eds) 2001 Apley's system of orthopaedics and fractures, 8th edn. Hodder Arnold, London
Orthoteers website: http://www.orthoteers.co.uk

Objectives

In this chapter you will learn:

- The conditions that predispose to carpal tunnel syndrome.
- To recognize the symptoms and signs of carpal tunnel syndrome.
- The clinical consequences of damage to the ulnar, radial and common peroneal nerves.

CARPAL TUNNEL SYNDROME

Definition

Carpal tunnel syndrome (CTS) results from compression of the median nerve as it passes through the carpal tunnel at the wrist. The carpal tunnel is formed by the space between the transverse carpal ligament and the carpal bones.

Incidence

CTS is common, especially in middle-aged and elderly women.

Aetiology

CTS is usually idiopathic, but can be associated with several underlying conditions (Fig. 25.1).

Clinical features

CTS presents with pain and/or paraesthesia in the median nerve distribution (Fig. 25.2). These symptoms can radiate proximally towards the elbow. They are often worse at night and classically wake the patient from sleep.

Examination may reveal sensory loss in the median nerve distribution, but can be unremarkable. The strength of the thenar muscles should be tested. These may be weak and wasted in advanced disease. The opponens pollicis muscle is tested by asking the patient to touch the thumb to the little finger and resist attempts to separate the two. Phalen's and Tinel's tests may reproduce the symptoms (Fig. 25.3).

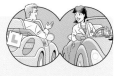

Don't expect every patient with carpal tunnel syndrome to complain of pain radiating from the wrist to their thumb, index and middle fingers. Patients often find it difficult to localize their symptoms and they may complain that their whole forearm and hand feel painful and/or numb.

Investigations

Nerve conduction studies show reduced nerve conduction velocities across the wrist. Investigations such as thyroid function tests should be performed to exclude underlying medical conditions.

Management

The most successful treatment is surgical decompression of the carpal tunnel by division of the transverse carpal ligament. This can be performed under local anaesthetic. Wrist splints may help nocturnal symptoms, and corticosteroid injection of the carpal tunnel may bring some relief.

ULNAR NERVE ENTRAPMENT

Definition

The ulnar nerve can become compressed as it passes behind the medial epicondyle or through Guyon's canal in the wrist.

Conditions predisposing to carpal tunnel syndrome

Diabetes mellitus
Hypothyroidism
Rheumatoid arthritis
Pregnancy
Acromegaly
Trauma, e.g. wrist fractures

Fig. 25.1 Conditions predisposing to carpal tunnel syndrome.

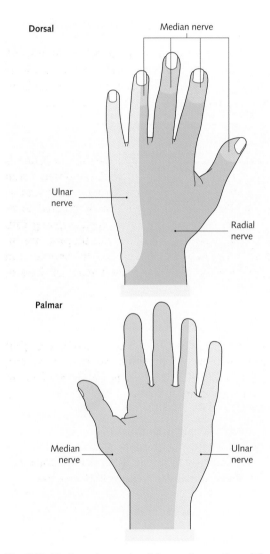

Fig. 25.2 Median, ulnar and radial nerve innervation of the hand.

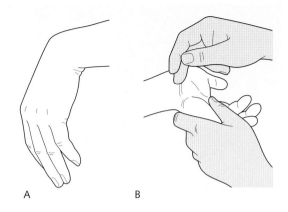

Fig. 25.3 Provocation tests for carpal tunnel syndrome may reproduce the patient's symptoms. (A) Phalen's test: the wrist is held in maximal palmar flexion. (B) Tinel's test: tap over the median nerve proximal to the transverse carpal ligament in the wrist.

Precipitating factors for ulnar nerve entrapment

Local trauma, e.g. fractures of the elbow
Prolonged leaning on the elbow
Elbow synovitis

Fig. 25.4 Precipitating factors for ulnar nerve entrapment.

Aetiology

Ulnar nerve entrapment may be idiopathic or due to a precipitating cause (see Fig. 25.4).

Clinical features

Patients develop pain and/or paraesthesiae in the medial side of the elbow, which radiates to the medial forearm and the ulnar nerve distribution in the hand (see Fig. 25.2). The pain is often exacerbated by elbow flexion.

Examination usually reveals reduced sensation in the ulnar nerve distribution. Palpation of the nerve behind the medial epicondyle may provoke the symptoms. Motor dysfunction may result in atrophy of the hypothenar eminence. Abduction and adduction of the fingers is weak. There may be clawing of the hand due to weakness of the intrinsic muscles (Fig. 25.5).

Investigations

Nerve conduction studies confirm the diagnosis and establish the site of compression.

Incidence

Ulnar nerve damage at the elbow is fairly common due to its superficial position.

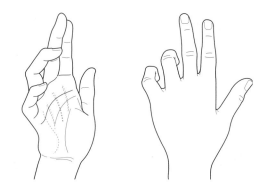

Fig. 25.5 Clawing of the hand due to ulnar nerve palsy.

Management

Ulnar nerve compression due to elbow synovitis may respond to corticosteroid injection of the elbow. Surgical decompression should be performed if sensory symptoms cannot be tolerated or if there is muscle weakness or wasting.

RADIAL NERVE INJURIES

Aetiology

Radial nerve compression at the axilla is typically seen in a drunk person who falls asleep with an arm hanging over the back of a chair ('Saturday night palsy'). The radial nerve may also be injured by fractures of the humerus.

Clinical features

The wrist extensors are paralysed, resulting in wrist drop. Grip strength is dramatically reduced, as the finger flexors do not function well with the wrist in a flexed position. Nerve injury in the axilla will also lead to paralysis of the triceps. Due to nerve overlap, sensory loss only affects a small area of skin on the dorsum of the hand between the first and second metacarpals.

Management

The wrist should be splinted immediately and the cause of the radial nerve palsy should be assessed. If there is no resolution, tendon transfer or nerve grafting may be indicated.

COMMON PERONEAL NERVE INJURIES

Aetiology

The common peroneal nerve winds around the neck of the fibula and is in a vulnerable position. It may be damaged by fractures of the neck of fibula or pressure from a tight bandage or plaster cast.

Clinical features

Common peroneal nerve injury results in paralysis of the ankle and foot extensors. Unopposed action of the foot flexors and inverters cause the foot to be plantar flexed and inverted. This is referred to as 'foot drop'. Patients develop a high-stepping gait, flicking the foot forwards to avoid tripping over it. There is also loss of sensation over the anterior and lateral sides of the leg and the dorsum of the foot and toes.

Management

Pressure on the nerve should be relieved and a splint should be applied. If the foot drop does not resolve, an ankle–foot orthosis can be used to maintain some degree of dorsiflexion.

Further reading

Nashel D J 2003 Entrapment neuropathies and compartment syndromes. In: Hochberg M C et al (eds) Rheumatology, 3rd edn. Mosby, London, p 713–724

Soft tissue disorders

Objectives

In this chapter you will learn:

- About problems affecting tendons (tendinopathy, tenosynovitis and tendon rupture).
- How to recognize, investigate and treat bursitis.
- Which factors predispose to Dupuytren's contracture.

Introduction

Soft tissue disorders are common. They are responsible for many days of absence from work and contribute significantly to the workload in primary care, accident and emergency departments, and rheumatology and orthopaedic clinics. This chapter will discuss the presentation, diagnosis and management of some common soft tissue lesions.

TENDON LESIONS

The three main pathologies that affect tendons are:

- Tendinopathy.
- Tenosynovitis.
- Rupture.

Tendinopathy

Definition

Pain arises from strain or injury to tendons and their insertions to bone. The term 'enthesopathy' is used to describe cases with a significant periosteal component, such as lateral epicondylitis (tennis elbow).

Aetiopathogenesis

The pathogenesis of tendinopathy is poorly understood. Some cases occur as part of a systemic inflammatory condition and others are related to injury from overuse. However, most cases of tendinopathy are idiopathic.

Clinical features

The most frequent sites of tendinopathy are the:

- Shoulder.
- Elbow.
- Achilles tendon.

Patients complain of pain that is worsened by active movement. Examination findings include:

- Tenderness of the tendon and its insertion.
- An increase in pain when active movement is performed against resistance.
- Soft tissue swelling (not always present).

An example: tennis elbow and golfer's elbow
In these conditions, pain is centred around the lateral and medial epicondyles respectively, although it may radiate distally from the elbow. The examination findings are as follows:

Tennis elbow   The origin of the forearm extensors is tender, and pain is exacerbated by resisted wrist extension (Fig. 26.1A). Pain on extension of the ring finger is particularly specific for tennis elbow.

Golfer's elbow   The origin of the forearm flexors is tender, and pain is exacerbated by resisted wrist flexion (Fig. 26.1B).

Investigation of tendinopathy

Tendinopathy can be diagnosed clinically and investigations are often unremarkable. Radiographs may show abnormalities, such as calcification in chronic rotator cuff disease. Ultrasound may also detect changes in the tendon and surrounding tissue.

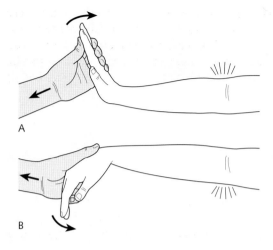

Fig. 26.1 The pain of tennis elbow is exacerbated by resisted wrist extension (A). The pain of golfer's elbow is exacerbated by resisted wrist flexion (B).

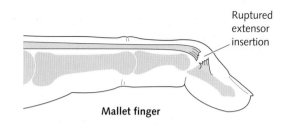

Fig. 26.2 'Mallet finger'.

Management of tendinopathy

The interventions shown below may lead to improvement of symptoms. The strategies at the top of the list should be employed early in the disease process, whilst those at the bottom should be reserved for resistant cases:

- Rest or avoidance of precipitating cause.
- Non-steroidal anti-inflammatory drug (NSAID) therapy.
- Local corticosteroid injection.
- Ultrasound therapy.
- Surgery.

Tenosynovitis

Definition

Tenosynovitis is inflammation of the synovial lining of a tendon sheath.

Aetiology

The two main causes are:

- Inflammatory arthritis.
- Trauma.

Trauma usually results from repetitive or unaccustomed movement.

Clinical features

Patients present with pain in the region of the affected tendon. Common sites of tenosynovitis are the abductor pollicis longus and extensor pollicis brevis tendons (De Quervain's tenosynovitis) and finger flexors. On examination, the tendon is swollen and tender, and crepitus may be felt on palpation.

A trigger finger or thumb results from tenosynovitis of the flexor tendons. A nodule can develop on the tendon in response to constriction of the tendon sheath. The nodule 'catches' as it enters or leaves the flexor tunnel and a 'snapping' or 'flicking' movement of the digit occurs on flexion or extension.

Management

Treatment includes rest, splinting and local corticosteroid injection. Surgical decompression of the tendon sheath may be required.

Tendon rupture

Aetiology

Tendon rupture may result from chronic inflammation and degeneration or trauma. For example, rupture of the extensor tendons of the fingers is often seen in rheumatoid arthritis.

Clinical features

The resulting clinical features are loss of movement at the joint to which the tendon provides power, deformity and sometimes swelling. After rupture of the biceps tendon, a bulge formed by the lateral muscle belly is seen in the upper arm. Extensor tendon rupture at the distal end of the finger can occur when catching a cricket ball. It results in flexion of the distal interphalangeal (DIP) joint ('Mallet finger') (Fig. 26.2).

Management

Surgery can often be performed to repair the tendon and restore function.

BURSITIS

Bursae are small sacs of fibrous tissue that are lined with synovial membrane, which secrete synovial fluid. They reduce friction where ligaments and tendons pass over bone. Inflammation of a bursa (bursitis) can be idiopathic, part of a systemic inflammatory disease or due to injury, infection or gout. Some types are notifiable industrial disorders (e.g. coal miner's 'beat' knee).

Olecranon bursitis and prepatellar bursitis are common and their clinical features and management are discussed below.

Olecranon bursitis

This can be precipitated by excessive friction at the elbow, for example by resting the elbow on a desk. Septic olecranon bursitis causes pain on elbow flexion. Idiopathic and traumatic cases are usually only painful when pressure is applied to the bursa; movement of the elbow is not usually uncomfortable or impaired. On examination the bursa is distended and tender.

Bursal fluid should be aspirated to exclude infection and improve symptoms. Local corticosteroid injection is effective in non-septic cases. Infection should be treated with appropriate antibiotics.

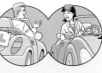

Soft tissue lesions are commonly precipitated by overuse injuries. It is therefore important to ask patients about their work and leisure activities.

Prepatellar or infrapatellar bursitis (housemaid's or carpet-fitter's knee)

This is common in people such as carpet fitters who spend a lot of time kneeling. A hot, red swelling develops over the front of the patella. Active knee extension is usually quite painful. Infection and gout should be excluded by aspirating fluid. Treatment involves rest. Recurrent episodes may require surgical excision of the bursa. Antibiotic therapy should be given for sepsis.

DUPUYTREN'S CONTRACTURE

Definition

Dupuytren's contracture is a common condition, characterized by nodular fibrosis of the palmar fascia, which draws one or more fingers into flexion.

Incidence

Before the age of 55, the incidence of Dupuytren's contracture is much higher in men than women. After this time the incidence is equal.

Aetiology

Several factors predispose to Dupuytren's contracture. These are shown in Figure 26.3.

Clinical features

The ulnar side of the hand is most commonly affected. Patients complain of inability to extend one or more fingers, usually the ring and little fingers. It is rarely painful. The fibrosis may remain stable or progress. Progressive cases can result in marked deformity and loss of function, with the fingers held in a fixed position curled into the palm.

In early cases, nodules may be felt in the palm or on the palmar surface of the finger. In more advanced cases, flexion at the metacarpophalangeal (MCP)

Factors associated with Dupuytren's contracture
Family history of Dupuytren's contracture
Hepatic cirrhosis
Peyronie's disease
Diabetes mellitus
Anticonvulsant therapy

Fig. 26.3 Factors associated with Dupuytren's contracture.

joints is seen (see Fig. 5.2) and the palm of the hand cannot be placed flat on a table (positive table top test).

Management

The most effective treatment is surgery. Palmar fasciectomy is the most commonly performed procedure. There is a risk of recurrence postoperatively.

Further reading

Hazleman B, Riley G, Speed C (eds) 2004 Soft tissue rheumatology. Oxford Universtiy Press, Oxford

HISTORY, EXAMINATION AND COMMON INVESTIGATIONS

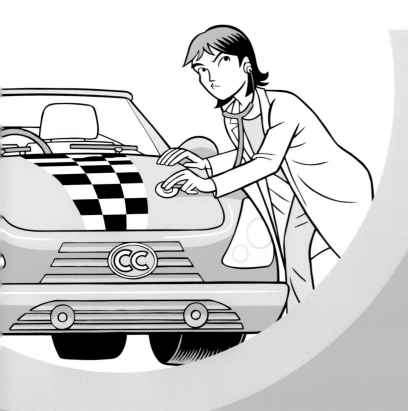

Good history taking is a valuable skill and crucial to making a correct diagnosis. It is important to establish a good rapport with patients. A relaxed, trusting patient will find it easier to share information with you and answer your questions.

The first things to document in your history are:

- The patient's name, age, date of birth, sex and hospital number.
- The date, time and place of the consultation (e.g. accident and emergency department).
- The patient's occupation and dominant hand.
- The source of referral, e.g. GP referral.

Problems affecting the dominant upper limb will be more disabling than those affecting the non-dominant side.

PRESENTING COMPLAINT

This should be a short statement, summarizing the patient's presenting symptoms. The following are some examples:

- Painful right knee.
- Pain and stiffness of both arms.

HISTORY OF THE PRESENTING COMPLAINT

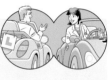

Begin your history with open questions, e.g. 'Tell me about your pain', then ask closed questions if necessary, e.g. 'Does your knee ever give way?'.

This should contain details of the patient's presenting symptoms from their onset to the current time. The following areas should be discussed when taking a rheumatological or orthopaedic history:

Symptom onset

- Date and time of symptom onset.
- Speed of onset—was it acute or gradual?
- Presence of any precipitating factors, such as trauma, commencement of a new drug, etc.

Pain, swelling and stiffness

Establish the following points:

- Site and radiation.
- Nature.
- Periodicity—is it continuous or intermittent?
- Exacerbating and relieving factors.
- Timing—is it worse at any particular time of day?

As a rule, pain and stiffness due to inflammatory conditions such as rheumatoid arthritis are worse first thing in the morning and improve as the day progresses. The duration of the early morning stiffness is quite a good guide to the severity of the inflammation. In contrast, pain due to a mechanical or degenerative problem tends to be worse later in the day and associated with a milder degree of stiffness.

Deformity

Some patients consult their doctor because they have developed a deformity and are concerned. This may or may not be associated with pain.

Weakness

It is important to ascertain whether this is localized or generalized. Localized weakness suggests a focal problem, such as a peripheral nerve lesion, whereas generalized weakness is more likely to have a systemic cause.

Numbness

The distribution of numbness or paraesthesia should be documented, as well as any precipitating factors. For example, if numbness affects the radial three and a half fingers, it is probably due to carpal tunnel syndrome. If it affects all the digits, is associated with pallor and provoked by cold weather, Raynaud's phenomenon is more likely.

Functional loss and disability

These are common in musculoskeletal disease and can be due to pain, weakness, deformity or any of the other problems discussed above. Loss of function refers to a person's inability to perform an action, such as gripping an object or walking. Disability is the result that functional loss has on the individual's ability to lead a full and active life.

Always record a patient's level of function in the notes. It is a good marker of progress.

Any restriction that a patient's disease has on their activities of daily living should be documented.

PAST MEDICAL HISTORY

Ask about all current and previous medical and surgical disorders, including any musculoskeletal problems. In certain situations, it is worth asking about specific illnesses. For example, a patient with carpal tunnel syndrome may have underlying hypothyroidism or diabetes mellitus.

DRUG HISTORY

The drug history is always important, but it sometimes has great relevance to orthopaedic and rheumatological problems. Acute gout can be precipitated by the initiation of diuretic therapy, and long-term corticosteroid use can cause osteoporosis.

SOCIAL HISTORY

Record relevant information about the patient's domestic situation, degree of independence, smoking and alcohol intake.

FAMILY HISTORY

Ask particularly about a family history of musculoskeletal disease.

SYSTEMIC ENQUIRY

This should include a brief review of any symptoms affecting other systems of the body. It is particularly relevant if you think the patient might have a connective tissue disease.

General principles of examining joints

Objectives

You should be able to:

- Establish a rapport with the patient and remember never to hurt the patient.
- Recognize pathological gait patterns.
- Develop a logical routine for examination of a joint.

GETTING OFF TO THE RIGHT START

It is important to establish a rapport with the patient, and you should look smart and be polite!

Always remember to introduce yourself and start by asking if any area is painful before you touch the patient. The last thing you want to do is hurt the patient. There are also specific marks for these acts of courtesy in the Objective Structured Clinical Examination (OSCE).

It is a cliché but the examination really does start when the patient enters the room. One of the first things to notice is how the patient walks. Pathological gait patterns are shown in Figure 28.1. Also note how the patient enters the room. The patient could be in a wheelchair, use a stick or walk unaided.

Watch how reliant patients are on relatives during simple tasks such as getting undressed or getting up from a chair.

As soon as you see the patient you should be making a mental note of any features on inspection such as typical features of rheumatoid arthritis in the hands.

Start your examination as you normally would, by looking at the hands first and then moving to the face and so on. Often the majority of features are normal, as in the case of a single osteoarthritic joint.

A thorough general examination is required for patients presenting with:

- Polyarthritis—these patients may have an inflammatory arthropathy, and a general

examination is tailored towards looking for extra-articular manifestations. Examination of the cardiovascular system, respiratory system and abdomen is required.
- Widespread aches and pains—these patients may have an inflammatory arthritis, connective tissue disorder or malignancy. Examination of other systems is required, such as the skin, eyes and other joints.

EXAMINING JOINTS

- Start with adequate exposure.
- Stand and walk the patient.
- Position the patient for the joint to be examined. Make the patient comfortable and make sure you can get to the correct side of the patient.

When examining joints make sure you stand on the side of the joint to be examined. Don't lean across the patient to examine the opposite hip or knee. A really nasty examiner might put the couch up against the wall and ask you to examine the knee that is beside the wall. If this happens move the couch to the centre of the room!

Fig. 28.1 Pathological patterns of gait.

Pathological patterns of gait		
Gait	**Features**	**Cause**
Trendelenburg	Waddling gait	Loss of abductor function
Antalgic (painful)	The patient tries to offload the painful limb by quickening and shortening the weight-bearing stance phase of the gait cycle	Any painful condition
Short leg gait	Dipping of shoulder on affected side	Any condition causing significant leg length discrepancy
High stepping	Knee is flexed and foot is lifted high to avoid foot dragging on the floor	Nerve palsy (peroneal or sciatic)
Stiff knee	Knee cleared of floor by swinging out away from the body	Fusion of knee

- LOOK:
  —Swelling, muscle wasting, scars, erythema, sinus or discharge.
- FEEL:
  —Palpate the joint systematically, noting any effusion and any tenderness over the joint line or other prominent features of the joint.
- MOVE:
  —Demonstrate joint movement actively and passively.
- Any special tests to remember?
- Examine the joints above and below.
- Don't forget peripheral pulses.

Practise a routine on your friends.

Using these basic principles of examining joints you can examine any joint.

For example, if asked, you could examine the temporomandibular joint (I don't expect you to be able to do it) by applying the basic rules.

Objectives

You should be able to:

- Know how to examine the major joints of the upper and lower limbs and spine.
- Describe special examination tests for each joint.
- Describe the MRC grading for assessment of power and be able to perform a full neurological examination of the limbs.

EXAMINATION OF THE HIP

Hip disease is common and examination involves the use of a few special tests that often cause confusion. Unlike with other joints the special tests are used first when examining the hip.

As a general principle always examine the joints above and below. Remember to examine the peripheral neurovascular system.

Gait

A Trendelenburg gait (waddling) is due to failure of the hip abductors to elevate the pelvis on weight bearing, causing a dipping or rolling gait. To compensate for this the trunk is swung over the weight-bearing hip, which maintains balance.

Failure of hip abduction can be due to pain or ineffectual muscle function following hip surgery (see Fig. 29.1).

The patient may also have an antalgic gait (see Fig. 28.1, p. 194).

Trendelenburg's test

This is used to assess the function of the hip abductors.

Stand face on to the patient and put your hands on the patient's pelvis, then ask the patient to place their hands on your forearms to steady themselves. Ask the patient then to lift each leg in turn and watch for pelvic tilt. Remember it is the standing leg you are testing and show the patient they should lift up the leg behing them by bending at the knee. (If the hip is flexed this can tilt the pelvis)

If the abductors are not functioning the pelvis tilts downwards towards the unsupported leg (Fig. 29.1B and D).

Thomas' test

This is a test for fixed flexion of the hip.

The idea of the test is to abolish the natural lumbar lordosis of the spine and visualize the true degree of flexion deformity at the hip.

To perform the test, the patient is positioned supine (flat on the back) and the opposite hip is flexed fully. This manoeuvre fully corrects the lordosis that is felt by placing a hand under the spine. Now simply observe the degree (if any) of hip flexion (Fig. 29.2).

Leg length discrepancy

Ensure the patient is lying comfortably on the examination couch with the knees straight.

Measure both limbs from the anterior superior iliac spine to the medial malleolus and compare the values.

An idea of where any leg length discrepancy lies can be obtained by flexing both hips and knees and placing them together. Look from the side and determine the relative positions of the knees.

If one knee is higher than the other then this suggests tibial shortness; however, if one knee lies

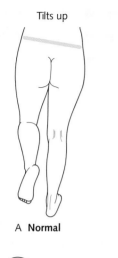

Tilts up

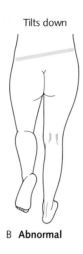

Tilts down

A **Normal**   B **Abnormal**

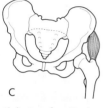

C   D

Abductors functioning
elevating pelvis

Abductors not functioning
pelvis tilts down

Fig. 29.1 The Trendelenburg test.

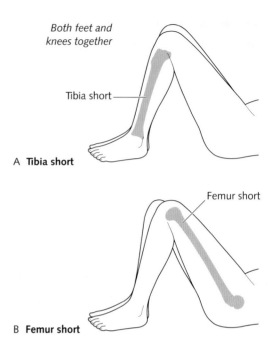

*Both feet and
knees together*

Tibia short

A **Tibia short**

Femur short

B **Femur short**

Fig. 29.3 Assessing leg length discrepancy.

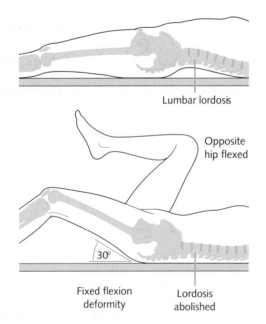

Lumbar lordosis

Opposite
hip flexed

30°

Fixed flexion
deformity

Lordosis
abolished

Fig. 29.2 The Thomas test for fixed flexion of the hip.

behind the other it suggests a femoral discrepancy (Fig. 29.3).

Inspection

Scars from previous surgery could be present anteriorly, laterally or medially. Look for erythema, sinuses and muscle wasting. Look at both sides of the hip by turning the patient to the prone position.

Palpation

The hip is deeply situated and few features are palpable.

The greater trochanter is easily felt laterally, over which bursitis may be present.

Movement

Normal movements are shown in Figure 29.4.

When assessing hip movements remember to stabilize the pelvis with a hand to ensure that pelvic tilting does not occur.

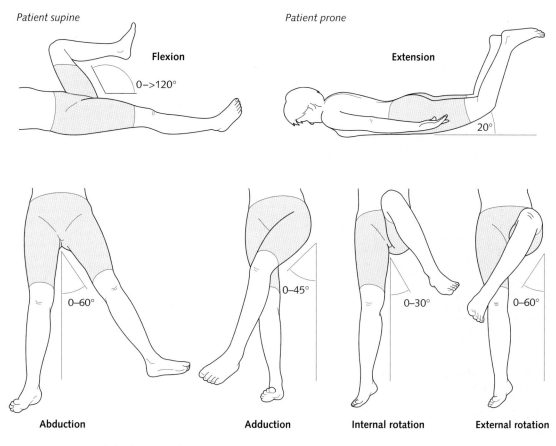

Patient supine

Flexion
0–>120°

Patient prone

Extension
20°

0–60°   0–45°   0–30°   0–60°

Abduction   Adduction   Internal rotation   External rotation

Fig. 29.4 Movements of the hip (note all ranges are approximate and vary from patient to patient.

EXAMINATION OF THE KNEE

The knee lies superficially and many landmarks are easily palpable.

Don't forget to examine the hip if asked to examine the knee.

Inspection

Ask the patient to stand and walk, and note any gait abnormality.

Deformities (varus, valgus and fixed flexion) are more obvious on standing.

Look for quadriceps wasting, which can be assessed by measuring the thigh circumference and comparing it with the measurement on the other side.

Localized swelling anteriorly or posteriorly may be visible (remember to inspect the back of the knee—this is easily done with the patient standing).

Note an effusion (which can be seen by loss of normal skin dimples at the joint line), scars, erythema or sinuses.

Palpation for an effusion

A knee effusion is important to recognize (Fig. 29.5) as it always indicates pathology. There are two tests commonly used.

Patella tap

Fluid is milked down from the suprapatellar pouch, which lifts the patella away from the femur. The patella is then pushed down onto the femur producing a 'tap' (Fig. 29.6).

197

Wipe test

Fluid is milked out of the medial dimple. The examining hand then sweeps the fluid from the lateral side of the knee, refilling the medial dimple with a visible bulge.

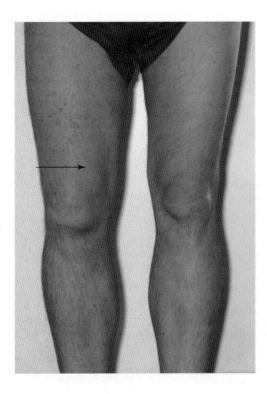

Fig. 29.5 Right knee effusion.

Palpation

Flexing the knee to 90° allows structures to be palpated more easily.

Be methodical, starting distally over the tibial tubercle and moving proximally, palpating in turn the patellar tendon, proximal tibia, medial and lateral joint lines, femoral condyles, patella, and quadriceps tendon (Fig. 29.7). The collateral ligaments are also palpable (the lateral collateral is a cord-like structure more easily felt with the knee in the figure of four position).

Remember to palpate the posterior aspect of the knee. A Baker's cyst or bursa may be present.

Movement

Both active and passive movement should be tested. The normal range is 0–150° (Fig. 29.8). Note any fixed flexion or hyperextension of the knee. Feel for patellar crepitus during flexion.

Special tests

Different patients have different degrees of laxity of the ligaments. It is therefore important to compare your examination with the normal side.

Collateral ligaments

This test should be performed in full extension and 30° flexion (instability in full extension is not present in an isolated ligament rupture and therefore indicates a much more severe injury).

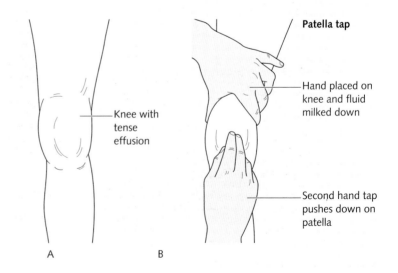

A   B

Fig. 29.6 Patella tap sign.

The foot is held between the examiner's elbow and body and both of the examiner's hands are placed on either side of the patient's knee (Fig. 29.9). A valgus or varus strain can then be placed on the knee and opening up of the joint noted.

Anterior cruciate ligament (ACL)

Lachman's test

This is the best for ACL deficiency. The idea of the test is to bring the tibia forward on a fixed femur.

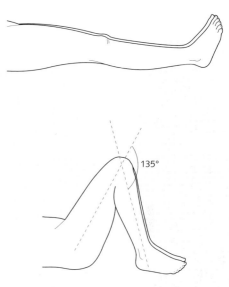

Fig. 29.8 Range of movement of the knee.

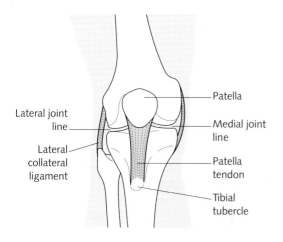

Fig. 29.7 Anatomical structures easily palpated around the knee.

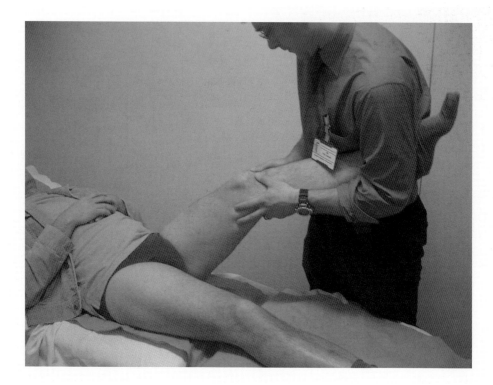

Fig. 29.9 Collateral ligament examination.

Flex the knee to 30°. Then, with the thumbs pointing towards the patient's hip, place one hand around the proximal tibia and stabilize the femur with the other. Lift up on the tibia seeing if there is abnormal forward movement (Fig. 29.10).

Anterior drawer test

This is also a test for ACL deficiency but can be misleading (the anterior drawer test can be positive

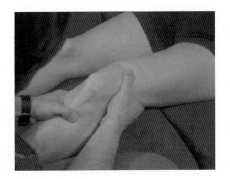

Fig. 29.10 Lachman's test for anterior cruciate ligament deficiency.

after medial meniscectomy or in posterior cruciate ligament (PCL) deficiency).

The knee is flexed to 90° and the hamstrings are relaxed. The examiner sits carefully on the patient's foot and both thumbs are placed on the proximal tibia and over both joint lines. The tibia is pulled forward and if movement is excessive the test is positive.

Pivot shift test

It can be a difficult test to perform, but the pivot shift is very useful in that it represents the way in which an ACL-deficient knee causes instability and hence gives way.

The test relies on the knee pivoting around the medial collateral ligament and uses the iliotibial band to move the tibia anteriorly.

The flexed knee is held in internal rotation with a valgus force applied as the knee is extended (Fig. 29.11). As the knee comes from flexion to extension at about 15° the tibia jumps forward into a subluxed position.

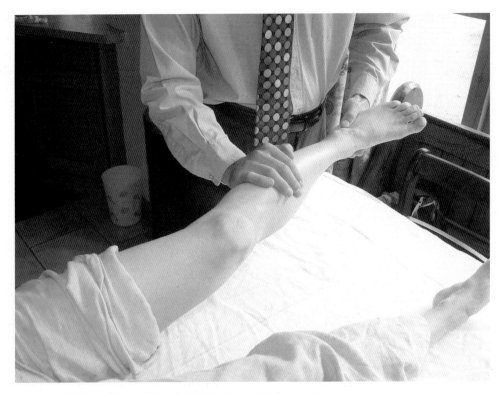

Fig. 29.11 The pivot shift test for instability of the anterior cruciate ligament.

Posterior cruciate ligament (PCL)

The posterior drawer test is performed exactly as the anterior drawer but the knee is pushed backwards.

The classic sign for a PCL rupture is the posterior sag. This is demonstrated by flexing both knees to 90° and comparing the knee contour (Fig. 29.12). A sag occurs as the tibia falls posteriorly and the tibial tubercle becomes less prominent.

Examining menisci

The most commonly used test is Mcmurray's test. It is difficult to perform and all surgeons have a different way of doing it!

The idea of the test is to 'catch' a torn meniscus between the tibial and femoral joint surface. Flex the affected knee as much as possible and load the medial or lateral compartment with a valgus or varus force, apply an axial load (i.e. push the two surfaces together) and rotate the leg as the knee is extended. A click may be heard or felt in the presence of a tear. Be careful or you can hurt the patient.

The patellofemoral joint

To examine the patellofemoral joint, sit the patient on the edge of the couch so that the legs are free to flex. Watch the patella carefully as the knee extends and look at how the patella tracks. Lateral maltracking is demonstrated as the patella deviates laterally towards the end of extension.

Patella apprehension is demonstrated when the examiner tries to push the patella laterally when the patient's knee is fully extended on the couch. If the patella is unstable the patient will grimace.

EXAMINATION OF THE ANKLE AND FOOT

Inspection

Inspect the ankle and foot with the patient in both resting and weight-bearing positions. Look at the distribution of any swelling. Synovitis of the ankle usually produces diffuse swelling, obscuring the contours of the medial and lateral malleoli. Swelling in the region of the Achilles tendon is more likely to be due to Achilles tendinopathy or tendon rupture.

Disease of the subtalar joint or abnormalities of the longitudinal arch of the foot may disrupt the alignment of the heel and Achilles tendon. This should be vertical and is seen easily from behind whilst the patient is standing. Pes planus (flat foot) can cause pronation of the foot and valgus deformity of the heel (Fig. 29.13).

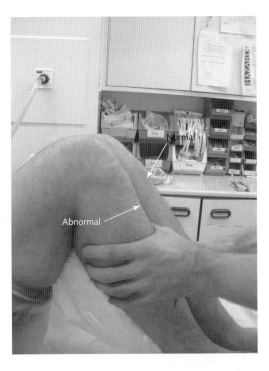

Fig. 29.12 Posterior sag sign. The right knee shows the positive sign. Note that the tibial tuberosity is more prominent on the left.

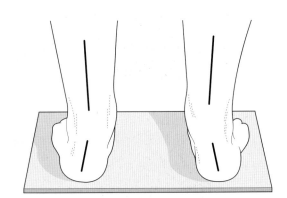

Fig. 29.13 Pes planus with pronation of the feet and hindfoot valgus.

201

Forefoot problems are common. Hallux valgus is a deformity of the great toe, which becomes abducted at the MTP joint. Excessive pressure on the medial side can lead to formation of a bursa, often referred to as a 'bunion'. Figure 29.14 shows some other deformities that commonly affect the forefoot.

The MTP joints are commonly affected by RA and may sublux. The metatarsal heads become prominent and callosities often form in the overlying skin.

Palpation

Palpate the joints of the ankle and foot with the foot in slight plantar flexion to assess for swelling and tenderness. Tenderness of the heel may be due to plantar fasciitis. Tenderness at the insertion of the Achilles tendon to the calcaneus occurs in Achilles tendinopathy.

Movement

Test plantar flexion and dorsiflexion of the ankle with the knee flexed. The subtalar joint allows inversion and eversion of the hindfoot. This is tested by stabilizing the tibia with one hand and turning the calcaneus inward and outward with the other. Midtarsal movements contribute to plantar flexion, dorsiflexion, inversion and eversion. These are tested by stabilizing the heel with one hand and moving the forefoot with the other. Movements of the MTP, PIP and DIP joints are best examined whilst the patient is lying or sitting.

EXAMINATION OF THE SPINE

When examining the spine always remember to also perform a peripheral nervous system examination.

Inspection

In acute conditions muscle spasm and loss of normal lumbar lordosis may be seen. Look at the posture of the patient. If the patient has sciatica the affected leg is often flexed and the patient is stooped.

Note any scars, erythema or deformity. Deformities of the spine such as scoliosis or kyphosis may be obvious on inspection.

- In scoliosis the rib hump deformity is more clearly seen when the patient bends forwards (see Fig. 23.12, p. 170).
- Kyphotic deformity is best visualized from the side (see Fig. 5.4, p. 36). A gibbus is a very pronounced kyphotic deformity caused by fracture, tumour or infection.

Remember the spine normally has a lumbar and cervical lordosis and a thoracic kyphosis.

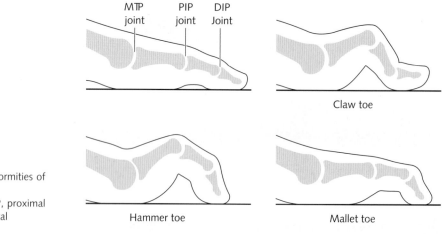

Fig. 29.14 Common deformities of the forefoot. MTP, metatarsophalangeal; PIP, proximal interphalangeal; DIP, distal interphalangeal.

Palpation

Palpation is performed standing and with the patient lying prone.

The C7 spinous process is a useful landmark (the most prominent in the upper spine).

Tenderness is elicited by palpation over the spinous processes.

Movement

Cervical spine

Movements of the cervical spine (Fig. 29.15) are usually stated as percentage loss when compared with normal, if possible.

Flexion

Ask the patient to bend the head forward to put the chin on the chest.

Extension

Ask the patient to look up at the ceiling.

Lateral flexion

Ask the patient to put the ear down to the shoulder.

Rotation

Ask the patient to look to either side.

Thoracolumbar spine (Fig. 29.16)

Flexion

Often patients are reluctant to flex the spine if it is acutely tender. Ask patients to bend over and reach as far as they can.

Look and feel for unfolding of the lumbar spine. This can be measured by marking two points on the lumbar spine and observing the increase in the distance between them on flexion.

Extension

Get the patient to arch the back backwards. In conditions such as spinal stenosis this can exacerbate the pain.

Rotation

Stabilize the pelvis by asking the patient to sit when examining rotation in order to abolish hip rotation.

Lateral flexion

Ask the patient to slide one hand down the side of the leg.

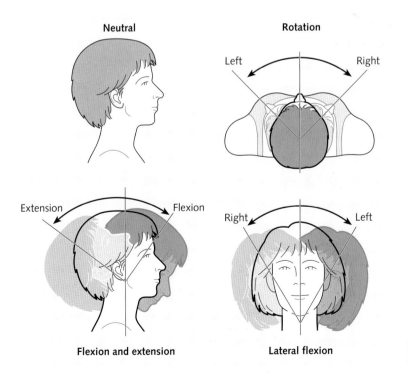

Fig. 29.15 Movements of the cervical spine.

Fig. 29.16 Thoracolumbar movements.

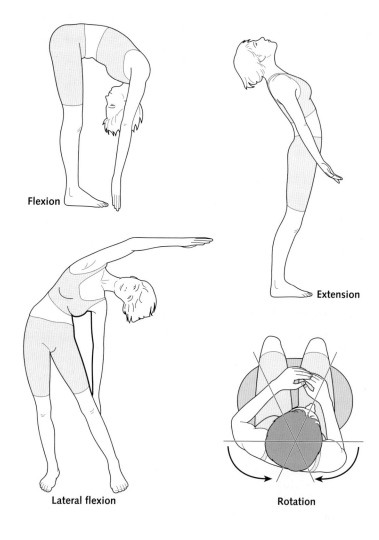

Flexion

Extension

Lateral flexion

Rotation

Special tests

Straight leg raising

Straight leg raising is a test for nerve root irritation (radiculopathy).

With the patient supine elevate the affected leg passively keeping it straight. If the patient complains of pain down the leg look at the angle that the leg makes with the couch, e.g. 30°. The next step is to bend the knee as this will abolish the symptoms by relieving tension on the nerve.

For the test to be positive the pain must radiate to the foot (often patients will complain of back pain when elevating the leg).

The crossover sign is present with severe acute prolapsed discs and occurs when the normal leg is elevated causing pain radiating down the opposite leg.

Peripheral nervous examination

Spinal cord conditions such as stenosis or prolapsed disc can cause abnormalities of the peripheral nervous system due to compression on nerve roots. The most commonly affected are the L5 and S1 nerve roots.

Lower limb

Tone

Lower limb tone is usually normal but is reduced in spinal cord compression (flaccid paralysis).

Power is assessed by Medical Research Council (MRC) grade:

Testing lower limb muscle function (myotomes)	
Muscle action	Nerve roots tested
Hip flexion (iliopsoas)	L1, L2
Knee flexion (quadriceps)	L3
Ankle dorsiflexion (tibialis anterior)	L4
Great toe extension (extensor hallucis longus)	L5
Ankle plantar flexion (soleus/gastrocnemius)	S1

Fig. 29.17 Testing lower limb muscle function.

0   Nothing.
1   Flicker.
2   Power to move limb with gravity eliminated.
3   Power to move limb against gravity.
4   Reduced from normal.
5   Normal.

Test muscle function as shown in Figure 29.17.

Reflexes
Always compare the reflexes with the opposite limb and make sure the patient is relaxed. Reflexes can be reduced, brisk or absent.

Three reflexes are commonly tested:

- Knee L3–L4: flex both knees over the couch and tap lightly on the patellar ligament.
- Ankle L5, S1: dorsiflex the ankle with the knees flexed and the leg externally rotated. Tap the Achilles tendon.
- Plantar: this is performed by stroking the plantar skin with the handle of the tendon hammer. If the toes extend this is abnormal and called 'up going', indicating an upper motor neuron lesion.

Sensation
Ask the patient if the sensation is normal and the same as on the other side. Dermatomes are shown in Figure 29.18.

Anal tone
In cauda equina syndrome anal tone is lost; therefore an examination per rectum (PR) is an important part of any spinal examination.

Perianal sensation
This is also reduced in cauda equina syndrome.

Chest expansion
Patients with severe scoliosis or ankylosing spondylitis have reduced lung function and may show reduced chest expansion.

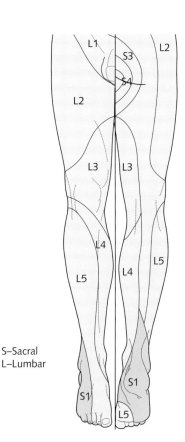

Fig. 29.18 Dermatomes of the lower limb.

EXAMINATION OF THE SHOULDER

Movement of the shoulder occurs at four joints (Fig. 29.19). The majority of the total range of movement arises from the glenohumeral and scapulothoracic joints.

Inspection

Look at the position and contours of the shoulder and compare with the opposite one.

Fig. 29.19 Anatomy of the shoulder.

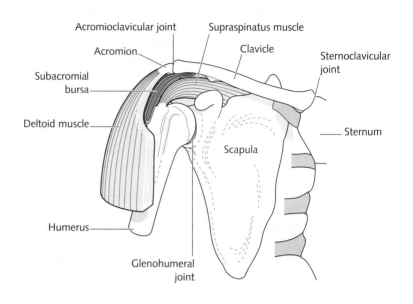

- Acromioclavicular joint
- Supraspinatus muscle
- Acromion
- Clavicle
- Sternoclavicular joint
- Subacromial bursa
- Deltoid muscle
- Sternum
- Scapula
- Humerus
- Glenohumeral joint

- Swelling of the shoulder is uncommon. When it does occur, it is best seen anteriorly.
- Muscle wasting may be due to chronic shoulder pathology, such as chronic rotator cuff tendinopathy.
- Rupture of the long head of biceps is usually obvious, as it produces a bulge anteriorly in the upper arm.
- Look for winging of the scapula by asking the patient to do a press-up against the wall. Weakness of the serratus anterior muscle causes the medial border to protrude backwards. This can occur in long thoracic nerve palsy or other causes of muscular weakness.
- Look for a step in the acromioclavicular joint due to dislocation. This is seen best whilst the patient's arm is hanging in a relaxed position.

Palpation

Feel for tenderness and swelling of the acromioclavicular, sternoclavicular and glenohumeral joints. A gap on palpation of the acromioclavicular joint indicates dislocation. Crepitus of the glenohumeral or acromioclavicular joints may be felt on shoulder movement. Palpate the muscles of the shoulder girdle and neck to identify any tender 'trigger' points of fibromyalgia (see Fig. 19.3, p. 140).

Movement

Examine active and passive movements, looking at the range of abduction, forward flexion, and internal and external rotation.

- A normal range of passive movements suggests that glenohumeral disease is very unlikely.
- Normal passive movements with painful or restricted active movements indicate a muscle or tendon problem.
- A 'hitch-up' of the shoulder on active abduction of the arm is a sign of reduced glenohumeral range (Fig. 29.20).
- Loss of passive external rotation, and abduction are highly indicative of adhesive capsulitis ('frozen shoulder').

A quick way to evaluate active shoulder movements is by asking patients to:

- Put their hands behind their head, with the elbows back.
- Reach behind their back, as if to fasten a bra strap.
- Raise their arms up to their sides and then above their head.

The rotator cuff

The supraspinatus, infraspinatus, teres minor and subscapularis muscles make up the rotator cuff.

They hold the head of the humerus in the glenoid cavity, maintain stability and initiate shoulder abduction. Rotator cuff inflammation, injury and degeneration are common. Disease of the supraspinatus especially, causes pain on abduction when the tendon becomes compressed under the acromion. The pain is felt at between 60° and 120° of abduction (Fig. 29.21). This is referred to as a 'painful arc'.

Resisted shoulder movements should be examined. Pain or weakness on resisted movements suggests involvement of the rotator cuff muscles and tendons.

- Supraspinatus is tested with the arm abducted to 30°, flexed to 30° and internally rotated with the thumb pointing downwards. Abduction is then resisted.
- Resisted internal rotation tests the subscapularis.
- Resisted external rotation tests the infraspinatus and teres minor.

Apprehension testing

An unstable shoulder makes the patient apprehensive when it is put into abduction and external rotation. The patient should be supine with the arms abducted to 90° and elbows flexed to 90°. Ask the patient to lower the hands backward (i.e. towards 90° of external rotation). The patient's apprehension will limit external rotation of a dislocation-prone shoulder.

Acromioclavicular joint testing

Pain arising from pathology of the acromioclavicular joint may be accentuated if the patient places the hand on the opposite shoulder and the examiner pulls the elbow in the same direction.

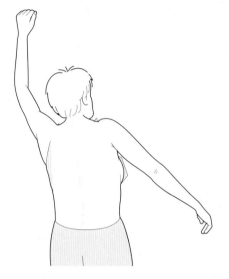

Fig. 29.20 A 'hitched' shoulder. The patient is unable to elevate her arm to the side properly, so is 'cheating' by shrugging her shoulder.

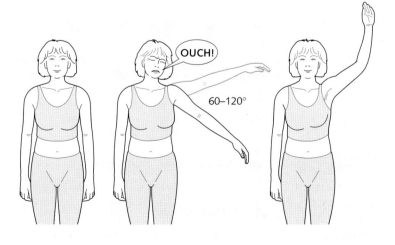

OUCH!

60–120°

Fig. 29.21 Demonstration of the painful arc.

EXAMINATION OF THE ELBOW

The elbow joint consists of two articulations:

- The first is between the humerus, radius and ulna, which allows flexion to a range of 150°.
- The second is the superior radioulnar joint, which allows rotation of the wrist through 180°.

Inspection

Inspect the elbow from behind with the patient's arm flexed and extended. The lateral infracondylar recess will be filled in if an effusion is present. Look also for swelling of the olecranon bursa and the presence of rheumatoid nodules along the border of the ulna.

Palpation

Palpate the olecranon process and medial and lateral epicondyles. The lateral epicondyle will be tender in tennis elbow. The radial head is usually felt easily in the lateral aspect of the joint and its movement can be assessed during pronation and supination.

Movement

Test flexion, extension, pronation and supination. Extension of the elbow is to 180° or beyond in almost all normal people. The inability to straighten the elbow to 180° is therefore considered pathological, even if it is pain-free and unnoticed by the patient. It will usually be a sign of arthritis. On the other hand, many people can extend another 5–10°, so hyperextension (as in hypermobility) is defined as extension beyond 190°.

It is best to assess pronation and supination with the elbow flexed to 90° and held close to the side of the body. If you suspect the patient may have epicondylitis, examine resisted movements of the wrist for pain (see Fig. 26.1, p. 186).

EXAMINATION OF THE WRIST AND HAND

Inspection

Inspection of the hands is an important part of the musculoskeletal examination. Look first at the skin and the nails.

- Pitting of the nails or onycholysis is commonly found in psoriatic arthritis.
- Nail fold infarcts and digital ulcers can occur as a consequence of vasculitis. A magnifying glass is useful when looking for nail fold infarcts.
- Telangiectasia and sclerodactyly are features of systemic sclerosis.
- Heberden's nodes, gouty tophi or rheumatoid nodules may develop in the fingers.

Look next for deformities, which are common in inflammatory arthritis. Arthritis mutilans is a rare, but severe type of joint destruction in psoriatic arthritis. Rheumatoid arthritis (RA) can cause many deformities in the hand and wrist, including:

- Volar subluxation and radial deviation of the carpus.
- Boutonnière and swan-neck deformities of the fingers (see Fig. 10.9, p. 62).
- Z-deformity of the thumb.

Look carefully for swelling. The distribution gives a good clue to the cause. For example, swelling of the metacarpophalangeal (MCP) and proximal interphalangeal (PIP) joints is common in RA, whereas distal interphalangeal (DIP) joint involvement is more typical of osteoarthritis (OA) or psoriatic arthritis. The swelling of tenosynovitis follows the route of the tendon.

It is also important to note any muscle wasting. Atrophy of the dorsal interossei occurs in RA. Carpal tunnel syndrome can lead to wasting of the muscles of the thenar eminence.

Palpation

Palpate any swellings to confirm whether they are hard due to bony overgrowth, or soft due to synovitis. Synovitis at the MCP joints is best felt with the patient's fingers semi-flexed and the examiner's fingertips placed at either side of the MCP joint, feeling for soft tissue swelling. With practice, it is easily detected, even in podgy hands. Synovitis at the PIP joint bulges out either side of the extensor expansion. Enthesitis at the DIP joint due to psoriatic arthritis is to be distinguished from Heberden's nodes; this is not always easy. Crepitus may be felt on palpation of the first carpometacarpal (CMC) joint in OA. Tenosynovitis of the finger flexors can be associated with tendon nodules, which can be felt moving on finger flexion.

Muscles responsible for hand and wrist movement	
Movement	Muscle(s) responsible (nerve supply)
Wrist flexion	Flexor carpi radialis (median) Flexor carpi ulnaris (ulnar) Palmaris longus (median)
Wrist extension	Extensor carpi radialis longus and brevis (both radial) Extensor carpi ulnaris (radial)
DIP joint flexion	Flexor digitorum profundus (median and ulnar)
PIP joint flexion	Flexor digitorum superficialis (median)
MCP joint flexion and IP joint extension	Lumbricals (median and ulnar)
Finger abduction	Dorsal interossei (ulnar)
Finger adduction	Palmar interossei (ulnar)
Extension of MCPs, PIPs and DIPs	Extensor digitorum (radial)
Thumb abduction	Abductor pollicis brevis (median)
Thumb adduction	Adductor pollicis (ulnar)
Thumb opposition	Opponens pollicis (median)
Thumb extension	Extensor pollicis longus (radial)

Fig. 29.22 Muscles responsible for hand and wrist movement.

Movement

It is important to assess hand function. Active and passive movement of the wrist and digits should be tested, as well as the patient's ability to perform certain tasks. The muscles responsible for various movements of the hand and wrist are shown in Figure 29.22.

The 'prayer' sign is useful when assessing hand and wrist function. Ask the patient to extend both wrists and place the palms of the hands flat against each other, as if praying (Fig. 29.23). Patients with limited wrist extension or deformities or synovitis of their MCP or PIP joints will find this difficult.

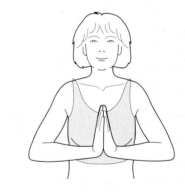

Fig. 29.23 The 'prayer' sign.

Ask the patient to pick a penny up from the table or fasten a button. This will give you a good idea of what their hand function is like. It is surprising how well some people can perform fiddly tasks, despite having hand deformities.

Special tests

Tinel's and Phalen's tests should be performed in patients who have symptoms suggestive of carpal tunnel syndrome. These tests are described in Chapter 25.

Writing up a medical clerking

Objectives

You should be able to:

- Understand the importance of clear and accurate documentation in the medical notes.
- Write up your medical clerking in a methodical and organized format.

INTRODUCTION

Patients with musculoskeletal problems usually present to hospital in one of two ways. Many are referred to the outpatient department by their family doctors. Those with more urgent problems attend the accident and emergency department.

The doctor clerking the patient should record the history and examination in the medical notes. Clear documentation will remind the doctor of the patient's problems and is valuable for other clinicians involved in their care. Good record keeping is also extremely important for medicolegal reasons.

PRESENTATION

Notes should be legible, easily understood and neatly filed. Only well-recognized abbreviations should be used. Diagrams may be helpful, particularly to illustrate examination findings, such as swellings, scars or rashes.

CONTENT

The patient's name and hospital number should be written on every page of the notes.

The date, time and place of the consultation should be recorded, followed by the details of the history and examination findings. Negative answers in the history and normal examination findings can be as helpful as positive ones in formulating a diagnosis. The investigations requested should be listed, as should the results when they arrive. A clear management plan should include details of all intended interventions. Every entry made in a patient's medical notes should finish with the doctor's signature, followed by his/her name, grade and bleep number.

Sample clerking

Figure 30.1 shows a typical clerking of a patient seen for the first time in a rheumatology clinic.

27/11/07

New patient

Orthopaedic outpatient dept

UNIT No. C99999

Carol Smith DOB 22/9/45

62 year old, retired shop assistant

PC   Painful right knee

> 1. Presenting complaint should be brief

HOPC   RA since age of 28

Worsening R knee pain for past 5 years

> 2. It is helpful to briefly mention relevant PMH, such as this lady's history of RA

No history of trauma

"Ache" in anterior aspect of knee

       Worst on exertion, but present all day and
       disturbs sleep at night
       Walks with a stick, ↓ exercise tolerance
       Naproxen and cocodamol help a little

Wrists, hands and feet ache and swell intermittently

No problems with other joints

Early morning stiffness variable - 30 to 60 mins

PMH   RA diagnosed in 1973
           ↑ BP
           Appendectomy 1962

DH   Methotrexate 15mg weekly
         Folic acid 5mg weekly
         Naproxen 500mg bd
         Cocodamol (8/500) 2 qds
         Bendroflumethiazide 2.5mg od
         No known allergies

SH   Lives with husband (fit and well) in house
         Struggles to climb the stairs and get in and
         out of bath

> 3. The social history is particularly important in patients with musculoskeletal diseases, as they can interfere greatly with patients activities of daily living

         Also has difficulty taking lids of bottles
         and jars
         Lifelong non-smoker
         4 units alcohol/week

FH   Father died of MI
         Mother had RA

SE   CVS - no chest pain/SOB/palpitations
         RS - no cough/phlegm/wheeze/haemoptysis
         AS - wt steady, no nausea/vomiting/abdo pain/CIBH/ PR bleeding
         GU - no frequency/urgency/dysuria/haematuria
         End - no DM
         CNS - no headache/LOC/paraesthesiae

Fig. 30.1 Sample clerking.

OE   No an/jau/cy/cl

CVS   Pulse 70 reg
        BP 150/80
        JVP
        HS I+II+0
        No ankle oedema

RS   Chest clear

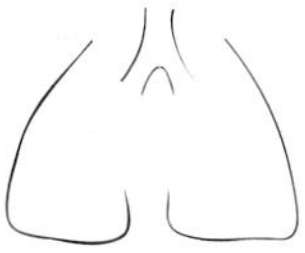

AS   Abdo soft and non-tender
        No LKKS

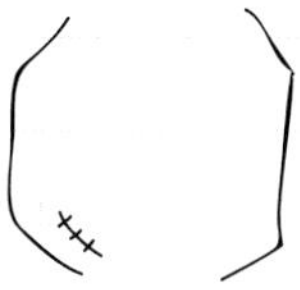

> 1. Diagrams are a useful way of recording your examination findings

Joints

R knee   small effusion, fixed in 10° flexion, crepitus on flexion/extension ++,
         wasting of quadriceps muscles   Range of motion
L knee   no effusion, mild crepitus   10-90%
Feet   MPTJs slightly tender, no swelling
Elbows   bilateral rheumatoid nodules\
Wrists   ↓ flexion/extension, mild synovitis
Hands   weak grip, mild synovitis of MCPJs all fingers
Other joints NAD
Neuro   Tone normal
        Power 4/5 flexion/extension R knee (limited by pain)
        Otherwise normal all 4 limbs
        Reflexes all present and symetrical, plantars downgoing

Summary
        A 62 year old lady with long standing Ra, presents with worsening R knee pain.
        Examination reveals a flexion deformity, small effusion and crepitus
Impression
        Degenerative disease R knee secondary to RA
Plan
Investigations

> 2. Always include a management plan - even when you are astudent. It might not be completely correct, but you need to train yourself to think like a doctor

        Weight-bearing-X-ray R knee
        FBC, ESR, CRP, U+E, RBS, LFT, Ca profile
Management
        Refer to physios and occupational therapists
        Give patient information on joint replcement surgery and list the R
        total knee replacement if she is willing to proceed

> 3. Sign, your notes, print your surname and record your bleep number if you have one

HORTON-SZAR   437

Objectives

You should be able to:

- Understand which general and specific blood tests are useful for various orthopaedic and rheumatological conditions.
- Describe what tests can be done on a joint fluid aspirate to help make a diagnosis.
- Describe some tests useful in the diagnosis of neuromuscular conditions.
- Describe common tests used to diagnose osteoporosis and understand the difference between an isotope and a DEXA bone scan.
- Understand the different uses and indications for X-ray imaging, CT and MRI.

BLOOD TESTS

The following blood tests are useful in the investigation of rheumatic disease.

Full blood count

- Anaemia may be due to chronic inflammatory disease or iron deficiency from non-steroidal anti-inflammatory drug (NSAID) therapy.
- A polymorphonuclear leucocytosis may be a consequence of infection, such as septic arthritis or osteomyelitis. It can also be a sign of inflammation or prolonged corticosteroid use.
- Leucopenia can be a feature of systemic lupus erythematosus (SLE) or bone marrow suppression from disease-modifying antirheumatic drugs (DMARDs).
- Thrombocytosis often occurs in active inflammatory disease. It is sometimes referred to as a 'reactive thrombocytosis'.

Chronic inflammatory disease can cause anaemia, but the haemoglobin rarely drops below 9 g/dL.

Erythrocyte sedimentation rate (ESR) and C-reactive protein (CRP)

- These are non-specific markers of inflammation and will rise in infectious and inflammatory disorders.
- The ESR measures aggregation of erythrocytes, which increases with the concentration of plasma proteins such as fibrinogen and immunoglobulins.
- The upper limit of normal for the ESR increases with age.
- CRP is synthesized by the liver and rises within 6–10 hours of an inflammatory event.

The CRP responds more rapidly than the ESR to inflammation.

Urea and electrolytes (U&E)

Renal impairment might occur in gout or connective tissue disease.

Liver function tests (LFTs)

- A raised level of alkaline phosphatase is seen in Paget's disease.

- Many drugs used for musculoskeletal problems can be hepatotoxic, such as methotrexate and NSAIDs.

Uric acid

- Prolonged hyperuricaemia predisposes to gout.
- Occasionally, uric acid levels are normal during an acute attack of gout.

Calcium

- Hypocalcaemia occurs in osteomalacia.
- Hypercalcaemia can be a feature of malignancy.

Creatine kinase (CK)

- This muscle enzyme exists as three isoenzymes (CK-MM, CK-MB and CK-BB).
- Elevated levels of CK-MM may be due to myositis or other causes of skeletal muscle damage.
- CK-BB is found in the brain and CK-MB in the myocardium.

Autoantibodies

These are found in many autoimmune rheumatic diseases. Medical students and doctors often find the results of autoantibody tests difficult to interpret, usually because they have been requested inappropriately. Some autoantibodies can occur in healthy people and tests for them have little diagnostic value unless they are done in appropriate circumstances.

Example

An elderly man visits his doctor complaining of pain in his knees that is worse in the evenings and has been present for several years. On examination, he has bilateral knee crepitus, without swelling, and Heberden's and Bouchard's nodes in his hands. His family doctor requests several investigations, including a test for rheumatoid factor, which is positive. There is now confusion as to the correct diagnosis. Does this man have osteoarthritis or rheumatoid arthritis?

The correct diagnosis is osteoarthritis. This man has no clinical features of rheumatoid arthritis. The prevalence of rheumatoid factor in the 'normal' population is at least 1% and this increases with age. The presence of rheumatoid factor in this case has no relevance.

Autoantibody tests should only be requested if there is real clinical suspicion of an autoimmune disease.

Rheumatoid factor

The definition of a rheumatoid factor is an antibody directed against the Fc fragment of human immunoglobulin G (IgG). Rheumatoid factors may be of any immunoglobulin class, although IgM anti-IgG is the rheumatoid factor that is most commonly measured. Patients who are rheumatoid factor-positive tend to have more aggressive disease.

Anti-cyclic citrullinated peptide (anti-CCP) antibodies

These antibodies are highly specific for RA and may be detected years before onset of the disease. They are associated with joint destruction and can be present in patients who are rheumatoid factor-negative.

Antinuclear antibodies (ANAs)

These are antibodies to nuclear antigens. They are detected by labelling methods, such as indirect immunofluorescence. A positive ANA simply indicates that the patient's blood contains antibodies, which will bind to the nuclei of a sample of cells used in the test.

If an ANA test is positive, it is important to examine which nuclear antigens the antibodies are binding to. The pattern of fluorescence gives a clue. ANAs are found in 5–10% of the normal population and 95% of SLE patients. They are also seen in other connective tissue diseases.

Figure 31.1 lists the ANAs against specific nuclear antigens and the diseases with which they are associated.

Antibodies to double-stranded DNA (dsDNA) are very specific for SLE. They are also useful measures of disease activity.

Antineutrophil cytoplasmic antibodies (ANCA)

These antibodies are directed against enzymes present in neutrophil granules. Two main patterns

ANAs against specific nuclear antigens and their associated diseases	
Autoantibodies	Disease
Histone	Drug-induced SLE
Double-stranded DNA (dsDNA)	SLE
Sm	SLE
Ro, La	Sjögren's syndrome
Scl-70 (topoisomerase)	Diffuse cutaneous scleroderma
Anti-centromere	Localized cutaneous scleroderma

Fig. 31.1 ANAs against specific nuclear antigens and their associated diseases.

Significance of changes in appearance of synovial fluid	
Synovial fluid appearance	Pathology
Yellow and clear	Normal
Blood-stained	Haemarthrosis or puncture of a blood vessel on aspiration
Cloudy	Increased cell count due to inflammation or septic arthritis
Frank pus	Septic arthritis or occasionally crystal arthritis

Fig. 31.2 Significance of changes in appearance of synovial fluid.

of immunofluorescence are seen: cytoplasmic (c-) and perinuclear (p-).

c-ANCA and p-ANCA bind to several proteins, the most common being proteinase 3 and myeloperoxidase, respectively. Antibodies to proteinase 3 are found in about 80% of patients with Wegener's granulomatosis. Those against myeloperoxidase are found in polyarteritis nodosa and rheumatoid and lupus vasculitis. A positive p-ANCA can also be found with malignancy and certain infections.

Antiphospholipid antibodies (APAs)

Lupus anticoagulant and anticardiolipin antibodies are found in the antiphospholipid syndrome. They are associated with venous and arterial thrombosis.

SYNOVIAL FLUID ANALYSIS

This is the most important investigation for suspected septic or crystal arthritis. Synovial fluid can be aspirated from most peripheral joints and only a small amount is needed for analysis.

Macroscopic appearance

Normal synovial fluid is pale yellow and clear. Changes in the macroscopic appearance can give clues to the underlying joint pathology (Fig. 31.2).

Gram stain and culture

This should be performed if there is any suspicion of septic arthritis. The absence of organisms on microscopy does not exclude infection.

Polarized light microscopy

For accurate identification of crystals, synovial fluid should be examined under a polarized light microscope. Urate crystals are needle-shaped and show strong negative birefringence. This means that crystals parallel to the plane of light appear yellow, whereas those at right angles are blue. Calcium pyrophosphate dihydrate (CPPD) crystals are either rhomboid or rod-shaped and show weak positive birefringence.

NERVE CONDUCTION STUDIES (NCS) AND ELECTROMYOGRAPHY (EMG)

These electrophysiological tests are used to diagnose and assess neuromuscular problems. They help to differentiate between primary muscle disease and neuropathic disorders. NCS measure the conduction velocity of motor and sensory nerves and can localize and assess the severity of peripheral nerve lesions. EMG records the spontaneous and voluntary electrical activity of muscle.

BIOPSY

Biopsies are occasionally performed in the investigation of musculoskeletal disease. Muscle is biopsied in cases of suspected myositis. Evidence of vasculitis can be obtained from biopsy of blood vessels, nerves and skin. Renal biopsies can assess the extent of renal involvement in connective tissue diseases and guide prognosis. Bone biopsy is necessary in the diagnosis of primary bone tumours.

IMAGING

X-rays

A plain X-ray (radiograph) is usually the first-line investigation of any musculoskeletal disease. X-rays are good at visualizing bone. Soft tissues can also be seen on X-ray and give valuable information (for example a lipohaemarthrosis in the knee) but for detail of ligamentous or cartilage structures other investigations are necessary.

A radiograph involves the use of electromagnetic radiation produced by electrons striking a rotating metal target in an X-ray tube. A narrow beam of X-rays is produced, which then passes through the patient, and the image is formed on an X-ray-sensitive film placed behind the patient (Fig. 31.3).

The amount of the X-ray beam absorbed by the tissues determines the overall appearance of the image. Bone absorbs the most and appears white on the image, muscle absorbs some and appears dark grey, fat is darker grey and air appears black (see Fig. 1.8).

The X-ray machine is controlled by a radiographer who will determine the amount of exposure and the correct position of the patient.

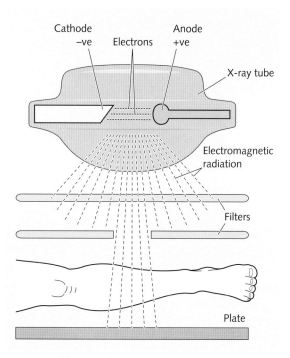

Fig. 31.3 Production of a radiographic image.

Any X-ray causes a small radiation exposure. This effect is cumulative and has been linked with the development of tumours. Avoid unnecessary X-rays to minimize risk. Avoid X-rays in pregnancy unless absolutely necessary.

Two views are required, taken at 90° to each other, of the joint or bone to be examined (usually anteroposterior (AP) and lateral). Sometimes special views are taken, such as scaphoid views when looking for a fracture.

Fluoroscopy (also known as screening) uses the same principles as radiography but the image is obtained on a screen and is in real time (i.e. moving). Screening is commonly used intraoperatively in orthopaedic surgery when fixing fractures and as guidance for joint injections.

Ultrasound

Ultrasound is used widely in orthopaedics and has the advantages of being cheap, portable and safe, and it allows dynamic images.

The image is produced using a transducer that emits a beam of high-frequency sound (ultrasound) and detects the sound waves reflected from the soft tissues of the patient. Different tissues absorb or reflect different amounts of the sound beam, and the reflections are analysed to produce a black and white image.

Areas commonly imaged in this way include the shoulder for rotator cuff tears, the hip for joint effusion, and extra-articular structures around the knee such as the patellar tendon.

Ultrasound can also be used for guidance, for example for joint aspiration.

Computed tomography (CT)

CT uses the basic principles of an X-ray machine but the image is obtained when the X-ray tube is circled around the patient in the scanner. Instead of an X-ray plate the CT scanner has detectors within the machine to collect images. A large number of images are acquired and processed by the computer and the resulting images are in the form of cross-sectional slices taken in different planes.

The main role for CT in orthopaedics is the study of bones, particularly complex fractures.

Remember that CT scans also produce a significant radiation exposure.

It is also possible to reconstruct images in three dimensions. Three-dimensional (3-D) reconstructions are useful in orthopaedics when planning complex pelvic or hip surgery.

Magnetic resonance imaging (MRI)

MRI gives excellent images of soft tissues and bone marrow.

The images are generated by the use of a powerful magnet, which aligns protons in the body with the electromagnetic field. A pulse of radiofrequency energy then causes the protons to 'flip' (change alignment) and images are acquired when energy is released as the protons realign themselves within the magnetic field. A coil collects data, which are then reconstructed with complex computer software to produce the image.

As a large magnet is used, any metal components or foreign bodies may become dislodged. Patients with cardiac pacemakers and intraocular metallic foreign bodies must not have an MRI scan.

MRI is commonly used around the knee to look for meniscal or ligamentous injuries (Fig. 31.4), the shoulder for capsule or rotator cuff lesions, and the spine for disc prolapse and nerve root compression.

MRI is also good at assessing bone changes such as in infection, tumour and osteonecrosis.

Isotope bone scan

An isotope bone scan involves the use of a radioactive tracer injected intravenously and taken up by physiologically active bone. The most commonly used is technetium-99m (^{99m}Tc) and its decay is measured with a gamma camera. The procedure is divided into three phases depending on the time after injection: blood flow (initial); blood pool (30 minutes); and delayed (4 hours).

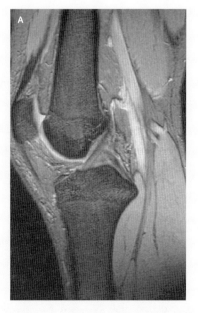
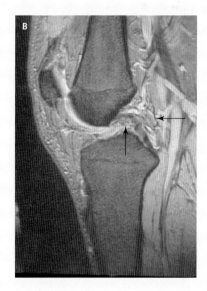

Fig. 31.4 MRI scans of the knee: (A) normal; (B) showing rupture of both cruciate ligaments.

The images obtained show an outline of the body with areas highlighted where the isotope has accumulated.

Bone scans are useful as a tool for identifying the presence of a disease process (sensitive) but not very good at telling you exactly what the disease is (non-specific). Increased uptake occurs typically in growth plates, arthritis, fractures, metastases (commonly used in malignancy), infection and Paget's disease. Decreased uptake occurs in some tumours (haemo-poietic) and also in avascular bone.

Measurement of bone mineral density

Bone mineral density is usually measured at the lumbar spine, femoral neck or wrist. There are several current methods in use for measurement. These include:

- Dual energy X-ray absorptiometry (DEXA).
- Quantitative computed tomography (QCT).
- Broad-band ultrasound attenuation (BUA).

Bone density is expressed in relation to a young adult mean.

- Osteoporosis is defined as bone mineral density of greater than 2.5 standard deviations below the mean.
- Osteopenia is defined as bone mineral density of between 1 and 2.5 standard deviations below the mean.

Arthrography

Arthrograms are investigations in which the patient also has contrast or air injected into the joint. Plain X-ray arthrograms have largely been superseded by other investigations but are still used for hip conditions in the child. CT and MRI arthrograms are now becoming widespread for the diagnosis of intra-articular pathology, particularly in the shoulder, such as a Bankart lesion.

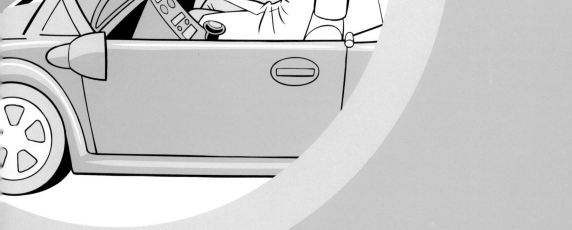

SELF-ASSESSMENT

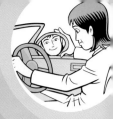

Indicate whether each answer is true or false.

Rheumatology

1. **Rheumatoid arthritis:**
   a. Is associated with the HLA-DR4 genotype.
   b. Rarely affects the hands.
   c. Affects women more commonly than it affects men.
   d. Is a disease that only affects the joints.
   e. Only occurs in people who have a positive serum rheumatoid factor.

2. **Gout:**
   a. Is more common in people with a low body mass index.
   b. Is a recognized cause of renal failure.
   c. Often causes X-ray changes after the first attack.
   d. Can be caused by high-dose salicylate therapy.
   e. Commonly affects the first metatarsophalangeal (MTP) joint.

3. **The following features are recognized complications of ankylosing spondylitis:**
   a. Atlantoaxial subluxation.
   b. Mitral stenosis. *Aortic regurg*
   c. Plantar fasciitis.
   d. Anterior uveitis.
   e. Pulmonary fibrosis.

4. **Psoriatic arthropathy:**
   a. Affects over 50% of people with psoriasis.
   b. May precede the development of psoriatic skin lesions.
   c. Tends to worsen in parallel with the skin disease.
   d. Often causes dactylitis. *- inflammation of entire digit*
   e. Does not cause erosions.

5. **Sjögren's syndrome:**
   a. Is characterized by inflammation of endocrine glands. *Exocrine*
   b. Is associated with an increase in autoantibody production.
   c. Can occur in patients with rheumatoid arthritis.
   d. Can affect the nervous system.
   e. Is associated with the development of carcinomas. *lymphomas.*

6. **Giant cell arteritis (GCA):**
   a. Is always associated with a high erythrocyte sedimentation rate (ESR). *can be normal.*
   b. Rarely affects the elderly.
   c. Can cause blindness.
   d. Can always be diagnosed with a temporal artery biopsy.
   e. Can occur in association with polymyalgia rheumatica (PMR).

7. **Fibromyalgia:**
   a. Affects men more commonly than it affects women.
   b. Causes joint inflammation.
   c. Is commonly associated with anxiety and depression.
   d. Causes soft tissue tenderness.
   e. Is usually cured by cognitive behavioural therapy.

8. **Systemic lupus erythematosus (SLE):**
   a. Can be induced by the drug minocycline.
   b. Often causes erosive damage to the joints.
   c. Is associated with a positive antinuclear antibody in 30–40% of patients.
   d. Only causes a raised erythrocyte sedimentation rate (ESR) if infection, serositis or synovitis is present.
   e. Is a recognized cause of seizures.

9. **Dermatomyositis:**
   a. Can develop in childhood. *proximal myopathy*
   b. Typically presents with distal muscle weakness.
   c. Is more likely than polymyositis to be associated with an underlying malignancy.
   d. Can cause a rash on the dorsum of the hands.
   e. Causes an elevated creatine kinase.

10. **Tennis elbow:**
    a. Only develops in tennis players. *lateral*
    b. Causes tenderness over the medial epicondyle.
    c. Pain is exacerbated by resisted wrist flexion.
    d. May be a feature of enteropathic arthritis.
    e. Often improves with rest.

— loss of lumbar lordosis
— kyphosis of thoracic + C spine.

11. **Carpal tunnel syndrome:**

a. Is due to compression of the median nerve.
b. Causes pain in the ring and little fingers.
c. May result in weakness of the thenar muscles.
d. May be associated with diabetes mellitus.
e. Is a common complication of rheumatoid arthritis.

12. **Disease-modifying antirheumatic drugs (DMARDs):**

a. Have a quick onset of action.
b. Are not usually prescribed in rheumatoid arthritis until patients have developed joint erosions.
c. Should never be used in conjunction with corticosteroids.
d. May suppress the immune system.
e. May cause bone marrow suppression.

13. **The following suggest that joint pain is due to an inflammatory cause:**

a. The pain is at its worst first thing in the morning.
b. The joints feel stiff for at least 30 minutes after rising from bed.
c. The pain is associated with fatigue.
d. There is associated 'boggy' swelling of the joints.
e. The joints feel warm on palpation.

14. **The erythrocyte sedimentation rate (ESR):**

a. Measures aggregation of erythrocytes.
b. Is always raised if the C-reactive protein (CRP) is elevated.
c. Has a normal range that changes with age.
d. Is always elevated in cases of inflammatory joint disease.
e. Increases with the concentration of plasma proteins.

15. **Determine whether the following statements regarding radiological investigations are true or false:**

a. The vertebrae become squared in ankylosing spondylitis.
b. Rheumatoid arthritis causes periarticular sclerosis of bone.
c. Sclerosis of the sacroiliac joints may be seen in psoriatic arthritis.
d. Calcification of cartilage in the menisci of the knee is a common feature of pyrophosphate arthropathy.
e. Magnetic resonance imaging is capable of detecting the bony erosions of rheumatoid arthritis before they are visible on plain X-rays.

16. **Reactive arthritis:**

a. Is a form of septic arthritis.
b. Is often triggered by a genitourinary infection.
c. Usually affects the joints symmetrically.
d. Never causes dactylitis.
e. Can cause symptoms for several months.

17. **Determine whether the following statements regarding musculoskeletal deformities are true or false:**

OA a. Bouchard's nodes are a feature of rheumatoid arthritis.
b. Ulnar deviation of the wrist occurs in rheumatoid arthritis. *SLE*
c. 'Jaccoud's arthritis' is the name used to describe the hand deformities of rheumatoid arthritis.
d. The 'question-mark' posture in ankylosing spondylitis describes the exaggerated lumbar lordosis and extension of the thoracic and cervical spines.
e. Arthritis mutilans is a severe deformity seen in the hands of some patients with psoriatic arthritis.

18. **Determine whether the following statements regarding the skin in musculoskeletal disease are true or false.**

a. Keratoderma blenorrhagica affects some patients with reactive arthritis.
b. A 'butterfly' rash is a common feature of systemic sclerosis. *SLE*
c. Vasculitis can present with urticarial lesions, ulceration, ischaemia, palpable purpura and splinter haemorrhages.
d. A lilac-coloured rash of the skin over the eyelids occurs in polymyositis. *= Dermatomyositis*
e. Telangiectasia are seen more commonly in limited than in diffuse systemic sclerosis.

19. **Dupuytren's contracture:**

a. Occurs more commonly in individuals who have a positive family history of the disease.
b. Is characterized by nodular fibrosis of the palmar fascia.
c. Affects the index finger more commonly than it affects the little finger. *ulnar side more*
d. Is more common in alcoholics than in people who abstain.
e. Can recur after surgical treatment.

20. **Regarding the antiphospholipid antibody syndrome:**

a. It can present with transient ischaemic *teratogenic* attacks.
b. It can present with migraine.
c. Female patients with antiphospholipid antibody syndrome should be strongly encouraged to take the combined oral contraceptive pill.
 *warfarin* d. A pregnant woman with the antiphospholipid antibody syndrome and a history of fetal loss should be fully anticoagulated with warfarin throughout her pregnancy.
e. Serological tests for syphilis (e.g. VDRL) may be falsely positive in patients with lupus anticoagulant or anticardiolipin antibodies.

21. Regarding synovial fluid:

a. Only infected joints produce cloudy synovial fluid.
b. Septic arthritis can be confidently excluded if no organisms are seen on microscopy of freshly aspirated synovial fluid.
c. For accurate identification of crystals, synovial fluid must be examined under a polarized light microscope.
d. Urate crystals are needle-shaped and show strong negative birefringence.
e. Calcium pyrophosphate dihydrate (CPPD) crystals are either rhomboid or rod-shaped and show negative birefringence. *weak +ve.*

22. The following can cause pain in the forefoot:

a. Morton's neuroma.
b. Pre-Achilles bursitis.
c. Hallux rigidus.
d. Acute gout.
e. Tarsal tunnel syndrome.

23. Regarding platelets:

a. Thrombocytopenia can occur in methotrexate toxicity. *↓ platelets.*
b. Thrombocytopenia can be a feature of systemic lupus erythematosus (SLE).
c. Thrombocytosis can be a feature of active vasculitis.
d. Thrombocytosis can be a feature of active rheumatoid arthritis.
e. The antiphospholipid antibody syndrome causes thrombocytosis. *Thrombocytopaenia.*

24. Regarding juvenile idiopathic arthritis:

a. It can cause growth retardation.
b. Splinting of joints may help prevent deformity.
c. Oligoarticular disease affects five or more *1–4* joints.
d. Children with enthesitis-related arthritis are often HLA-DR4 positive. *HLA B27*
e. A positive antinuclear antibody is associated with a reduced risk of uveitis. *↑*

25. Regarding systemic sclerosis:

a. It is more common in men than in women.
b. Raynaud's phenomenon is a common feature.
c. Gastrointestinal complications are the most frequent cause of death.
d. Pulmonary hypertension is a recognized complication.
e. It can involve the myocardium, leading to cardiac failure.

26. Vasculitis: *high doses long term.*

a. Is often cured by a short course of low-dose oral corticosteroids.
b. Can cause infarction due to stenosis of blood vessels.
c. Can cause haemorrhage due to rupture of blood vessels.
d. Is rarely symptomatic if it affects small blood vessels.
e. Can complicate HIV infection.

27. Sensory loss in the foot may be caused by:

a. Diabetes mellitus.
b. Plantar fasciitis.
c. Tarsal tunnel syndrome.
d. Morton's neuroma.
e. Achilles tendinitis.

28. The following may be manifestations of systemic lupus erythematosus (SLE):

a. Fever.
b. Calcinosis.
c. Photosensitivity.
d. Hepatic cirrhosis.
e. Conjunctivitis.

29. The following are recognized causes of secondary Sjögren's syndrome:

a. Osteoarthritis.
b. Paget's disease.
c. Polymyositis.
d. Chronic active hepatitis.
e. Multiple sclerosis.

30. Decide whether the statements below concerning autoantibodies are true or false:

a. Titres of anti-double-stranded DNA antibodies rise during a flare of rheumatoid arthritis (RA).
b. Rheumatoid factor antibodies may be detected in patients with primary Sjögren's syndrome.
c. Antihistone antibodies are associated with drug-induced systemic lupus erythematosus (SLE).
d. Antibodies to serine proteinase 3 are found in patients with Wegener's granulomatosis.
e. Antinuclear antibodies are found in 40% of the normal population.

31. The following may be extra-articular features of rheumatoid arthritis (RA):

a. Anterior uveitis.
b. Pericarditis.
c. Pleural effusion.
d. Hypothyroidism.
e. Pulmonary fibrosis.

32. **Felty's syndrome:**

    a. Is an extra-articular manifestation of rheumatoid arthritis.
    b. Causes hepatomegaly. *Splenomegaly*
    c. Is associated with a neutrophil leucocytosis. *leucopenia*
    d. Makes patients prone to bacterial infections.
    e. Usually affects patients who are rheumatoid factor negative.

33. **Regarding calcium pyrophosphate dihydrate crystals:**

    a. They may be deposited in tendons.
    b. They can cause acute gout. *pseudogout*
    c. They can cause a chronic arthropathy.
    d. Deposition is more common in patients with haemochromatosis.
    e. They may be detected in synovial fluid that also contains monosodium urate crystals.

34. **Regarding histopathology:**

    a. Pannus is chronically inflamed tissue found in the joints of patients with systemic lupus erythematosus (SLE).
    b. Skin biopsy from a patient with cutaneous SLE shows deposition of IgG and complement at the dermal–epidermal junction.
    c. It is possible to make a diagnosis of vasculitis from histological examination of a nerve biopsy.
    d. Giant cells are seen on examination of the temporal artery in giant cell arteritis.
    e. Skin biopsy from a patient with dermatomyositis shows deposition of IgG and complement at the dermal–epidermal junction.

35. **Regarding uric acid:**

    a. It is formed from breakdown of nucleic acids.
    b. It is predominantly excreted via the gastrointestinal (GI) tract.
    c. Before the menopause, women have higher serum levels than men.
    d. Hyperuricaemia is most often due to increased production of uric acid.
    e. Hyperuricaemia can be caused by chemotherapy for malignant disease.

36. **Rheumatoid nodules can occur in:**

    a. Pleura.
    b. Pericardium.
    c. Myocardium.
    d. Subcutaneous tissue.
    e. Epidermis.

37. **Recognized features of polyarteritis nodosa include:**

    a. It affects women more frequently than it affects men.
    b. It is associated with aneurysm formation.
    c. It can be diagnosed from sural nerve biopsy.
    d. Some cases are associated with hepatitis C *hepB* infection.
    e. It is usually associated with a positive p-ANCA.

38. **Conditions that may arise from repetitive manual work include:**

    a. Tennis elbow.
    b. Tenosynovitis.
    c. Carpal tunnel syndrome.
    d. Gout.
    e. Rheumatoid arthritis.

39. **The following are features of systemic-onset juvenile idiopathic arthritis (Still's disease):**

    a. Hepatomegaly.
    b. Splenomegaly.
    c. Pericarditis.
    d. Lymphadenopathy.
    e. Anaemia.

40. **The following metabolic diseases may predispose to calcium pyrophosphate dihydrate (CPPD) crystal deposition:**

    a. Thyrotoxicosis.
    b. Hypoparathyroidism.
    c. Acromegaly.
    d. Diabetes insipidus.
    e. Addison's disease.

41. **The following are associated with HLA-B27:**

    a. Reiter's syndrome.
    b. Psoriatic arthropathy.
    c. Wegener's granulomatosis.
    d. Ankylosing spondylitis.
    e. Pyrophosphate arthropathy.

42. **The following are radiological features of rheumatoid arthritis (RA):**

    a. Osteophytes.
    b. Erosions.
    c. Joint space narrowing.
    d. Periostitis.
    e. Ankylosis.

43. **Osteoporosis:**

    a. Can be diagnosed by a plain radiograph of the hip.
    b. Is more likely to develop in women who have a premature menopause.
    c. Can present with a kyphosis of the spine.
    d. Is defined as bone mineral density of greater than 1.5 standard deviations below the mean.
    e. Is a common cause of femoral neck fractures.

44. **The following may be complications of Paget's disease of bone:**

    a. Cardiac failure.
    b. Deafness.
    c. Osteosarcoma.
    d. Spastic paraparesis.
    e. Osteoarthritis.

45. The following radiological signs may be seen in psoriatic arthropathy:

a. Periostitis.
b. Looser's zones.
c. Pencil-in-cup deformities.
d. Reabsorption of the terminal phalanges.
e. Erosions.

46. Raynaud's disease can be caused by:

a. Cervical rib. — *Raynaud's phenom*
b. Systemic sclerosis.
c. SLE.
d. Syringomyelia.
e. Pneumatic drill.

47. In ankylosing spondylitis:

a. There is a family history in 25% of cases.
b. It is more common in females.
c. There is an association with lung fibrosis.
d. There is an increased risk of leukaemia.
e. There is an association with cardiac conduction defects.

48. Sarcoidosis is associated with:

a. Erythema multiforme.
b. Hypercalcaemia.
c. Proteinuria.
d. Keratoconjunctivitis sicca.
e. Diarrhoea.

49. Causes of osteoporosis are:

a. Heparin.
b. Steroids. *?*
c. Marfan's syndrome.
d. Thyrotoxicosis.
e. Alcohol.

50. Paget's disease:

a. Is usually associated with increased serum calcium.
b Is common in Africa.
c. Is associated with cardiac failure.
d. Bisphosphonates may be used for severe back pain.
e. Is associated with deafness.

Orthopaedics

1. When treating osteoarthritis (OA):

a. Surgery is usually necessary.
b. Methotrexate has a beneficial effect.
c. Physiotherapy is useful to improve muscle strength and function.
d. Non-steroidal anti-inflammatory drugs (NSAIDs) give relief of symptoms.
e. Joint fusion is commonly used around the foot and ankle.

— internal rotation in flexion usually first movement

2. Osteoarthritis:

a. Is an inflammatory arthropathy.
b. Typically has radiographic features of loss of joint space, cysts, sclerosis and osteophytes.
c. Can be due to lower limb deformity.
d. Is a degenerative synovial joint disease.
e. Is characterized by decreased water content in cartilage.

3. Joints commonly affected by osteoarthritis include:

a. Atlantoaxial.
b. Distal interphalangeal (DIP) joint of the finger.
c. Hip.
d. Patellofemoral.
e. Carpometacarpal joint of the thumb.

4. Clinical features of osteoarthritis:

a. Include crepitus of the joint.
b. Usually get worse with activity.
c. Of the hip include a loss of external rotation before other movements are diminished.
d. Include general ill-health.
e. Tend to deteriorate over time.

5. Surgical options for the treatment of arthritis include:

a. Joint arthrodesis.
b. Carpal tunnel release.
c. Joint replacement.
d. Open reduction and internal fixation (ORIF).
e. Osteotomy.

6. The following conditions are associated with septic arthritis:

a. Intravenous drug use.
b. Sickle cell disease.
c. Carcinoma of the bowel.
d. Chronic renal failure.
e. Asthma.

7. The differential diagnosis of an acutely hot swollen joint includes:

a. Gout.
b. Inflammatory arthropathy.
c. Septic arthritis.
d. Discitis.
e. Developmental dysplasia of the hip (DDH).

8. Osteomyelitis:

a. Is only found in children. *— Surgery/trauma*
b. Is usually from haematogenous infection.
c. Following surgery is best treated with antibiotics alone.
d. Is common after closed tibial fractures. *open*
e. Is usually due to infection with streptococci.
staph aureus

dead bone needs to be removed.

9. **Tuberculosis:**
   a. Is becoming less common in the UK.
   b. Can spread to the spine, hip or knee.
   c. Is caused by mycobacterium infection.
   d. Can cause collapse of a vertebra.
   e. Is easy to diagnose by culture and microscopy.

   — may take 6 weeks to culture

10. **The anterior cruciate ligament (ACL):**
    a. Is the primary restraint to forward motion of the tibia.
    b. Is commonly injured in skiers.
    c. Usually heals without too much trouble.
    d. Chronically gives pain rather than instability if injured. *instability = main problem*
    e. Can be reconstructed.

    — bleeding into joint.

11. **Causes of a knee haemarthrosis include:**
    a. Anterior cruciate ligament (ACL) rupture.
    b. Posterior cruciate ligament (PCL) rupture.
    c. Peripheral meniscal tear.
    d. Osteochondral fracture.
    e. Patellar dislocation.

12. **Meniscal tears:**
    a. Are more common in the lateral meniscus.
    b. Can cause locking of the knee.
    c. Can be produced by relatively minor injury.
    d. Are more likely in an anterior cruciate ligament (ACL)-deficient knee.
    e. Are usually repaired. *— excised majority*

13. **Osteoporosis can be due to:**
    a. Prolonged use of steroids.
    b. Ageing.
    c. Lack of circulating oestrogen following the menopause.
    d. Disuse.
    e. Endocrine disorders.

14. **Osteomalacia:**
    a. Results from decreased calcium intake.
    b. Can be diagnosed by Looser's zones on X-ray.
    c. Weakens bony structure.
    d. Is caused by increased activity of osteoblasts.
    e. Is usually treated with vitamin D supplements.

15. **Paget's disease of bone:**
    a. Can weaken bone, predisposing to pathological fractures.
    b. Presents with bone pain in the majority of patients.
    c. Is treated with bisphosphonates.
    d. Is associated with very vascular bone.
    e. Often produces deformity.

    Most patients pain.

16. **Spinal stenosis:**
    a. Is due to narrowing of the spinal canal.
    b. Causes symptoms which are worse after walking and relieved by rest.
    c. Is thought to be due to ischaemia of the nerve roots. *aching radiates to leg*
    d. Always gives sharp shooting pain into the foot.
    e. Is usually a disease of older men with manual jobs.

17. **A lesion in bone on X-ray is likely to be malignant if:**
    a. There is a history of recent breast cancer.
    b. The lesion has destroyed the cortex and is not well defined.
    c. The appearances are of a clear isolated defect with a distinct zone of transition.
    d. There is periosteal elevation, Codman's triangle and sunray spicules.
    e. Onion skinning is present.

18. **Metastatic bone deposits are:**
    a. Commonly from a liver primary.
    b. Embolic through the venous system.
    c. Lytic if from a prostate primary. *— sclerotic*
    d. Usually located centrally in the skeleton.
    e. Associated with a fracture risk.

19. **Dislocation of the shoulder:**
    a. Is usually posterior. *anterior*
    b. If anterior will usually heal and not re-dislocate.
    c. Is usually caused by forced internal rotation.
    d. Can be reduced in the A&E department.
    e. May cause neurological deficit.

20. **Patellar dislocation:**
    a. Is prevented by a large lateral femoral condyle.
    b. May cause an osteochondral fracture.
    c. If recurrent may require surgical realignment.
    d. Usually occurs medially.
    e. Is treated with early surgical repair. *rest + physio*

21. **Ankle sprains:**
    a. Are very common.
    b. Damage the deltoid ligament. *lateral ligament*
    c. Should be treated with a plaster cast for 6 weeks. *early mobilisation*
    d. Are diagnosed on X-ray. *clinically*
    e. Often result in chronic instability. *rare.*

22. **Symptoms suggestive of nerve root compression include:**
    a. Back pain worse on movement. *— leg pain*
    b. Pain shooting down the leg into the foot.
    c. Bladder or bowel dysfunction if the cauda equina is involved.
    d. Tingling and numbness in the foot.
    e. Complete loss of power and sensation in the lower limbs (flaccid paralysis).

    spinal cord compression

23. Regarding postoperative complications:
a. They only occur in unfit old patients.
b. Fat embolus can cause confusion.
c. They can be reduced with preoperative antibiotics.
d. They are minimized by early mobilization.
e. Deep vein thrombosis (DVT) tends to occur in the first 24 hours after surgery. *2 weeks.*

24. Concerning fractures: *— scaphoid.*
a. Those of the radius have a high incidence of avascular necrosis.
b. They are termed pathological if through abnormal bone. *urgent debridement + stabilisen*
c. Open fractures should be treated with plaster immobilization and antibiotics.
d. Displaced intracapsular hip fractures in the elderly are treated with open reduction and internal fixation (ORIF). *hemiarthroplasty*
e. Those of the wrist are usually displaced in a volar (palmar) direction. *dorsally.*

25. Children with Perthes disease:
a. Often present with knee pain.
b. Are usually teenage girls.
c. Are more commonly from lower socioeconomic groups.
d. Have avascular necrosis of the femoral head.
e. Often have diminished hip abduction.

26. Developmental dysplasia of the hip (DDH):
a. Can present late with a limp.
b. Is diagnosed clinically by performing Barlow's and Ortolani's tests.
c. Is more common in Afro-Caribbean races.
d. Results in a shallow poorly developed acetabulum.
e. Is more common in patients with a family history.

27. Slipped upper femoral epiphysis: *groin radiates down front of thigh into knee*
a. Presents with pain radiating down the back of the leg and into the foot.
b. Usually occurs in infants. *adolescent*
c. Occurs through the physis.
d. Is a very common cause of pain and limp in children. *rare.*
e. Can present over a long period.

28. A prolapsed intervertebral disc:
a. Most commonly causes compression of the L4 nerve root. *S1 + L5.*
b. Produces symptoms that are worse on sitting.
c. Usually settles without needing surgery.
d. Is common in the elderly.
e. Occurs through a weakness in the annulus fibrosis.

29. Scoliosis:
a. May be secondary to neurological conditions.
b. Causes a rib hump deformity.
c. Usually needs surgical correction.
d. If severe can cause reduced lung volume.
e. Surgery is relatively simple with no significant risks to the patient.

30. Back pain:
a. Is a very common condition affecting over half of the population at some time in their lives.
b. Is always due to disc prolapse.
c. Can be a presentation of malignancy.
d. In young patients does not need investigation.
e. Is treated with prolonged bed rest.

31. Deep vein thrombosis (DVT):
a. Is a common complication after orthopaedic surgery.
b. Risk can be reduced with mechanical (graduated compression stockings) and chemical (e.g. aspirin or heparin) measures.
c. May be fatal if pulmonary embolus results.
d. Is treated with warfarin.
e. Can result in long-term swelling and pain in the limb.

32. Magnetic resonance imaging (MRI): *pacemaker.*
a. Is a safe but expensive investigation for all patients.
b. Produces images by relaxation of electrons within a magnetic field.
c. Is particularly useful when looking for meniscal or ligamentous injuries to the knee.
d. Is more sensitive than plain X-rays for detecting metastases.
e. Can be used to detect occult fractures.

33. Regarding joint replacements:
a. They are carried out to relieve pain and improve function of an arthritic joint.
b. Those of the hip can dislocate if the patient is not careful getting up from a chair.
c. They are at risk of infection unless strict asepsis is routine in theatre.
d. The most common cause of failure is loosening.
e. They are generally successful 90–95% of the time.

34. Ganglions:
a. If aspirated contain jelly-like fluid.
b. Are commonly found around the wrist.
c. May spontaneously disappear.
d. Never recur following surgery. *60%*
e. May be asymptomatic and left alone.

35. Easily palpable features when examining the knee include:

a. Menisci.
b. Anterior cruciate ligament (ACL).
c. Lateral collateral ligament (LCL).
d. Posterior cruciate ligament (PCL).
e. Patellar ligament.

36. Pain in the foot can be due to:

a. Prolapsed intervertebral disc.
b. Morton's neuroma.
c. Hallux valgus.
d. Stress fracture.
e. Gout.

37. Clinical features of early primary osteoarthritis include:

a. Deformity.
b. Instability.
c. Swelling.
d. Muscle wasting.
e. Effusion.

sensitive but not specific

38. An isotope bone scan:

a. Is a useful screening test looking for metastases.
b. Is a specific test but not a sensitive one.
c. Is performed in three phases.
d. Requires a small dose of radioactive tracer.
e. Shows increased uptake in the growth plates of children.

39. Methods of preventing osteoporotic fractures include:

a. Calcium and vitamin D supplements.
b. Glucosamine tablets.
c. Hip protectors.
d. Bisphosphonates.
e. Falls clinics.

40. Concerning proximal femoral fractures:

a. Extracapsular fractures are treated with hip hemiarthroplasty. *internal fixation*
b. The mortality rate is 80% in the year after hip fracture. *30 ~50.*
c. Undisplaced intracapsular hip fractures can be treated with operative fixation.
d. Patients having one hip fracture are at increased risk of a second.
e. Subtrochanteric fractures are often pathological.

41. The following are operations used for patients with rheumatoid arthritis:

a. Synovectomy.
b. Ankle replacement.
c. High tibial osteotomy.
d. Shoulder replacement.
e. Triple fusion.

42. When assessing a patient preoperatively:

a. It is important to inspect the skin over the operation site.
b. Heart murmurs should be investigated.
c. A haemoglobin should be checked on all patients. *not in young fit*
d. For joint replacement it is important to test the urine.
e. Distal pulses should be palpable.

43. Concerning primary bone tumours:

a. An osteosarcoma is a benign slow-growing tumour.
b. Enchondromas are often found in the hand.
c. A Ewing's tumour is a rare but highly malignant tumour.
d. Patients present with a painful swelling.
e. Treatment of malignant lesions includes chemotherapy and surgery.

44. Immediate postoperative care includes:

a. Elevation of the operated limb.
b. Analgesia.
c. Sedation.
d. Distal and general observations.
e. Pulse oximetry to measure PO_2.

45. Concerning gait patterns:

a. High-stepping gait is due to peroneal nerve palsy.
b. Trendelenburg gait is due to failure of hip adductors. *abd.*
c. An antalgic gait is due to pain.
d. A Trendelenburg gait may be present after total hip replacement.
e. A short-leg gait is characterized by dipping of the opposite shoulder. *shoulder on short side.*

46. Causes of postoperative shortness of breath include:

a. Atelectasis.
b. Deep vein thrombosis (DVT). *- PE.*
c. Fluid overload.
d. Renal failure.
e. Shock.

47. Special examination tests in orthopaedics include:

a. The pivot shift for posterior cruciate ligament (PCL) instability. *ACL*
b. Thomas' test for fixed flexion of the hip.
c. Trendelenburg test for hip abductor function.
d. Sciatic stretch test for nerve root irritation.
e. Lachman's test for anterior cruciate ligament (ACL) deficiency.

48. Normal variants in a child's development include:

a. Genu varum. *- bowed*
b. Genu valgum. *- knock knees*
c. Cubitus varus.
d. Developmental dysplasia of the hip (DDH).
e. Rigid flat foot.

49. Causes of a painful joint include:

  a. Rheumatoid arthritis.
  b. Pseudogout.
  c. Tuberculosis.
  d. Avascular necrosis.
  e. Tarsal tunnel syndrome.

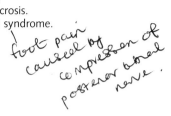

foot pain caused by compression of posterior tibial nerve.

50. Causes of swellings around the knee include:

  a. Baker's cyst.
  b. Olecranon bursitis. *— tip of elbow*
  c. Meniscal cyst.
  d. Osteochondroma.
  e. Osteosarcoma.

Short-answer questions (SAQs)

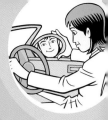

Rheumatology

1. List five causes of anaemia in rheumatoid arthritis (RA).

2. A 23-year-old man consults you with a 2- to 3-year history of gradually worsening lower back pain. The pain is worse first thing in the morning and he feels very stiff for the first 1–2 hours. This stiffness often returns if he sits for long periods. The patient has found that swimming and non-steroidal anti-inflammatory drugs (NSAIDs) help his symptoms. Based on the history, what is the most likely diagnosis, what investigations would you recommend and what results would you expect?

3. What clinical signs might you see in the hands of a patient with limited systemic sclerosis?

4. What is rheumatoid factor?

5. List three factors capable of triggering a flare of systemic lupus erythematosus (SLE).

6. A paediatric rheumatologist sees a 3-year-old girl with a 4-month history of joint pain and swelling. On examination, she is limping and has synovitis of both ankles and her right knee. The child's family doctor has enclosed the results of some blood tests, which show her to have a positive antinuclear antibody (ANA) and raised erythrocyte sedimentation rate (ESR). The rheumatologist makes a diagnosis of juvenile idiopathic arthritis (JIA) and initiates appropriate treatment. What other specialist in the hospital should the rheumatologist refer the patient to and why?

7. What are the main clinical features of antiphospholipid antibody syndrome?

8. A 70-year-old woman consults you complaining of a headache. She rarely suffers with headaches and is concerned, because this one started a week ago and is worsening. What features of the history would point towards a diagnosis of giant cell arteritis?

9. What triad of clinical features is described by Reiter's syndrome?

10. Describe the gait of a patient with a common peroneal nerve injury. At what site is the nerve most vulnerable to injury?

Orthopaedics

1. How can postoperative complications be classified? What systems can be affected by complications?

2. Why do elderly people fall? What are the three typical osteoporotic fractures?

3. Describe the pathology of osteoporosis and list the risk factors.

4. What are the X-ray features of osteoarthritis and what treatment options are available?

5. What features might be present in the history and on examination of a patient with a rupture of the anterior cruciate ligament?

6. What features of an X-ray lesion would make you suspicious of malignancy? List malignant diseases that can present in such a way?

7. How do you differentiate between patients with musculoskeletal back pain and those with a prolapsed intervertebral disc?

8. What is the most important investigation when assessing a patient with an acutely hot swollen joint? Why? List a differential diagnosis.

9. Outline the pathology in haematogenous osteomyelitis.

10. What conditions should be considered when examining a child with a limp and at what age do they present?

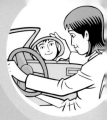

Extended matching questions (EMQs)

Rheumatology

1.

A. Osteoarthritis
B. Carpal tunnel syndrome
C. Gout
D. Trigger finger
E. Dupuytren's contracture
F. Ulnar nerve palsy
G. Pyrophosphate arthropathy
H. Complex regional pain syndrome
I. De Quervain's tenosynovitis
J. Radial nerve palsy
K. Psoriatic arthropathy

Instruction: You are examining the right hand of the patients below. Look at the description of the clinical findings and choose the most appropriate diagnosis from the list above.

1. The muscles of the hypothenar eminence are wasted. Abduction and adduction of the fingers is weak. Sensation over the little finger is reduced. **F**

2. There is pitting of the fingernails. On palpation of the distal interphalangeal (DIP) joints of the middle and ring fingers, there is tender, boggy swelling. The whole length of the index finger is swollen and tender. **K**

3. There is mild generalized swelling of the hand. The skin is pale, cool and extremely hypersensitive, to the extent that light touch produces severe pain. The radial and ulnar pulses are easily palpable. **H**

4. When the patient opens his fist to extend his fingers, the middle finger responds more slowly than the others. In order to fully straighten the digit, the patient has to pull it with his other hand. The palm at the base of the finger feels lumpy. **D**

5. There is bony swelling of all the DIP joints and the base of the thumb. Crepitus can be felt on movements of the thumb. **A**

2.

A. Serum urate level
B. Temporal artery biopsy
C. Measurement of lupus anticoagulant and anticardiolipin antibodies
D. Synovial fluid aspiration, Gram stain and culture
E. Nerve conduction studies and electromyography
F. Erythrocyte sedimentation rate (ESR)
G. Full blood count
H. Plain X-ray of the hand and wrist
I. Thyroid function test
J. Plain X-ray of the knee

Instruction: What single investigation from the above list would be the most useful when trying to make a diagnosis in the following situations?

1. A 63-year-old woman, who is taking low-dose oral corticosteroids and methotrexate for her rheumatoid arthritis, develops swelling and severe pain in her wrist. She is febrile with a temperature of 38.2° and feels generally unwell. **D**

2. A 28-year-old woman is admitted to hospital as an emergency with pleuritic chest pain. She is proven to have a pulmonary embolus and treated accordingly. She has no obvious risk factors for venous thromboembolism. Her past medical history includes recurrent migraines and three previous miscarriages. **C**

3. A 72-year-old man presents with a headache and pain in his jaw when chewing food. He has noticed that the right side of his scalp is tender when he combs his hair. **B**

4. A 36-year-old diabetic man complains of pain and tingling in his left thumb, index and middle fingers. This seems to be worse at night and stops him sleeping. **E**

5. A 65-year-old man who has had one previous attack of gout develops severe pain in his knee. On examination, the joint is hot, swollen and tender. The patient is reluctant to weight bear. **D**

Extended-matching questions (EMQs)

3.

A. Rheumatoid arthritis
B. Systemic sclerosis
C. Systemic lupus erythematosus
D. Polymyositis
E. Polymyalgia rheumatica
F. Kawasaki's disease
G. Primary Sjögren's syndrome
h. Takayasu's arteritis
I. Giant cell arteritis
J. Wegener's granulomatosis

Instruction: Read the clinical details of each patient below and decide which is the most appropriate diagnosis from the list above.

1. A 3-year-old boy develops an acute febrile illness. On examination, he is obviously unwell and has marked cervical lymphadenopathy, an oligoarthritis and desquamation of the skin of his hands and feet.

2. A 44-year-old woman complains that her hands have become slightly swollen and feel tight and itchy. She also finds that her fingers become blue and painful in the cold weather. Apart from heartburn, for which she takes regular antacids, she was previously fit and well. The first thing that her family doctor notices when she walks into his consulting room, is that she has a few telangiectasia on her face.

3. A 48-year-old man becomes acutely breathless and is admitted to hospital as an emergency. He deteriorates rapidly and is intubated and transferred to the intensive care unit for ventilation. A chest X-ray shows multiple shadows in both lung fields, consistent with severe infection or pulmonary haemorrhage. The patient's wife explains to the on-call doctor that he has been unwell for several months with symptoms of joint pain and intermittent skin rashes. He is under regular follow-up with an ear, nose and throat specialist because of recurrent epistaxis.

4. A 56-year-old woman consults her doctor with a 3-month history of weakness of her limbs. She is finding it increasingly difficult to climb the stairs and can no longer carry heavy bags of shopping. She has no pain, but feels very lethargic. Neurological examination of her limbs reveals normal tone and muscle bulk with no fasciculation. Proximal power is reduced at 3/5 in all four limbs. All reflexes are present and normal. Her plantar responses are flexor. Sensory examination is normal.

5. A 45-year-old woman is concerned because her eyes feel dry and gritty and are often red. Her mouth is also dry and she has to take frequent sips of water with her meals. Apart from occasional joint pain, she is otherwise well and has no significant past medical history. Her doctor organizes some blood tests, which reveal a mild normocytic anaemia with a slightly elevated ESR. An autoantibody profile shows the presence of anti-Ro and anti-La antibodies.

4.

A. Rotator cuff tendinitis
B. Capsulitis
C. Osteoarthritis
D. Polymyalgia rheumatica
E. Gout
F. Ruptured long head of biceps
G. Pancoast tumour
H. Acute myocardial infarction
I. Rheumatoid arthritis
J. Bicipital tendinitis

Instruction: Read the clinical details of each patient below and decide which is the most appropriate diagnosis from the list above.

1. A 31-year-old woman presents with a 2-month history of left shoulder pain, which is gradually worsening. The pain is in the region of her deltoid muscle and is exacerbated by arm movements and lying on her left side. She is now struggling to reach behind her back to fasten her bra strap. On examination, the shoulder looks normal and has a full range of passive movement. However, active movements are painful, and the patient has a painful arc on abduction. **A**

2. A 65-year-old diabetic man develops acute severe pain in his left shoulder whilst walking home from the pub. His wife is worried because he looks grey and sweaty and is slightly short of breath. He seems able to move his arm normally. **H**

3. A doctor is called to a nursing home to visit an elderly woman with advanced dementia. The staff are concerned because they have noticed a swelling in her upper arm. On examination, the swelling is more obvious when the patient flexes her elbow. It feels soft on palpation and does not appear to be tender. **F**

4. A 73-year-old woman presents with a 4-day history of pain in both shoulders. Her arms feel weak and extremely stiff. She has also had some pain in her thighs. The patient's doctor arranges some blood tests, which show that she has a normal full blood count and a very high erythrocyte sedimentation rate (ESR). **D**

5. A 58-year-old man who suffers with chronic obstructive pulmonary disease is admitted to hospital for investigations. Over the past few weeks, he has developed severe pain in his right shoulder and upper arm. The pain is continuous, day and night, and has not responded to any analgesia. The patient complains that he has been losing weight, is more breathless than usual and has coughed up a small amount of blood. **G**

5.

A. Anti-dsDNA
B. c-ANCA
C. p-ANCA
D. Anti-Sm
E. Anticentromere
F. Antigliadin
G. Anticardiolipin
H. Anti-Jo1
I. ~~Antihistone~~

Instruction: For each of the following patients, select the most characteristic autoantibody profile from the list above.

1. A 59-year-old woman presents with symptoms of Raynaud's phenomenon and dysphagia. On examination, she has painful lesions on her fingers and facial telangiectasia. **E**

2. A 23-year-old man consults his doctor complaining of joint pains, mouth ulcers, lethargy and a rash. His only past medical history is of severe acne, for which he takes minocycline. **I**

3. A 60-year-old man develops acute renal failure. He has been unwell for some time with symptoms of joint pain, skin rashes and several episodes of haemoptysis. On examination, he has a saddle nose deformity. **B**

4. A 45-year-old man presents with abdominal pain, weight loss and a skin rash. On examination, he has wasting of the small muscles of his hands and a purpuric rash on his legs. **C**

5. A 30-year-old woman is admitted to hospital as an emergency with a left hemiparesis. She has a history of recurrent severe migraines, but does not have a headache at present. The doctor examining her notices the rash of livedo reticularis on her lower limbs. **G**

6.

A. Gout
B. RA
C. Pseudogout
D. Haemophilia
E. Septic arthritis
F. Reactive arthritis
G. Haemachromatosis
H. Haemarthrosis

Instruction: The most likely diagnosis from the above list is

1. A 68-year-old lady presents with a sore throat that she has had for a few days. She has been feeling generally unwell for the last 2 weeks. She has a swollen left wrist and swollen tender right knee and right ankle. She has a normal WCC, high ESR and high CRP. **F**

2. An 84-year-old lady with osteoarthritis develops a swollen warm right wrist. She has no other joint swelling and is otherwise well. **C**

3. A 42-year-old man develops swelling of his 2nd and 3rd MCPs. He has no other swelling but has chondrocalcinosis on an X-ray. **G**

4. A 65-year-old lady who has had a recent MI develops an acutely swollen painful right knee. **H**

5. A 70-year-old lady with inflammatory arthritis develops an acutely swollen painful left knee. She is systemically unwell. **E**

7.

  A. OA
  B. RA
  C. Psoriatic arthritis
  D. Ankylosing spondylitis
  E. DISH
  F. Gout
  G. Enteropathic arthritis
  H. Reactive arthritis

Instruction: The most likely diagnosis from the list above is

1. A 30-year-old gentleman presents with back pain and stiffness. It is worse in the morning and better by the end of the day.   **D**

2. An 80-year-old lady presents with swelling and pain of her PIPs and DIPs of her hands. She has noticed that her joints are changing shape and that she is finding it more difficult to open bottles. Her mother also had similar shaped hands.   **A**

3. A 64-year-old lady has abnormally shaped fingers and some fingers are shorter than others. She also has pitting of her nails.   **C**

4. A 40-year-old man has a painful swollen 1st MTP joint. He has abnormal areas on his ears and a normal serum uric acid level.   **F**

5. A 42-year-old man has a swollen left knee and ulcerative colitis.   **G**

8.

  A. Osteoporosis
  B. Paget's disease
  C. Osteopaenia
  D. Osteomalacia
  E. Rickets
  F. Hyperparathyroidism
  G. Lymphoma
  H. Myeloma

Instruction: The most likely diagnosis from the list above is

1. A 7-year-old Asian boy presents with pain in his hips and knees. He has abnormally shaped legs, decreased serum calcium and raised ALP.   **E**

2. A 70-year-old man has hip pain and hearing problems. He has a raised ALP and high calcium.   **B**

3. A 60-year-old man presents with back pain, weight loss, raised calcium and high ESR.   **H**

4. An 80-year-old lady with RA presents with back pain and height loss.   **A**

5. A 60-year-old lady presents with renal failure, bone pain and low calcium.   **D**

9.

A. Churg–Strauss disease
B. PAN
C. Wegener's granulomatosis
D. Polymyositis
E. Dermatomyositis
F. Microscopic polyangitis
G. SLE
H. Systemic sclerosis
I. Behçet's disease

Instruction: The most likely diagnosis from the list above is

1. A 42-year-old man has asthma, proteinuria and a raised WCC. **A**

2. A 40-year-old man presents with weakness of his hands, abdominal pain and blood in his urine. His ANCA is negative. **B**

3. A 40-year-old Turkish man has mouth and scrotal ulcers. He has problems with his vision. **I**

4. A 60-year-old man has a rash on his fingers and around his eyes. He is finding it difficult to stand from sitting and is losing weight. **E**

5. A 60-year-old lady presents with chest pain, swollen painful joints and protein in her urine. Her ANCA is negative but she is ANA positive. **G**

10.

A. RA
B. OA
C. Fibromyalgia
D. Psoriatic arthritis
E. Gout
F. Pseudogout
G. Enteropathic arthritis

Instruction: The most likely diagnosis from the list above is

1. A 60-year-old lady has painful joints, no swelling, normal ESR and normal CRP. **C**

2. A 70-year-old lady who is overweight has painful knees. She is finding it difficult to climb stairs and finds that her knees lock and creak. Her ESR and CRP are normal. **B**

3. A 60-year-old man has a swollen painful right knee. He has chondrocalcinosis on an X-ray. **F**

4. A 68-year-old lady has swollen MCPs bilaterally. She has stiffness in the morning for about an hour. She has raised ESR and CRP. **A**

5. A 50-year-old man has a swollen left elbow and swollen right knee. He has stiffness for 2 hours in the morning. He has a raised ESR and CRP with a normal rheumatoid factor. **D**

11.

A. Polymyositis
B. Polymyalgia rheumatica
C. Myasthenia gravis
D. Muscular dystrophy
E. RA
F. Cervical spondylosis
G. Small cell lung cancer

Instruction: The most likely diagnosis from the list above is

1. A 68-year-old lady has stiffness of both shoulders in the morning. She has difficulty brushing her hair. She has a raised ESR. She has had no weight loss or weakness. **B**

2. A 50-year-old lady has tenderness of her shoulders and thighs. She has weakness of her proximal muscles, raised inflammatory markers and no wasting. **A**

3. A man has weakness of his arms and eyes. He gets weaker during the day. He has a normal ESR and CRP. **C**

4. A 40-year-old man has weakness of his arms. He has proximal muscle wasting. His brother had similar symptoms. **D**

5. A 40-year-old lady has pain and stiffness of both shoulders. She has swollen knees and hands. She has raised ESR and CRP. **E**

12.

A. Wrist
B. Knee
C. CPs
D. MTPs
E. DIPs
F. Shoulder
G. Elbow

Instruction: The most likely joint to be affected in the below conditions from the above list is

1. Rheumatoid arthritis. **C**
2. Gout. **D**
3. Pseudogout. **D**
4. Osteoarthritis. **E**
5. Septic arthritis. **B**

13.

A. Low C3, low C4
B. Rheumatoid factor
C. ANCA
D. Anti centromere
E. Anti RNP
F. SS DNA
G. Anti Jo-1

Instruction: The most appropriate antibody profile from the list above for the following conditions is

1. Polymyositis. **G**
2. SLE. **A**
3. Sjögren's syndrome. **B**
4. Mixed connective tissue disease. **E**
5. Wegener's granulomatosis. **C**

14.

A. Heberden's nodes
B. Photosensitive rash
C. Telangiectasia
D. Eosinophilia
E. Back pain
F. Onycholysis
G. Nail pitting

Instruction: The most likely sign from the above list for the following conditions is

1. Ankylosing spondylitis. **E** ☐
2. Osteoarthritis. **A** ☐
3. SLE. **B** ☐
4. CREST. **C** ☐
5. Churg–Strauss disease. **D** ☐

15.

A. Methotrexate
B. Sulfaslazine
C. Azathioprine
D. Infliximab
E. Hydroxychloroquine
F. Cyclophosphamide
G. Rituximab

Instruction: Which drug from the above list is most likely to cause the following complications?

1. Haemorrhagic cystitis. *Cyclophosphande* E
2. Bronchiolitis obliterans. *Methotrexate* A
3. Hepatitis. *Methotrexate* A
4. Optic neuritis. *Hydrochloroquine* E
5. TB. *Infliximab* . D

Orthopaedics

1.

A. Prostate metastasis
B. Lung metastasis
C. Myeloma
D. Kidney metastasis
E. Bowel metastasis
F. Breast metastasis
G. Osteosarcoma
H. Thyroid metastasis
I. Osteochondroma

Instruction: Read the clinical details of each patient below and decide which is the most appropriate diagnosis from the list above.

1. An 80-year-old man presents with pain in the hip. An X-ray shows a sclerotic lesion in the proximal femur with a poorly defined zone of transition. He has a history of hesitancy and poor stream. A

2. A 10-year-old boy presents with a short history of severe pain around the knee. Examination reveals a tender mass just below the joint in the proximal tibia. An X-ray shows cortical destruction and periosteal elevation. G

3. A 55-year-old man presents with a pathological fracture of his left clavicle after lifting a suitcase. On the X-ray there is a diffuse area of abnormal bone. The skull shows numerous lytic lesions and his erythrocyte sedimentation rate (ESR) is 130. C

4. A 15-year-old girl presents with a gradual swelling around the knee. It occasionally gives a little discomfort. Examination reveals a hard mass over the distal femur. X-ray shows a pedunculated well-defined lesion in continuity with the cortex of the bone. I

5. A 60-year-old woman presents with a complete flaccid paralysis of the legs. Prior to this she had 3 weeks of severe back pain. X-rays show complete collapse of T12 vertebra. Chest X-ray, abdominal and thyroid ultrasound scans are normal. The ESR is 30 and serum electrophoresis is normal. E

6. A 66-year-old man who has been a lifelong smoker has pain in his right arm. A lesion is present in the proximal humerus on X-ray and his chest X-ray is abnormal. B

2.

A. Anterior cruciate ligament rupture
B. Medial meniscal tear
C. Osteoarthritis
D. Pseudogout
E. Medial collateral ligament sprain
F. Osteochondritis dissecans
G. Patella dislocation
H. Tibial fracture
I. Posterior cruciate ligament injury
J. Patella tendon rupture

Instruction: Read the clinical details of each patient below and decide which is the most appropriate diagnosis from the list above.

1. A 30-year-old patient presents after a road traffic accident. The only injury is to the left knee which hit the dashboard of the car on impact. The knee is generally tender, has a large effusion and a posterior sag. X-ray shows no obvious fractures.

2. A 25-year-old woman is playing netball and twists her knee with the foot on the ground. The 'knee went in'. She hobbled off the court but was able to weight bear. Examination shows no effusion but tenderness medially above the joint line. Lachman's test is negative. *E*

3. A 55-year-old man presents with gradually increasing left knee pain over 6 months. He played football as a young man and has always had 'dodgy knees'. He remembers a few injuries but simply bandaged his knee and played again the week after. He stands with a varus deformity, and has a mild effusion with reduced range of movement and crepitus.

4. A 30-year-old woman has an accident on her first skiing holiday when her ski is caught in the snow at slow speed. The boot stays in the ski and the right knee is twisted. She feels something go and the knee swells up immediately. Clinical examination is difficult due to pain but she does have an effusion.

5. A 35-year-old man presents with knee pain after a relatively minor injury at work several months ago. The knee was bent and twisted when carrying something down stairs. The knee was very sore initially but settled to some extent. He still has the feeling of something catching and doesn't fully trust the knee. Examination is normal apart from medial joint line tenderness and a small effusion.

6. A 36-year-old man suffers an injury playing rugby. He is not sure what happened exactly but was tackled and felt severe pain in his right knee. Examination shows swelling and tenderness below the patella. He is unable to straight leg raise.

3.

A. Paget's disease
B. Osteomalacia
C. Rickets
D. Osteoporosis
E. Myeloma
F. Leukaemia
G. Lymphoma
H. Osteogenesis imperfecta
I. Osteoid osteoma
J. Hypercalcaemia

Instruction: Read the clinical details of each patient below and decide which is the most appropriate diagnosis from the list above.

1. A 70-year-old man presents with pain in both hips and thighs. The history is gradual but night pain is now a feature. Examination shows a normal gait but some restriction of hip movements, particularly hip internal rotation. His X-ray shows some early osteoarthritis of the hip but also areas of abnormal bone architecture in the pelvis and left femur. His alkaline phosphatase is 250 U/L. *A*

2. A 12-year-old boy of Asian origin presents with joint aches and pains, particularly of the wrists. He a small and has some diffuse swelling over the wrists with tenderness. X-rays show widened epiphyses with cupping of the physis. *C*

3. A 72-year-old woman presents with back pain and an obvious kyphosis. She had a fall several months ago, which made matters worse. She has no history of previous fractures. X-rays show loss of height in several thoracic vertebral bodies but the pedicles are intact. All blood tests are normal. *D*

4. A 7-year-old boy presents with severe right hip pain. He has been unwell for several weeks with weight loss and various aches and pains but the hip pain has come on over the last 24 hours. Clinically the child looks unwell and any movement of the hip is extremely painful. He is apyrexial and his white cell count (WCC) is abnormal at 1.2×10^9/L. The orthopaedic registrar is worried about septic arthritis and takes the patient to theatre for a washout of the right hip. The culture from theatre is negative. *F*

5. A 10-month-old baby is brought to the casualty department for the fourth time unsettled and in pain. The child appears to localize pain to the right arm. The mother is sure she has not dropped the baby and has supervised the baby well. The A&E senior house officer thinks she might have a case of non-accidental injury and refers the baby to the paediatric doctors who admit the child. A full skeletal X-ray shows several rib fractures and a humeral fracture with a thin cortex and osteopenia. *H*

6. A 14-year-old boy presents with severe right lower leg pain which has been getting worse over 2 months. The pain is present at rest, and night pain is a feature. The pain is relieved by ibuprofen prescribed by the GP. X-rays show a thickened cortex of the distal shaft of the tibia. A CT scan shows a nidus within a cortical lesion. *I*

4.

A. Osteoarthritis
B. Rheumatoid arthritis
C. Reiter's syndrome
D. Septic arthritis
E. Gout
F. Avascular necrosis
G. Ankylosing spondylitis
H. Enteropathic arthritis
I. Psoriatic arthropathy

Instruction: Read the clinical details of each patient below and decide which is the most appropriate diagnosis from the list above.

1. A 65-year-old woman presents with a gradual history of pain in the first metatarsophalangeal (MTP) joint. The pain is worse on walking, particularly when she pushes off from that foot. She is only able to wear certain shoes and finds her walking boots surprisingly comfortable. Examination shoes a bony lump over the dorsum of the metatarsal and diminished movements of the joint with crepitus. She has no other joint problems. **A**

2. A 25-year-old soldier comes home for some leave after being on duty for 3 months. She has been complaining of knee pain and swelling for several weeks. She has also recently been diagnosed by her GP as having conjunctivitis. Examination reveals a diffusely swollen knee with a large effusion and bilateral eye redness. She has recently also had dysuria. **C**

3. A 40-year-old man presents with pain and swelling of his right hand with multiple swollen joints, particularly the metacarpophalangeal (MCP) joints. He has had a rash over the extensor part of the arm, which has itched a bit but has never really troubled him. **I**

4. An 80-year-old woman, a resident of a nursing home, is normally pleasantly confused and mobile around the home. Over the last few days she has been unwell and has not used her right arm. She has become drowsy and listless and it is very difficult to obtain a history from her. There is swelling of her right shoulder which she holds close to her body. Her temperature is 38.6°C and her white cell count is 19×10^9/L. **D**

5. A 40-year-old man presents with an acutely inflamed left first MTP joint. He is a heavy drinker and works as a sales representative, entertaining clients a lot in the evenings. He is apyrexial and an X-ray is normal. His serum uric acid is normal. **E**

6. A 28-year-old man presents with back pain over several months. He was a keen cricketer but is now unable to do the sports he enjoys because of pain and stiffness. The stiffness is worse in the morning. Clinically he has diminished movement of the lumbar spine as demonstrated by Schober's test. The sacroiliac joints are also tender. X-rays show calcification between vertebral bodies. **G**

5.

A. Spondylolisthesis
B. Spinal stenosis
C. Prolapsed intervertebral disc
D. Discitis
E. Chronic musculoskeletal back pain
F. Spinal metastases
G. Acute low back pain
H. Ankylosing spondylitis
I. Abdominal aortic aneurysm
J. Cauda equina syndrome

Instruction: Read the clinical details of each patient below and decide which is the most appropriate diagnosis from the list above.

1. A 60-year-old man presents with low back pain and aching in both legs. The pain is worse on walking and relieved by rest. The leg pain radiates down the leg and into both calves. Examination shows reduced movements of the spine and pain on extension. Sciatic stretch testing is normal. X-rays show osteoarthritis of the spine. **B**

2. A 60-year-old woman has unrelenting low back pain which is not mechanical in nature. Night pain is severe and not relieved by simple analgesia. On examination she is pale and thin. Her abdominal system reveals a palpable liver edge. X-rays of her lumbar spine show loss of a pedicle (winking owl sign). **F**

3. A 56-year-old diabetic patient with chronic renal failure is admitted for dialysis. He also complains of new back pain. The patient becomes unwell with a raised temperature, a white cell count of 22.5×10^9/L, C-reactive protein (CRP) 125 mg/L, and erythrocyte sedimentation rate (ESR) 79 mm/h. The renal physicians treat him for line sepsis but he fails to respond. An X-ray of the lumbar spine 1 week later shows loss of disc space between L3–L4 with bony destruction of the end plates. **D**

4. A 32-year-old GP presents with a short history of back pain after straining in the garden. He has bilateral leg symptoms with pain radiating down both legs into the feet. He says the saddle area of his bottom feels odd when sitting down and he has difficulty passing urine. When he arrives in A&E he is in acute urinary retention and the crossover sign is positive. **J**

5. A 30-year-old man complains of low back pain after digging at work. The pain does not radiate and is worse on movement. He feels well and examination shows muscle spasm, reduced movements and some tenderness across the lower lumbar spine. **G**

6. A 15-year-old boy presents with increasing low back pain for 1 year. He is a county level fast bowler and big things are expected of him. The pain does not radiate and is worse after prolonged activity. Examination shows a well boy with well-maintained spinal movements and normal neurology. Pain is significant on extension. Oblique X-rays of the lumbar spine show a typical Scottie dog appearance with a pars defect at L5–S1. **A**

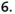

6.

A. Perthes disease
B. Juvenile idiopathic arthritis
C. Developmental dysplasia of the hip
D. Congenital talipes equinovarus
E. Slipped upper femoral epiphysis
F. Septic arthritis
G. Osteomyelitis
H. Reactive arthritis
I. Ewing's tumour.
J. Osgood–Schlatter disease

Instruction: Read the clinical details of each patient below and decide which is the most appropriate diagnosis from the list above.

1. A 13-month-old baby presents with a limp as the child begins to walk. The left leg looks short when compared with the right. The child has a waddling gait but is not in obvious discomfort. **C**

2. A 13-year-old boy presents with a 1-week history of left leg pain radiating from the groin down the thigh and into the knee. The pain is worse on activity and partially relieved by rest. Clinically he has an externally rotated left leg with pain on all movements. The AP X-ray of the hip shows a smaller epiphysis than on the right. The frog lateral view clinches the diagnosis. **E**

3. A 12-year-old boy has been unwell for a few months with pain and swelling in his right knee. He has also been more tired than usual and not himself. On further questioning it becomes clear that other joints are involved. The right knee is swollen with a small effusion. At presentation he is noted to have decreased visual acuity in his right eye. **B**

4. A 14-year-old boy is a keen footballer and presents with bilateral knee pain worse on movement and very tender if touched. On examination he is well and has tenderness over the tibial tubercle just beneath the patellar ligament. **J**

5. A 7-year-old boy presents with a 1-year history of right knee pain gradually increasing. He has a pronounced limp and has been off school for 1 month. On examination the right knee is normal but the hip is irritable and abduction is markedly decreased. X-rays show sclerosis of the femoral head. **A**

6. An 8-week-old baby girl is very ill on the paediatric intensive care unit. She has features of sepsis including a raised temperature and white cell count (WCC), and blood cultures have grown *Staphylococcus aureus*. There is no obvious focus of infection. An ultrasound scan of both hips is normal. **G**

7.

A. Tension pneumothorax
B. Pelvic fracture
C. Fracture/dislocation lumbar spine
D. Wedge fracture lumbar spine
E. Haemothorax
F. Fracture 7th cervical vertebra
G. Neck sprain
H. Hip dislocation
I. Osteomyelitis

Instruction: Read the clinical details of each patient below and decide which is the most appropriate diagnosis from the list above.

1. A 30-year old man falls 20 feet from some scaffolding. On admission to the Emergency Room he complains of shortness of breath and chest pain. On examination he is cyanosed and unable to complete sentences. His trachea is deviated to the right, and he has absent breath sounds on the left side. Blood pressure is low, pulse rate is 120/ minute and oxygen sats are only 80% on high flow oxygen.   A

2. A heavy steel girder falls directly onto a 45-year-old man on a construction site, crushing his lower abdomen. He is rushed to the Emergency Room and is noted to have bruising around his lower abdomen and groin. His airway and breathing are stable, but his blood pressure is low and he has a tachycardia. Intravenous fluids are started, which corrects the hypotension. On secondary survey, a doctor finds blood at the urethral meatus, and notes that the man has not passed urine.   B

3. A 23-year old woman loses control of her car at high speed and crashes. Unfortunately she is not wearing her seat belt and is ejected from the vehicle. When the paramedic arrives she complains of severe lower back pain, but says that she cannot feel her legs. When he examines her lower back he can feel a step in her lumbar spine. Later in hospital she is unable to pass urine, so a catheter is passed which drains 1000 mL of clear urine.   C

4. An 80-year-old man loses balance and falls on to his bottom on the pavement. He complains of lower back pain but is just about able to walk. His legs feel normal and he has normal bladder and bowel function. After 1 week the pain has not gone so he attends his general practice, and is sent for an X-ray.   D

5. A 32-year-old mountain biker goes over his handlebars and lands head first on the ground. He feels immediate neck pain but otherwise normal. He rides home, but the pain is severe so his wife brings him to casualty. He tells the doctor that he remembers hitting his chin against his chest quite hard. Examination reveals tenderness at the level of C7. Neurological examination is normal. A lateral X-ray of the man's neck shows from C1 to C6 and is normal. He therefore reassures the man and discharges him. On the way home the man develops tingling in his right little finger.   F

6. A 40-year-old lawyer is stationary in his car at the traffic lights. He is wearing his seatbelt. Suddenly he feels a shunt from behind as a van crashes into him at moderate speed. He gets out of his car. The back bumper has been damaged but otherwise the car is untouched. After 10 minutes he notices that his neck feels stiff. He goes home, but during the night his neck becomes very painful, and he develops a headache.   G

8.

A. Physiotherapy
B. Anti-inflammatory tablets
C. Unicompartmental knee replacement
D. Total knee replacement
E. X-ray of the hip
F. X-ray of the spine
G. Realignment surgery
H. Arthroscopy

Instruction: Read the clinical details of each patient below and decide which is the most appropriate action from the list above.

1. A 40-year-old heavy manual worker presents with a 2-year history of painful right knee. He says the pain is always on the inside of his knee and is worse after activity. He also gets stiffness and finds that the pain is starting to affect his ability to work. Examination reveals severe varus deformity of the knee. X-rays show arthritis in the medial compartment with a normal lateral compartment. **G**

2. A 35-year-old plumber presents to clinic with pain in his right knee. This occurred after he stood up from a squatting position. His knee swelled over 24 hours. The pain is on the medial aspect of his knee and he cannot fully straighten his knee. On examination he has a moderate effusion and has lost 20 degrees of extension. **H**

3. A 67-year-old male farmer presents with constant pain on the inside of his left knee. He still works as a farmer, but his pain is making it difficult. The pain is worse after walking, and despite painkillers he gets night pain which affects his sleep. On examination he has a swollen left knee, tenderness over the medial joint line and mild varus deforimity with a good range of movement. Radiographs show osteoarthritis confined to the medial compartment. **C**

4. A 55-year-old patient has been referred by her GP for a total hip replacement. She complains of left hip pain but also complains of numbness in her buttock that radiates down into her foot. Pain is relatively constant but she does not find that hip movements worsen her symptoms. She has a good range of hip movement on examination. X-rays of her hip show mild osteoarthritis. **F**

5. A 78-year-old retired miner presents with right knee pain. This is all over his knee associated with swelling and clicking. He has not slept properly because of the pain for the last 6 months and he can no longer cope with his symptoms. He has mild chronic obstructive airways disease, but is relatively fit otherwise. He lives alone, has stairs and normally walks with a stick. Examination reveals a fixed flexion deformity of 10 degrees and a Baker's cyst in the popliteal fossa. X-rays reveal loss of joint space, subchondral sclerosis and cyst, with large osteophytes. He would like an operation to help his pain. **D**

9.

A. Hypovolaemia
B. Sepsis
C. Anaphylaxis
D. Neurogenic shock
E. Cardiogenic shock
F. Drugs
G. Epidural anaesthesia

Instruction: Read the clinical details of each patient below and decide which is the most appropriate diagnosis from the list above.

1. A fit 65-year-old lady returns to the ward 2 hours after a total hip replacement. The nurse is worried because her blood pressure is only 90/60 mmHg. Her pulse rate is 74/min and she has a good urine output. She feels well and capillary refill is 2 seconds. Her legs feel numb but sensation is slowly returning. **G**

2. A 60-year-old man presents with a very painful right hip and feeling unwell. He has a history of type 2 diabetes mellitus and chronic obstructive airways disease for which he takes oral steroids. Recently he has had a 'bad chest' for which the GP gave antibiotics. On examination his hip is held in fixed flexion and he will not move it. His temperature is 38°C. Pulse is 120 beats per min and blood pressure records 80/40. His veins are distended and he has warm peripheries. **B**

3. A 25-year-old kitchen fitter is ejected from his van at high speed when he crashes on a motorway. He has lower back pain but is alarmed because he can no longer feel his legs. When he arrives in the emergency department he is fully examined by the doctor including a log roll and per rectal examination. This is normal apart from a boggy swelling at the level of L1 and loss of sensation and power in his legs. Pulse rate is 60/min and blood pressure is 100/50 mmHg. **D**

4. The night doctor is called urgently to review an 80-year-old lady on the ward 4 days after a hemiarthroplasty for a fractured neck of femur. She looks very unwell. On examination she has a pulse of 110 bpm, shallow and rapid breathing with crepitations at the bases, a raised JVP and is sweaty and clammy. Blood pressure is only 84/40. The ECG shows ST elevation in the lateral leads which is new compared with the preoperative ECG. **E**

5. A 40-year-old is being nursed in the recovery room in theatre after having a complex total hip replacement. His blood pressure is 90/50 mmHg despite 2 litres of intravenous fluids. His pulse rate is 120 bpm. His urine output is poor and he looks pale, sweaty and anxious. Capillary refill time is 5 seconds and his peripheries are cool. **A**

10.

A. Anterior dislocation
B. Posterior dislocation
C. Bankart lesion
D. Fracture of proximal humerus
E. Rotator cuff tear
F. Axillary nerve palsy

Instruction: Read the clinical details of each patient below and decide which is the most appropriate diagnosis from the list above.

1. A 25-year-old woman attends casualty holding her right arm. She landed awkwardly on her shoulder which at the time was abducted. It is now very painful and she can barely move it. On examination there is loss of the normal shoulder contour and X-ray of the shoulder confirms the diagnosis. **A**

2. A 20-year-old man is admitted to a medical ward following a prolonged epileptic seizure. As he regains consciousness he complains that his left shoulder is very painful. **B**

3. A 45-year-old man attends clinic complaining that his shoulder 'clunks' when he moves it in certain positions. He has a history of an anterior shoulder dislocation 6 months ago. **D**

4. A 65-year-old lady attends A&E; she fell on to her outstretched right arm after tripping on a kerb. Her shoulder is very painful and she has not been able to move it since. Examination reveals swelling and bruising over the shoulder. No movements are possible. **D**

5. A 45-year-old man injures his right arm after falling off his mountain bike. Initially it was stiff and painful but improved with physio after a few weeks. He now has difficulty lifting anything heavy and his arm is weak when testing initial abduction. **E**

11.

A. *Staph. aureus*
B. Anaerobic bacteria
C. Mycobacterium tuberculosis
D. Methicillin Resistant *Staph. aureus* (MRSA)
E. *Haemophilus influenzae*
F. *Neisseria gonorrhoeae*
G. *E. coli*

Instruction: Read the clinical details of each patient below and decide which is the most appropriate diagnosis from the list above.

1. A 2-year-old child is admitted with a hot, painful swollen left knee associated with a high fever. She will not move the knee because of pain. On further questioning it turns out that the child has never had any vaccinations because the mother has read in the newspapers that vaccinations are dangerous. **E**

2. A 60-year-old lady with known osteoarthritis of her left hip is admitted feeling unwell with a high temperature. Her hip is now very painful and she will not allow the doctor to move it. She says she has been unwell recently with a 'water infection'. **G**

3. A 51-year-old caucasian lady presents with back pain. She has not been well for the last 3 months. Recently she has lost weight and had night sweats. She mentions that she lived in India for 10 years when she was 20. On examination she has a gibbus in the mid part of the thoracic spine and has tenderness on palpation. **C**

4. A 10-year-old girl is admitted with pain in her left tibia and a fever. There is no history of recent illness. X-rays show osteomyelitis in the proximal tibia. **A**

5. A farmer falls 10 feet from a ladder in his cattle yard. He sustains an open fracture of his tibia which is heavily contaminated. **B**

12.

A. Salter–Harris fracture
B. Simple fracture
C. Pathological fracture
D. Open fracture
E. Complex Regional Pain Syndrome (CRPS)
F. Compartment syndrome
G. Non-accidental injury

Instruction: Read the clinical details of each patient below and decide which is the most appropriate diagnosis from the list above.

1. A 10-year-old boy falls out of a tree and lands on his left wrist. He cries immediately and his mother brings him to A&E because his wrist is deformed. When the doctor takes an X-ray he explains that the child has a fracture. **A**

2. A 50-year-old man suddenly feels pain in his right thigh and falls to the ground. He is alarmed to find that his leg is badly angulated and X-ray in casualty confirms a fracture. He explains that he has had pain in this leg for some time, and over the last few months has had weight loss. He also mentions that he has been coughing up blood and worries that his lifelong smoking habit is the cause. **C**

3. A 30-year-old footballer is kicked hard in his shin during a game. He doesn't feel too uncomfortable initially and can weight bear, but over the next 3 hours his pain becomes severe. The team doctor examines his leg and finds that his leg is swollen and tense. He has altered sensation over the dorsum of his foot and passive movement of his toes is extremely painful. Foot pulses are normal. **F**

4. An 18-month-old girl is brought to A&E by her mother following a fall off the settee at home. She has a painful swollen forearm. Radiographs show a transverse fracture of the forearm with callus formation. The grandmother says that the arm hurt a few days ago. **G**

5. A 46-year-old secretary falls from some ladders on to her forearm. Her arm is badly angulated and there is a tiny wound over the mid part of the forearm. The junior doctor straightens her arm and places it in to a cast and brings her back to clinic 2 days later. His consultant reviews the case and is very angry. **D**

13.

A. CT
B. MRI
C. Plain X-ray
D. Bone scan
E. Nerve conduction study
F. Ultrasound scan
G. Venous Doppler scan

Instruction: Read the clinical details of each patient below and decide which is the most appropriate investigation according to what you think the most likely diagnosis is.

1. A 56-year-old housewife says she gets pins and needles and pain, especially at night in her index, middle and half her ring fingers. This is relieved by hanging her hand over the end of the bed. She has a history of type 2 diabetes. **E**

2. A 40-year-old lady reports a 6-month history of shooting pains from her left buttock, radiating down the back of her leg into her foot. She has altered sensation over the lateral aspect of her lower leg and the sole of her foot. **B**

3. A 68-year-old man attends casualty with a swollen, tender left leg. He had a left total knee replacement 6 weeks ago. Movements of his ankle are quite painful. **G**

4. A 30-year-old man presents with a lump on the palmar aspect of his left wrist. He has had this for many years but recently it has slightly increased in size and can be painful as it catches on his watch. On examination it is mobile to the skin and underlying muscle and soft and has smooth round borders. It is not pulsatile. **F**

5. A 56-year-old man has renal cell carcinoma. He complains of pain in his right forearm. **C**

14.

A. Ulnar nerve compression
B. Cervical rib
C. Pancoast's tumour
D. Carpal tunnel syndrome
E. Axillary nerve palsy
F. Radial nerve palsy
G. C6/C7 cervical disc prolapse
H. Peripheral neuropathy

Instruction: Read the clinical details of each patient below and decide which is the most likely diagnosis from the list above.

1. A 21-year-old man complains of numbness in his little and ring fingers and over the medial aspect of his forearm with weakness of his hand. This only seems to occur in certain positions especially when his arm is raised above his head. His hand also turns white on occasions. There is wasting of the small muscles of the hand. **B**

2. A 65-year-old heavy smoker complains of weakness in his left hand. He has had a persistent cough for the last 3 months and has lost 2 stones in weight. On examination he has wasting of the small muscles of the hand. The doctor also notes that he has a constricted pupil on the left side with drooping of the eyelid and dry skin over the left side of his forehead. **C**

3. A 26-year-old man crashes his motorbike at 40 mph. He sustains a spiral fracture to the mid shaft of his right humerus. He has altered sensation over the first dorsal web space of his right hand and has weakness of extension of his wrist, fingers and thumb. **F**

4. A 40-year-old lady develops a sudden onset of severe neck pain after turning suddenly. This is associated with pain in her middle finger and weakness straightening her arm. She has no significant past medical history. **G**

5. A 40-year-old man is tackled heavily during a rugby game and lands awkwardly on his left shoulder. His shoulder has lost its normal contour and he finds all movements painful. He notices some tingling over the outer aspect of his upper arm. **E**

15.

A. Ataxic
B. Trendelenburg
C. Waddling
D. Antalgic
E. Foot drop
F. High stepping
G. Shuffling
H. Spastic

Instruction: Read the clinical details of each patient below and decide which is the most likely gait pattern from the list above.

1. A 62-year-old man presents with pain is his left hip which he has suffered with for many years. X-rays show osteoarthritis. When asked to stand on his left leg his pelvis drops. When standing on his right leg his pelvis tilts up. **B**

2. A 35-year-old football hooligan is seen in clinic saying that he can't walk properly. He was involved in a fight 6 weeks ago and says the policeman hit him very hard just below his right knee with a truncheon. He has some numbness over the dorsum of his foot but has no pain. When he walks he brings his right knee much higher than the left. **F**

3. A 10-year-old boy is seen in the orthopaedic clinic for review. When walking he displays muscular incoordination and has his feet quite wide apart. His old notes state that he had meningitis as an infant. **A**

4. A 30-year-old woman is seen in clinic with a painful ankle after she twisted it falling down a kerb. When walking she hobbles and has a reduced stance phase on the affected side. **D**

5. An 8-year-old boy is seen in clinic with his mother. His lower limb function has worsened over the last few years. He has flexed and adducted hips and walks with a stiff gait. His feet are in equinus. **H**

MCQ answers

Rheumatology

1. a. T—Several subtypes of HLA-DR4 are associated with susceptibility to RA.
    b. F—The hands are commonly involved in RA.
    c. T—The male:female ratio is approximately 1:3.
    d. F—RA is a multisystem disorder.
    e. F—10–30% of RA patients do not carry rheumatoid factor antibodies.

2. a. F—Obesity is associated with gout.
    b. T—Urate deposition in the renal interstitium and collecting tubules can cause a nephropathy. Urate stones can cause urinary tract obstruction.
    c. F—Radiological changes develop after several years of recurrent gouty attacks.
    d. F—Low-dose salicylate therapy reduces the renal excretion of uric acid and predisposes to gout.
    e. T—This is the commonest joint to be affected by acute gout.

3. a. T—This can complicate severe spinal diseases.
    b. F—Aortic regurgitation can occur.
    c. T—This and other types of peripheral enthesitis are common in AS.
    d. T—This occurs in approximately one-third of patients with AS.
    e. T—This tends to be a late feature of AS.

4. a. F—It affects approximately 10% of patients with psoriasis.
    b. T—Some people with psoriatic arthritis never develop psoriasis.
    c. F—There is no correlation between the severity of the arthritis and that of the skin disease.
    d. T—This is a common feature of psoriatic arthropathy.
    e. F—Erosions do occur.

5. a. F—It affects exocrine glands.
    b. T—B-lymphocytes are activated, resulting in an increase in immunoglobulin production.
    c. T—Rheumatoid arthritis, systemic lupus erythematosus, systemic sclerosis and polymyositis are all causes of secondary Sjögren's syndrome.
    d. T—Neurological manifestations include neuropathies, seizures and hemiparesis.
    e. F—Patients are at an increased risk of developing lymphomas compared to the general population.

6. a. F—The ESR can be normal.
    b. F—It predominantly targets people over the age of 60 years.
    c. T—This is due to ischaemic optic neuritis, caused by arteritis of the posterior ciliary artery and branches of the ophthalmic arteries.
    d. F—The arteritis is patchy and it is possible to obtain a segment of non-inflamed artery on biopsy.
    e. T—Approximately 50% of patients with GCA have symptoms of PMR.

7. a. F—It is much more common in women.
    b. F—The joints are normal in fibromyalgia.
    c. T—Approximately 20% of patients with fibromyalgia suffer with anxiety or depression.
    d. T—Patients usually have multiple areas of soft tissue tenderness over the upper and lower body.
    e. F—Cognitive behavioural therapy is not a cure for fibromyalgia, but it can help patients to cope with their symptoms.

8. a. T—The antibiotic minocycline can trigger drug-induced lupus.
    b. F—The arthritis of SLE is non-erosive.
    c. F—Antinuclear antibodies are detected in more than 95% of patients with SLE.
    d. F—The ESR usually rises during any flare of SLE. The C-reactive protein tends to remain normal unless infection, serositis or synovitis is present.
    e. T—SLE can involve the nervous system, causing seizures, headaches, neuropathies or psychiatric problems.

9.
a. T—It can affect children as well as adults.
b. F—It causes a proximal myopathy.
c. T—Up to 15% of adults with inflammatory muscle disease have an underlying malignancy. The association is thought to be much stronger for dermatomyositis than for polymyositis.
d. T—Scaly, erythematous, papules or plaques called Gottron's papules may develop over the metacarpophalangeal (MCP) and proximal interphalangeal (PIP) joints.
e. T—This enzyme is released from damaged muscle and is usually at least 10 times the upper limit of normal in active myositis.

10.
a. F—It may be precipitated by overuse of the elbow in any way and is sometimes idiopathic.
b. F—Pain and tenderness are over the lateral epicondyle at the origin of the forearm extensors.
c. F—Wrist extension against resistance exacerbates the pain.
d. T—Enthesitis at any site may be seen, in addition to axial and peripheral joint disease.
e. T—Symptoms may resolve after rest and avoidance of any precipitating causes.

11.
a. T—The median nerve becomes compressed as it passes through the carpal tunnel at the wrist.
b. F—Pain is felt in the thumb, index and middle fingers and the radial half of the ring finger.
c. T—Weakness and wasting of the thenar muscles may be seen in advanced cases.
d. T—Several endocrine diseases can predispose to carpal tunnel syndrome, including diabetes mellitus, hypothyroidism and acromegaly.
e. T—Patients with wrist synovitis are particularly prone to carpal tunnel syndrome.

12.
a. F—They are slow-acting drugs.
b. F—They are started soon after diagnosis with the aim of controlling disease activity and delaying the progression of erosive joint damage.
c. F—Corticosteroids are often used to suppress disease activity in patients who have not yet responded to their disease-modifying therapy.
d. T—Some DMARDs are immunosuppressants.
e. T—Most DMARDs have the potential to cause bone marrow suppression.

13.
a. T—Inflammatory joint pain tends to be worse in the morning and improve as the day progresses.
b. T—Stiffness that is worse first thing in the morning or after periods of rest is typical of inflammatory arthritis.
c. T—Patients with inflammatory arthritis often suffer with constitutional symptoms such as fatigue, fever and weight loss.
d. T—Inflammatory arthritis causes 'boggy' joint swelling in contrast to the hard, bony swelling of osteoarthritis.
e. T—The increased blood flow to inflamed joints often produces erythema and warmth of the overlying skin.

14.
a. T—It is the rate at which erythrocytes aggregate.
b. F—The CRP responds to inflammation faster than the ESR.
c. T—The upper limit of normal for the ESR increases with age.
d. F—Some patients with definite joint inflammation have a normal ESR.
e. T

15.
a. T—This is due to erosive damage.
b. F—Periarticular osteoporosis is one of the earliest radiological signs.
c. T—Sacroiliitis is found in up to 30% of cases and is usually asymmetrical.
d. T—Chondrocalcinosis may also be seen in the triangular cartilage of the wrist.
e. T—Early erosions can also be detected using ultrasound.

16.
a. F—It is an aseptic arthritis that develops after a distant infection.
b. T—Infections of the gastrointestinal tract are also common triggers.
c. F—It is usually an asymmetrical arthritis.
d. F—Dactylitis is common.
e. T—Symptoms can last for months and relapses are common.

17.
a. F—They are seen in osteoarthritis.
b. F—Patients usually develop ulnar deviation at the metacarpophalangeal (MCP) joints and radial deviation at the wrist.
c. F—It refers to the hand deformities seen in systemic lupus erythematosus, which result from tenosynovitis rather than erosive damage.
d. F—It describes the loss of lumbar lordosis and kyphosis of the thoracic and cervical spines.
e. T—Reabsorption of bone at the metacarpals and phalanges causes telescoping of the digits.

18.
a. T—This is a sterile pustular rash on the palms of the hands and soles of the feet.
b. F—This rash is a feature of systemic lupus erythematosus.
c. T—These are all manifestations of cutaneous vasculitis.
d. F—This heliotrope rash is a feature of dermatomyositis. Polymyositis does not affect the skin.
e. T—They are often seen on the hands and face of patients with limited systemic sclerosis.

19.
a. T—A positive family history is a risk factor for developing Dupuytren's contracture.
b. T—This results in flexion of the fingers.
c. F—The ulnar side of the hand is most commonly affected.
d. T—Cirrhosis of the liver is a risk factor for Dupuytren's contracture.
e. T—There is a risk of recurrence after partial fasciectomy.

20.
a. T—This is due to arterial thrombosis.
b. T—Migraines are common.
c. F—They should avoid oral contraceptives, which increase thrombotic risk.
d. F—Warfarin is teratogenic. Subcutaneous heparin should be used instead.
e. T

21.
a. F—Synovial fluid has a cloudy appearance if the cell count is high. This can be due to septic arthritis or joint inflammation. Infection should always be excluded.
b. F—The absence of organisms on microscopy does not exclude infection. Gram stain and culture should be performed.
c. T—Polarized light is required to examine the birefringence of crystals.
d. T
e. F—They show weak positive birefringence.

22.
a. T—Pain is felt in between the metatarsal heads and often radiates along the adjacent borders of the two affected toes.
b. F—This causes pain in the region of the Achilles tendon.
c. T—Pain is felt in the great toe.
d. T—This commonly affects the first metatarsophalangeal (MTP) joint.
e. T—This can, but does not always, cause forefoot pain.

23.
a. T—It can be a consequence of bone marrow suppression.
b. T—This is due to autoimmune destruction of platelets.
c. T—Active inflammation due to any cause can cause a reactive thrombocytosis.
d. T—As above.
e. F—It causes thrombocytopenia.

24.
a. T—Any prolonged, severe illness in childhood can delay growth.
b. T
c. F—It affects between one and four joints.
d. F—They are often HLA-B27 positive.
e. F—It is associated with an increased risk of uveitis.

25.
a. F—Women are affected more commonly than men.
b. T—This can be severe and lead to ischaemic changes of the digits.
c. F—Pulmonary or renal involvement is most likely to be fatal.
d. T—This can be primary or secondary to pulmonary fibrosis.
e. T—The pericardium can also be affected.

26.
a. F—High doses of corticosteroids are usually required initially and treatment often has to be continued for months or years.
b. T
c. T
d. F—The small vessel vasculitides (such as Wegener's granulomatosis and microscopic polyangiitis) cause significant morbidity and mortality.
e. T

27.
a. T—This can cause a symmetrical peripheral neuropathy, with a 'glove and stocking' distribution.
b. F
c. T—This results from posterior tibial nerve compression.
d. T—This usually affects the borders of adjacent toes.
e. F

28.
a. T—Fever may be a feature of active SLE and is often present in the absence of infection.
b. F—This occurs in systemic sclerosis.
c. T—Patients may develop rashes on light-exposed areas.
d. F—This is not a recognized feature of SLE.
e. F—This is not a recognized feature of SLE.

29.
a. F
b. F
c. T
d. T
e. F

Please see Figure 12.9 (p. 82) for the diseases associated with secondary Sjögren's syndrome.

30.
a. F—They reflect the disease activity of SLE, not RA.
b. T—Patients with primary Sjögren's syndrome can have very high titres of rheumatoid factor.
c. T—Although they are not present in all cases.
d. T—They are found in 80% of patients with active Wegener's granulomatosis.
e. F—They are found in 5–10% of the normal population.

31.
a. F
b. T
c. T
d. F
e. T

Please see Figure 10.11 (p. 64) for the extra-articular features of RA.

32.
a. T
b. F—It causes splenomegaly.
c. F—It causes leucopenia rather than a leucocytosis.
d. T—This is a consequence of leucopenia.
e. F—Patients are usually rheumatoid factor positive.

33.
a. T
b. F—They are the cause of pseudogout.
c. T—They can cause pyrophosphate arthropathy.
d. T—Haemochromatosis predisposes to pseudogout and pyrophosphate arthropathy.
e. T—Monosodium urate and calcium pyrophosphate dihydrate can coexist in some joints.

34.
a. F—Pannus is found in rheumatoid arthritis.
b. T—This is known as the lupus 'band' test.
c. T—The sural nerve is sometimes biopsied.
d. T
e. T—The findings are similar to those of SLE.

35.
a. T—It is derived from the breakdown of purine bases, which are components of nucleic acids.
b. F—Approximately two-thirds is renally excreted.
c. F—Levels are higher in males than in females from puberty until the menopause.
d. F—It is usually due to reduced uric acid breakdown.
e. T—This causes a massive increase in cell breakdown and, therefore, uric acid synthesis.

36.
a. T
b. T
c. T
d. T
e. F

37.
a. F—It presents most commonly in middle-aged men.
b. T—Microaneurysms are commonly found in the renal arteries and the coeliac axis.
c. T—Polyarteritis nodosa commonly affects the peripheral nerves.
d. F—There is an association with hepatitis B antigenaemia.
e. T

38.
a. T
b. T
c. T
d. F
e. F

All these conditions can result from overuse.

39.
a. T
b. T
c. T
d. T
e. T

Fever and rashes are also common symptoms.

40.
a. F—Hypothyroidism may be associated with CPPD deposition.
b. F—Hyperparathyroidism may be associated with CPPD deposition.
c. T—See Figure 14.7 (p. 106) for other predisposing diseases.
d. F
e. F

41. a. T
b. T
c. F
d. T
e. F

42. a. F
b. T
c. T Please see Figure 10.12 (p. 65) for the
d. F radiological signs of RA.
e. F

43. a. F—It is not possible to accurately estimate bone mineral density from radiographs. However, they can give an indication of osteopenia.
b. T—An early menopause results in a longer duration of relative oestrogen deficiency.
c. T—This is secondary to vertebral wedge compression fractures.
d. F—It Is defined as bone mineral density of greater than 2.5 standard deviations below the mean.
e. T

44. a. T—Vascular shunting of blood through diseased bone may occasionally lead to high output cardiac failure.
b. T—Bony expansion of the skull can cause compression of the eighth cranial nerve or conductive deafness.
c. T—This develops in less than 1% of cases.
d. T—This is a rare complication of vertebral Paget's disease.
e. T—Secondary osteoarthritis can occur.

45. a. T
b. F—These are a feature of osteomalacia.
c. T
d. T
e. T

46. a. F
b. F
c. F
d. F
e. F

Raynaud's disease means that the aetiology is idiopathic. Raynaud's phenomenon is associated with several things such as connective tissue disease.

47. a. T
b. F
c. T
d. F
e. T

48. a. F—Sarcoidosis is associated with erythema nodosum.
b. T
c. T
d. T
e. F

49. a. T
b. F
c. T
d. T
e. T

50. a. F—You get hypercalcaemia occasionally with immobility.
b. F
c. T
d. T
e. T

Orthopaedics

1. a. F—OA is very common and can normally be managed without surgery.
b. F—Methotrexate is a disease-modifying drug used in rheumatoid arthritis.
c. T—Early treatment of OA should include physiotherapy to maintain function.
d. T—NSAIDs are useful in controlling symptoms of OA.
e. T—Fusion is commonly performed around the foot and ankle for OA.

2. a. F—OA is a degenerative arthritis.
b. T—These are the four classical features of OA on X-ray.
c. T—Severe lower limb deformities cause abnormal loading of joints and predispose to OA.
d. T
e. F—Water content increases in OA and decreases in ageing.

3. a. F—It is often affected by rheumatoid arthritis.
    b. T—Herberden's nodes occur here.
    c. T
    d. T
    e. T

4. a. T—Patellar crepitus can be felt (and sometimes heard) when examining an arthritic knee.
    b. T—Walking distance is reduced.
    c. F—Internal rotation in flexion is usually the first movement lost.
    d. F—OA is not a systemic disorder.
    e. T—OA is a degenerative disorder.

5. a. T—Arthrodesis is often performed around the foot and ankle.
    b. F—This is performed for carpal tunnel syndrome.
    c. T—Replacement is now routine for the hip, knee, shoulder and elbow.
    d. F—This procedure is for fractures.
    e. T—Osteotomy is usually performed around the knee to correct a deformity and redistribute load.

6. a. T—This is due to the use of contaminated needles.
    b. F—These patients are at risk of salmonella osteomyelitis.
    c. F
    d. T—Patients with chronic renal disease have a reduced immune response.
    e. F

7. a. T—It is often difficult to distinguish between them.
    b. T—Although not common, inflammatory conditions can present with an acutely painful joint.
    c. T—This is the most important diagnosis to exclude.
    d. F—Discitis is an infection in the intervertebral disc.
    e. F—DDH presents with hip pain.

8. a. F—It can present at any age.
    b. F—It usually occurs following surgery or trauma.
    c. F—In post-surgical osteomyelitis there is usually dead bone present which acts as a nidus for infection and needs to be removed.
    d. F—Osteomyelitis can occur after open fractures.
    e. F—The most common infecting organism is *Staphylococcus aureus*.

9. a. F—It is becoming more common, partly due to immigration and increasing HIV/AIDS.
    b. T—Spread can occur throughout the body
    c. T
    d. T—This is called vertebra plana.
    e. F—Mycobacteria are notoriously difficult to culture and it may take 6 weeks.

10. a. T—ACL-deficient knees show abnormal forward movement.
    b. T—The ACL is frequently injured in this way.
    c. F—If completely ruptured, the ACL does not heal.
    d. F—Instability is the main symptom with patient complaining of the knee 'giving way'.
    e. T—Using either the hamstring tendons or patellar ligament (bone–patella–bone).

11. a. T—Swelling develops quickly.
    b. T—The PCL is another intra-articular ligament.
    c. T—The peripheral rim of the meniscus has a blood supply and therefore bleeding and a haemarthrosis can result.
    d. T—Bleeding occurs after fracture.
    e. T—It may be associated with osteochondral fragments.

12. a. F—They are more common in the medial meniscus.
    b. T—Large bucket handle tears often cause locking of the knee.
    c. T—Particularly in older patients.
    d. T—Unstable knees predispose to meniscal tears.
    e. F—Some can be repaired but the majority are excised.

13. a. T
    b. T—Primary osteoporosis is age related.
    c. T—This is the most important cause of osteoporosis.
    d. T—Immobilized patients develop osteoporosis.
    e. T—These are an important cause of secondary osteoporosis, e.g. hyperparathyroidism.

14. a. F—It is usually due to lack of vitamin D.
    b. T—These are stress fractures that are often seen around the hip or pelvis.
    c. T—Due to lack of mineralization.
    d. F
    e. T—Symptoms resolve with this treatment.

15. a. T—The patient may present with a fracture.
    b. F—Increased bone turnover, abnormal bony architecture and impending fractures cause pain but most patients do not have pain.
    c. T—They are effective at reducing pain.
    d. T—Bleeding is often significant at surgery.
    e. T—Sabre tibia is classical.

16. a. T
    b. T—So-called spinal claudication is typical of spinal stenosis.
    c. T
    d. F—The pain tends to be aching and radiates into the leg.
    e. T—It is more common in these patients.

17. a. T—A history of previous cancer is important.
    b. T—A poorly defined zone of transition is suspicious.
    c. F—These appearances suggest a benign lesion.
    d. T—These are the classic X-ray features of a primary malignant bone tumour.
    e. T—This is another feature associated with malignancy.

18. a. F—Bone metastases are usually from lung, breast, prostate, kidney or thyroid.
    b. T—Metastases spread to the axial skeleton through a plexus of veins.
    c. F—Prostatic metastases tend to be sclerotic.
    d. T—The spine, pelvis and proximal femur are common sites.
    e. T—A patient may present with a pathological fracture secondary to metastasis.

19. a. F—Anterior dislocation is much more common.
    b. F—There is a 70–80% chance of re-dislocation in young active patients.
    c. F—The arm is in the overhead position of abduction and external rotation.
    d. T—There are many techniques described and this is a very satisfying procedure for junior doctors to perform.
    e. T—A traction injury can occur to the axillary or musculocutaneous nerve.

20. a. T—This normal anatomical feature helps to prevent dislocation.
    b. T—A fragment of bone and cartilage may be 'knocked off' during dislocation and may require fixation.
    c. T—Recurrent dislocation can be treated with surgical realignment of the tibial tubercle.
    d. F—It occurs laterally.
    e. F—It is primarily treated with rest initially and then physiotherapy.

21. a. T—Ankle sprains are one of the most common injuries.
    b. F—The lateral ligament is injured.
    c. F—Early mobilization is now the treatment option for ankle sprains.
    d. F—The diagnosis is made clinically; X-rays may be taken to exclude a fracture.
    e. F—Instability is a rare complication of ankle sprains and may require reconstruction.

22. a. F—Leg pain is more suggestive of nerve root compression.
    b. T—This is classic sciatica.
    c. T—This is a worrying symptom and requires urgent investigation.
    d. T—It is usually due to L5 or S1 compression.
    e. F—This is due to spinal cord compression.

23. a. F—Any patient regardless of age can experience complications.
    b. T—Fat embolus causes hypoxia, which can lead to confusion.
    c. T—The incidence of infection is lower with preoperative antibiotics.
    d. T—General complications such as chest, thromboembolic and pressure sores are reduced in this way.
    e. F—DVT tends to occur later.

24. a. F—It is the scaphoid that has a poor blood supply and is at risk of this complication.
    b. T—For example, Paget's disease or tumour.
    c. F—These fractures need urgent debridement and stabilization.
    d. F—These fractures are usually treated with hemiarthroplasty to avoid the complication of avascular necrosis.
    e. F—The most common fracture is displaced dorsally.

25. a. T—Any child with knee pain must be examined for hip pathology.
    b. F—The child is usually male aged between 4 and 7 years.
    c. T
    d. T—A variable amount of the head suffers necrosis.
    e. T—This is one of the first clinical signs and if completely absent suggests subluxation of the joint.

26.
 a. T—A child with late-presenting DDH will have a Trendelenburg gait.
 b. T—Barlow's test is an attempt to dislocate a hip and Ortolani's test is an attempt to reduce a dislocated hip.
 c. F—It is more common in certain races, notably Northern Italy, and North American natives.
 d. T
 e. T—Family history is important.

27.
 a. F—The pain is usually felt in the groin and radiates down the front of the thigh and into the knee.
 b. F—It occurs in adolescents.
 c. T—The growth plate is an area of weakness.
 d. F—It is a rare but important cause of pain and limp in children.
 e. T—Often children's complaints are ignored by parents or GPs as growing pains.

28.
 a. F—The nerve roots most commonly affected are the S1 and L5.
 b. T—The disc pressure increases with this manoeuvre.
 c. T—70% of acute discs will settle with conservative treatment.
 d. F—Disc prolapse is more common in adult life.
 e. T—This tends to be laterally, as posteriorly the annulus is thickened by ligament attachment.

29.
 a. T—Due to abnormal forces acting on the spine, e.g. in spina bifida or cerebral palsy.
 b. T—It is more prominent on forward flexion.
 c. F—Most curves are mild and do not need treatment.
 d. T—Very severe scoliotic deformities cause chest complications.
 e. F—Scoliosis surgery is complex and associated with a small risk of complete paraplegia.

30.
 a. T—The vast majority of episodes settle with conservative treatment.
 b. F—Back pain can be due to many different pathologies including facet joint disease, disc degeneration and muscle spasm. It is often very difficult to be certain of the exact pathology involved.
 c. T—Particularly in the elderly.
 d. T—X-rays are rarely helpful initially. Further investigations are warranted for persistent symptoms or sinister features.
 e. F—A short period of bed rest followed by early rehabilitation is now recommended.

31.
 a. T—Very high rates of DVT occur after lower limb surgery.
 b. T—All patients routinely receive DVT prophylaxis, which reduces but does not abolish the risk.
 c. T—Most postoperative deaths are due to pulmonary embolus.
 d. T
 e. T—This is post-thrombotic syndrome.

32.
 a. F—MRI scanning is safe for most people but not for people with pacemakers or intraorbital metal foreign bodies.
 b. F—Protons are the important particle.
 c. T—It is now the investigation of choice for soft tissue injuries around the knee.
 d. T—MRI is much more sensitive than other methods.
 e. T—MRI is a useful investigation for suspected fractures of the scaphoid or neck of femur.

33.
 a. T—The main reason is always pain relief.
 b. T—This movement can dislocate the hip, particularly if the chair is low.
 c. T—In orthopaedic theatres a number of additional measures are used to prevent infection.
 d. T
 e. T—Most patients are very happy with the results of surgery.

34.
 a. T—This is a good diagnostic test.
 b. T—Dorsal or volar ganglions are common.
 c. T—Often they vary in size.
 d. F—Surgery is successful 60% of the time.
 e. T—Often this is the case.

35.
 a. T—The menisci are palpable along the medial and lateral joint lines.
 b. F—The ACL is not palpable.
 c. T—The LCL is palpable as a cord-like structure and is attached to the fibular head. The ligament is more prominent when the leg is in the figure of 4 position.
 d. F—It lies behind the ACL and is too deep to palpate.
 e. T—The patellar ligament is easily palpable at the front of the knee.

36. a. T—A disc pressing on the L5 or S1 nerve root will cause pain in the foot.

b. T—A swelling of the nerve commonly found in the web spaces of the foot.

c. T—'Bunions' are often painful due to pressure on footwear.

d. T—Stress fractures of the metatarsals are also known as march fractures.

e. T—Gout commonly affects the first metatarsophalangeal joint.

37. a. F—Deformity tends to occur later in the disease process.

b. F—The joint becomes stiffer.

c. T—An effusion may be palpable clinically.

d. T—Quadriceps wasting is common in knee osteoarthritis.

e. T—An effusion may be present.

38. a. T—'Hot spots' will be seen on the scan.

b. F—A bone scan is sensitive (i.e. good at detecting pathology) but not specific in terms of telling you what the pathology is.

c. T—Often referred to as a triple phase scan.

d. T—This is taken up by active bone.

e. T—Increased uptake is due to the area being metabolically active.

39. a. T—Simple dietary supplementation reduces the fracture risk.

b. F—Treatment of early osteoarthritis includes glucosamine.

c. T—But they are cumbersome, have poor compliance and are rarely used in clinical practice.

d. T—Patients with severe osteoporosis are treated with these drugs to reduce further bone loss.

e. T—An elderly patient who falls regularly has a high chance of fracture. Falls clinics are run by physicians to see if there is a treatable cause for recurrent falls. If so, treatment will reduce the chance of injury.

40. a. F—Extracapsular fractures are treated with internal fixation.

b. F—There is a significant mortality but it is between 30 and 50% at 1 year.

c. T—The risk of avascular necrosis is much lower in undisplaced fractures, and fixation is often performed.

d. T—The risk is higher after one fracture.

e. T—This area is a common place for metastasis.

41. a. T—Most commonly performed around the wrist.

b. T—The ankle is usually fused but replacements are gaining popularity.

c. F—For an osteotomy to work, part of the joint should be normal and this is not the case in rheumatoid patients. Arthroplasty is performed instead.

d. T—Good results are obtained in most patients.

e. T—This involves fusing three joints of the hindfoot: subtalar joint, talonavicular joint and calcaneocuboid joint.

42. a. T—If there is a rash or superficial infection the operation should be postponed until this has settled.

b. T—Patients may be at increased risk from the anaesthetic if, for example, they have aortic stenosis. An echocardiogram is the usual investigation requested.

c. F—Young fit patients may not require any investigations.

d. T—Any concurrent infection should be treated.

e. T—Adequate perfusion is required prior to any orthopaedic intervention.

43. a. F—Osteosarcomas are highly malignant.

b. T—Although they are not common overall, the hand is the usual place to find one.

c. T—The prognosis is poor: survival at 5 years is 60%.

d. T

e. T—Often radiotherapy is included.

44. a. T—On a Braun's frame or in a Bradford sling.

b. T—A comfortable pain-free patient is the goal.

c. F—Sedation is not given postoperatively as this will lower the conscious level further.

d. T—General: pulse, temperature, and blood pressure. Distal: neurovascular status.

e. F—The pulse oximeter measures oxygen saturation, not the PO_2.

45. a. T—This is due to foot drop; the patient must lift the leg high to avoid dragging it on the floor.

b. F—It is due to failure of hip abductors.

c. T—The patient quickens and shortens the step on the painful limb.

d. T—The abductor can be defunctioned.

e. F—It is the shoulder on the short side that dips.

46. a. T—Reduced numbers of functioning alveoli may result in shortness of breath.
    b. F—Unless the DVT becomes a pulmonary embolism.
    c. T—Fluid overload can cause pulmonary oedema.
    d. T—Renal failure may cause a metabolic acidosis, and in response to this the respiratory rate is increased to 'blow off' the excess CO_2.
    e. T—Shock is an important cause of increased respiratory rate because of inadequate tissue perfusion.

47. a. F—The pivot shift is a test for ACL deficiency.
    b. T—By abolishing the lumbar lordosis, the true degree of fixed flexion is observed.
    c. T—The pelvis tilts towards the unsupported leg.
    d. T—Commonly L5 or S1.
    e. T—The tibia moves forward on a fixed femur.

48. a. T—As infants, children are 'bow legged'.
    b. T—Later, as children grow, they become more 'knock kneed'.
    c. F—Normally the elbow is in valgus. A varus carrying angle usually results from a fracture.
    d. F—This is pathological.
    e. F—Flexible flat feet are common but a rigid one suggests a pathological cause.

49. a. T—Patients can present with a single joint arthritis.
    b. T—This is a common cause of joint pain and swelling.
    c. T—Tuberculosis can spread to joints.
    d. T—It usually occurs in the hip but is also found in the knee.
    e. F—Tarsal tunnel syndrome is a cause of foot pain caused by compression of the posterior tibial nerve.

50. a. T—The cyst is felt behind the knee and is usually due to degenerative disease.
    b. F—This bursa is over the tip of the elbow.
    c. T—Meniscal cysts are more common laterally and are due to meniscal tears that have a valve-like action, allowing synovial fluid to be pumped out.
    d. T—Osteochondromas are benign tumours that are often found around the knee.
    e. T—These are very rare tumours but they can occur here.

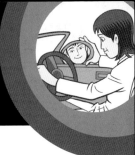

Rheumatology

1. • Chronic disease.
   • Autoimmune haemolysis.
   • Felty's syndrome.
   • Iron deficiency secondary to gastrointestinal blood loss from non-steroidal anti-inflammatory drugs (NSAIDs).
   • Bone marrow suppression secondary to disease-modifying antirheumatic drugs (DMARDs).

2. The history is suggestive of ankylosing spondylitis. Plain X-rays of the patient's lumbar spine and pelvis should be requested. There may be sclerosis of the sacroiliac joints and squaring of the vertebral bodies, with or without syndesmophyte formation. A full blood count may reveal a mild anaemia and the erythrocyte sedimentation rate (ESR) and C-reactive protein (CRP) will be raised during active disease.

3. • Sclerodactyly.
   • Telangiectasia.
   • Calcinosis.
   • Ischaemic changes, such as gangrene.

4. Rheumatoid factor is an antibody directed against the Fc fragment of IgG antibody. Rheumatoid factors may be of any immunoglobulin class, although IgM is the rheumatoid factor that is most commonly measured.

5. • Overexposure to sunlight.
   • Oral contraceptive pill.
   • Infection.
   • Stress.

6. An ophthalmologist should examine the child's eyes with a slit-lamp to look for signs of chronic anterior uveitis. She has oligoarticular JIA and a positive ANA, which means she has a significant risk of developing eye disease.

7. • Arterial and venous thrombosis.
   • Recurrent fetal loss.
   • Thrombocytopenia.

8. A history of scalp tenderness, jaw claudication or visual disturbance raises suspicion of giant cell arteritis. Approximately 50% of patients have symptoms of polymyalgia rheumatica, so pain and stiffness in the shoulder and pelvic girdles are also suggestive.

9. Arthritis, urethritis and conjunctivitis.

10. The foot is plantar flexed and inverted ('foot drop'). The patient takes high steps, flicking the foot forwards to avoid tripping over it. The common peroneal nerve is most vulnerable to injury where it winds around the neck of the fibula.

Orthopaedics

1. Any postoperative complications can be:
   • Immediate (within hours).
   • Early (days).
   • Late (months).

   and:
   • Local (i.e. related to that specific operation).
   • General (simply because the patient is having an operation).

   Any system can be affected by postoperative complications:
   • Respiratory: e.g. chest infection.
   • Cardiovascular: e.g. left ventricular failure (LVF) or myocardial infarction (MI).
   • Gastrointestinal (GI): ileus or upper GI bleeding.
   • Genitourinary: urinary retention.
   • Skin: pressure sores.

2. Elderly people fall because of:
   • Intrinsic factors:
     —Acute medical conditions: e.g. cerebrovascular accident (CVA), transient ischaemic attack (TIA), atrial fibrillation (AF)
     —Diminished senses: e.g. poor eyesight
     —Reduced reflexes: ageing produces an inability to recover from a slight stumble increasing falls
     —Poor mobility: e.g. arthritis or previous CVA.
   • Extrinsic factors:
     —Poor housing
     —Lack of social services.
   When elderly people do fall the three typical osteoporotic fractures are:
   1. Spine.
   2. Wrist.
   3. Hip.

3. Osteoporosis results from an imbalance of osteoblastic and osteoclastic activity. If the osteoclasts remove more bone than is being laid down by the osteoblasts then a net loss of bone results. The bony trabeculae become thinner with a decreased number of connections.

Risk factors for developing osteoporosis include:
- Age.
- Female sex.
- Family history.
- Small size.
- Caucasian race.
- Early menopause.
- Smoking.
- Alcoholism.
- Lack of weight-bearing activity.

4. The X-ray features of osteoarthritis (OA) are:
- Decreased joint space.
- Subchondral sclerosis.
- Cysts.
- Osteophytes.

Treatment options available for OA can be conservative or operative.
- Conservative: weight loss, modification of activity, analgesia, non-steroidal anti-inflammatory drugs (NSAIDs), physiotherapy, glucosamine, steroid injections.
- Operative: debridement and washout, fusion, joint excision, osteotomy, joint replacement.

5. Features in the history of an anterior cruciate ligament (ACL) rupture are as follows. Usually the patient is a young adult involved in sporting activity or skiing. A twisting injury or valgus force is usually reported; the patient may feel or hear a 'pop' and swelling is rapid. Once the initial injury has settled the patient will complain of the knee 'giving way', particularly on turning.

Initial examination may be difficult due to pain but a large effusion is typical.

The anterior drawer, Lachman's and pivot shift tests are positive in ACL rupture.

6. Features suggestive of malignancy are:
- Cortical destruction.
- A poorly defined zone of transition.
- Periosteal reaction (Codman's triangle).
- Sunray spicules.
- Onion skinning.

Possible causes of malignancy presenting in bone:
1. Metastatic bone tumours: from breast, lung, prostate, kidney, thyroid.
2. Primary bone tumours: osteosarcoma, Ewing's sarcoma, chondrosarcoma.
3. Haemopoietic disorders: myeloma, lymphoma, leukaemia.

7. Features in the history, examination, and investigations are as follows:
- History:
  —In musculoskeletal back pain the pain is a dull ache across the back with some radiation to the thighs.
  —A prolapsed disc causes severe sharp shooting leg pain. Back pain may be a secondary feature.
- Examination:
  —In a patient with musculoskeletal back pain there are few positive signs on examination apart from reduced range of movement (ROM).
  —A patient with disc prolapse which is compressing a nerve root will have a diminished straight leg raise with positive nerve root tension signs. Lower limb neurological examination may show weakness with diminished sensation in a dermatomal distribution.
- Investigation:
  —Most patients with back pain do not need further investigation.
  —An MRI will show a prolapsed disc.

8. Aspiration should be performed for any hot swollen joint to exclude septic arthritis.

The differential diagnosis includes:
- Septic arthritis.
- Crystal arthritis (gout, pseudogout).
- Inflammatory arthritis (including Reiter's syndrome).
- Haemarthrosis.

9. Acute haematogenous osteomyelitis usually occurs in children.
1. There may be a history of minor trauma.
2. A bacteraemia settles in the metaphysis of a long bone, which is susceptible due to its blood supply and lack of phagocytes.
3. Bacteria multiply and an abscess forms.
4. If pus escapes through small holes in bone (haversian canals) a periosteal abscess is formed.
5. Pus is now present on both sides of the bone, causing this part of the bone to die.
6. Dead bone now called the sequestrum harbours infection.
7. Periosteal new bone called involucrum forms as the body tries to fight the infection.
8. If dead bone is present this needs to be removed to cure the infection.

10. Think of diagnosis by age of child. Infection can present at any age. Also remember occult trauma, particularly non-accidental injury.

- Infant (always exclude infection):
  —Transient synovitis
  —Irritable hip
  —Developmental dysplasia of the hip.
- Child:
  —Irritable hip
  —Perthes disease
  —Juvenile idiopathic arthritis.

- Adolescent:
  —Hip disorders: slipped upper femoral epiphysis (SUFE)
  —Knee disorders: Osgood–Schlatter disease; osteochondritis dissecans
  —General disorders: juvenile idiopathic arthritis.

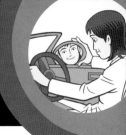

Rheumatology

1.

1. F   Ulnar nerve palsy. The ulnar nerve supplies the muscles of the hypothenar eminence, including the interossei, which are responsible for finger abduction and adduction. See Figure 25.2 (p. 182) for the sensory distribution of the ulnar nerve in the hand.

2. K   Psoriatic arthropathy. The patient has inflammatory arthritis affecting the DIP joints and causing a dactylitis of the index finger. This is typical of a spondyloarthropathy. The nail changes are suggestive of psoriasis.

3. H   Complex regional pain syndrome. These are classical signs of complex regional pain syndrome. The skin may undergo dramatic colour changes from white to purple, and growth of hair and nails may be affected.

4. D   Trigger finger. This results from tenosynovitis of the flexor tendon.

5. A   Osteoarthritis. The first carpometacarpal (CMC) joint and DIP joints are classical sites for OA. The bony swellings of the DIP joints are called 'Heberden's nodes'.

2.

1. D   Synovial fluid aspiration, Gram stain and culture. This woman has septic arthritis until proven otherwise. Her risk factors for this include rheumatoid arthritis and corticosteroid therapy.

2. C   Measurement of lupus anticoagulant and anticardiolipin antibodies. The patient's venous thromboembolism, recurrent miscarriages and migraine may well be manifestations of the antiphospholipid antibody syndrome.

3. B   Temporal artery biopsy. The symptoms are suggestive of giant cell arteritis, and a temporal artery biopsy is the investigation of choice. The patient's ESR is likely to be high, but this is a non-specific rather than a diagnostic finding.

4. E   Nerve conduction studies and electromyography. These are classical symptoms of carpal tunnel syndrome.

5. D   Synovial fluid aspiration, Gram stain and culture. The first and most important step is to exclude septic arthritis in this man. It would be dangerous to assume that this is just another attack of gout.

3.

1. F   Kawasaki's disease. This is a rare form of vasculitis that predominantly affects young children. Other clinical features include conjunctival congestion and coronary arteritis, which can lead to acute myocardial infarction.

2. B   Systemic sclerosis. This woman describes the early changes of scleroderma in her hands. She also has Raynaud's phenomenon, symptoms of oesophageal involvement and telangiectasia, which are all features of limited systemic sclerosis.

3. J   Wegener's granulomatosis. This is a small vessel vasculitis that had a very high mortality rate before the introduction of cyclophosphamide. This patient has had a life-threatening pulmonary haemorrhage. Renal complications can also be very serious. Please see Figure 12.19 (p. 92) for details of other clinical features of Wegener's granulomatosis.

4. D   Polymyositis. This painless, symmetrical proximal myopathy is consistent with polymyositis. Polymyalgia rheumatica causes proximal pain and stiffness, so is less likely.

5. G   Primary Sjögren's syndrome. Dryness of the eyes and mouth, arthralgia and positive anti-Ro and anti-La antibodies are all features of Sjögren's syndrome.

4.

1. A   Rotator cuff tendinitis. The site of the pain is typical of a rotator cuff problem. Passive movements of the joint are full, making glenohumeral arthritis or capsulitis unlikely. A painful arc is often seen with supraspinatus tendinitis.

2. H   Acute myocardial infarction. Cardiac pain is often referred to the shoulder and is not always felt in the anterior chest. This man's pain is unaffected by movements of the joint, making a musculoskeletal cause less likely. He is diabetic, so has at least one risk factor for ischaemic heart disease. The sweating and shortness of breath are common symptoms of cardiac ischaemia.

3. F   Ruptured long head of biceps. This is more common in the elderly and may follow only minimal trauma. It is painless and produces a bulge anteriorly in the upper arm.

4. D   Polymyalgia rheumatica. This patient is elderly and has proximal pain in both her shoulder and pelvic girdles, associated with stiffness and weakness. These symptoms are consistent with PMR, a diagnosis which is supported by the raised ESR.

5. G   Pancoast tumour. A Pancoast tumour is a carcinoma of the lung that invades the brachial plexus, causing pain in the upper limb. This man has chronic lung disease and is likely to be a smoker. The fact that his pain continues through the night and is unresponsive to analgesia raises the suspicion of malignancy. Weight loss and haemoptysis are both symptoms seen with lung carcinoma.

5.

1. E   Anticentromere. This patient has limited systemic sclerosis, which is strongly associated with anticentromere antibodies.

2. I   Antihistone. This man has drug-induced systemic lupus erythematosus, as a consequence of his minocycline therapy. Antihistone antibodies are commonly found in this condition.

3. B   c-ANCA. This man has Wegener's granulomatosis. 80% of patients are c-ANCA positive.

4. C   p-ANCA. This patient has polyarteritis nodosa, which is associated with p-ANCA.

5. G   Anticardiolipin. This patient has antiphospholipid antibody syndrome.

6.

1. F   Reactive arthritis. This patient has had a preceding infection and there is a short history of the swollen joints.

2. C   Pseudogout. Wrist is a common presentation and this is the right age group.

3. G   Haemachromatosis. Typically affects these joints. Must check ferritin.

4. H   Haemarthrosis. Recent MI therefore several antiplatelet drugs.

5. E   Septic arthritis. Patients with RA can have septic joints.

7.

1. D   Ankylosing spondylitis.
2. A   OA. Classical nodal OA.
3. C   Psoriatic arthritis. This lady has a severe form of psoriatic arthritis called arthritis mutilans.
4. F   Gout. Uric acid can often be normal.
5. G   Enteropathic arthritis.

8.

1. E   Rickets. This is due to low vitamin D.
2. B   Paget's disease.
3. H   Myeloma. Often presents with bone pain. Must check protein electrophoresis.
4. A   Osteoporosis. Patients with RA often have steroids which are a risk factor for osteoporosis.
5. D   Osteomalacia. This is like rickets but in adults.

9.

1. A   Churg–Strauss disease. Classically presents with eosinophilia.
2. B   PAN. Due to microaneurysms.
3. I   Behçet's disease. More common in the Mediterranean.
4. E   Dermatomyositis. Classical heliotopic rash and goitrons papules, proximal weakness. Related to malignancy.
5. G   SLE.

10.

1. C   Fibromyalgia. Diagnosis of exclusion. No joint swelling and normal inflammatory markers.
2. B   OA.
3. F   Pseudogout.
4. A   RA. Symmetrical distribution and most commonly affects MCPs.
5. D   Psoriatic arthritis. Inflammatory history with asymmetrical distribution.

11.

1. B   Polymyalgia rheumatica.
2. A   Polymyositis.
3. C   Myasthenia gravis. Weakness worse with exercise and affects all muscles.
4. D   Muscular dystrophy. Genetic.
5. E   RA.

12.

1. C MCPs.
2. D MTPs.
3. B Knee.
4. B Knee. Weight-bearing joint.
5. B Knee.

13.

1. G Anti Jo-1.
2. A Low C3, low C4.
3. B Rheumatoid factor. 100% of patients are positive for rheumatoid factor.
4. E Anti RNP.
5. C ANCA. Classically c-ANCA.

14.

1. E Back pain.
2. A Heberden's nodes. Bony swelling of DIPs.
3. B Photosensitive rash.
4. C Telangiectasia.
5. D Eosinophilia.

15.

1. F Cyclophosphamide. Therefore given with mesna.
2. A Methotrexate. Therefore baseline CXR required.
3. A Methotrexate. Therefore regular monitoring of LFTs.
4. E Hydroxychloroquine.
5. D Infliximab.

Orthopaedics

1.

1. A Prostate metastasis. The history of urinary dysfunction suggests prostate. Metastases from prostate cancer are sclerotic (the others being lytic).
2. G Osteosarcoma. Although rare, primary malignant tumours do occur in children and metastases are unheard of in this age group. The level of pain is suspicious but it is the X-ray features that give away the diagnosis.
3. C Myeloma. The fracture under normal loads should raise suspicion. The X-ray features are typical of myeloma as are the high ESR and skull lesions.
4. I Osteochondroma. The history is benign, of mild discomfort over long periods, and the X-ray appearance is typical of a benign lesion, in this case an osteochondroma.
5. F Breast metastasis. You were not told that she had a breast lump. She has a malignant spinal lesion causing spinal cord compression. The normal investigations exclude all the other potential sources of primary malignancy (except bowel carcinoma, but this rarely metastasizes to the spine) leaving breast carcinoma as the most likely.
6. B Lung metastasis. The history of smoking and an abnormal chest X-ray give away the diagnosis.

2.

1. I   Posterior cruciate ligament rupture. The history is typical with a backwardly directed force on the tibia. The posterior sag is pathognomonic for PCL rupture.
2. E   Medial collateral sprain. The history suggests medial ligament sprain and the fact that she could bear weight afterwards suggests a less serious injury. Tenderness at the joint line would be the meniscus but above is more likely to be medial collateral. The absence of an effusion excludes an anterior cruciate ligament rupture.
3. C   Osteoarthritis. The history is typical for OA with gradually increasing pain, a varus deformity and crepitus.
4. A   Anterior cruciate ligament rupture. The history of a skiing injury and the patient hearing a pop or feeling something go is typical. The presence of an effusion makes it more likely. Often knees such as these are difficult to examine initially but later will have positive Lachmann's and pivot shift tests.
5. B   Medial meniscal tear. The history of twisting injury, things settling but persistent niggling symptoms is typical. Joint line tenderness and an effusion also suggest meniscal injury.
6. J   Patellar tendon rupture. In this case the history is not helpful but examination findings of loss of straight leg raise with swelling and tenderness below the patella give the diagnosis.

3.

1. A   Paget's disease. The abnormal bony architecture and high alkaline phosphatase give the diagnosis.
2. C   Rickets. The history is typical for rickets, as are the clinical and X-ray features.
3. D   Osteoporosis, presenting with vertebral fractures. The history with deformity and X-ray features all point to osteoporotic vertebral fractures. The normal blood tests exclude pathological causes of fractures.
4. F   Leukaemia. The history of prolonged illness with aches and pains suggests a generalized disorder. The low WCC is also suggestive of a haematological disorder and a sterile hip washout makes septic arthritis very unlikely. Leukaemia does occasionally present with musculoskeletal symptoms.
5. H   Osteogenesis imperfecta. The history of 'spontaneous' or low-violence fractures is typical. These cases are often initially diagnosed as non-accidental injury but here the X-ray shows abnormal bone.
6. I   Osteoid osteoma. The history is typical with intense pain relieved by NSAIDs. The X-ray and CT finding are typical.

4.

1. A   Osteoarthritis of the first MTP joint (hallux rigidus). The pain in the toe-off stage is typical as the patient has lost extension. Walking boots can relieve the pain by minimizing this movement. Clinical features are typical of OA anywhere, with osteophytes (dorsal bump) and crepitus.
2. C   Reiter's syndrome. A syndrome of arthritis, conjunctivitis and urethritis. It is more common in men but does occur in women.
3. I   Psoriatic arthropathy. Commonly affects the hands which can be significantly deformed.
4. D   Septic arthritis. Can be a difficult diagnosis to make in the elderly. Her raised WCC and temperature point to an infective cause.
5. E   Gout. Typical history and the usual joint. The serum uric acid is often normal during an acute episode.
6. G   Ankylosing spondylitis. The condition tends to present in early adult life and the spine is commonly affected and stiffens, eventually ankylosing. The sacroiliac joints are commonly involved.

5.

1. B   Spinal stenosis. The history is typical and pain is often worse on extension. The X-ray often only shows osteoarthritis and a CT or MRI scan will confirm the presence of spinal stenosis.
2. F   Spinal metastases. The history sounds sinister, with unrelenting pain. The X-ray showing loss of the pedicle (winking owl) means bony destruction by tumour.
3. D   Discitis. Often this condition presents late after the patient has had a number of normal investigations. This patient is at risk of sepsis, having diabetes and chronic renal failure. The X-ray shows the typical features of long-standing discitis.
4. J   Cauda equina syndrome. This is a typical history. Bilateral symptoms are suspicious. Any patient with sciatica and new urinary or bowel disturbance should be investigated urgently.
5. G   Acute low back pain. Very common and usually resolves. Note the absence of leg pain.
6. A   Spondylolisthesis. Fast bowlers in cricket are at increased risk. The X-ray features in this case are diagnostic.

6.

1. C   Developmental dysplasia of the hip. Late-presenting DDH presents with a painless limp and leg length discrepancy. All the other conditions on the list will present with pain.

2. E   Slipped upper femoral epiphysis. The patient is the correct age and the history of pain is typical. The femoral head in SUFE rotates posteriorly and leaves an externally rotated leg. The frog lateral X-ray shows the slip more obviously than the AP X-ray.

3. B   Juvenile idiopathic arthritis. Presentation with a monoarthritis is common, with other joints involved later. Generalized symptoms suggest a systemic disorder. The presence of eye symptoms is worrying as blindness can result.

4. J   Osgood–Schlatter disease. The disease is often bilateral and occurs during the adolescent years. Tender swollen tibial tuberosities are present bilaterally.

5. A   Perthes disease. The boy is the right age to have Perthes and the history of knee pain is typical. The loss of abduction is worrying as it could mean impending joint subluxation. The sclerosis of the femoral head is due to avascular necrosis.

6. G   Osteomyelitis. Diagnosis is difficult in the very young child. In this case the child obviously has an infection. In the absence of an obviously swollen joint and with a normal hip ultrasound scan the most likely cause is osteomyelitis.

7.

1. A   Tension pneumothorax. This occurs after trauma creates a one-way valve in the lung or chest wall. This means that air flows into the chest cavity, but not out again, which collapses the lung causing hypoxia. The mediastinum is displaced to one side, which reduces venous return to the heart and therefore cardiac output. This causes hypotension. This is life threatening and requires immediate decompression with a large-bore needle (before a chest X-ray is sought!), followed by insertion of a chest drain.

2. B   Pelvic fracture. The mechanism here suggests that this poor man has had a heavy crush injury to his pelvis. Venous bleeding can be massive with pelvic fractures, and can even be fatal. The man's hypotension and tachycardia are signs of hypovolaemic shock. Associated bladder and urethral injuries are not uncommon, and this man may have either a ruptured bladder or a urethral tear, which would explain the blood at his urethral meatus, and inability to pass urine. He should have a retrograde urethrogram before attempted catheterization.

3. C   Lumbar spine fracture/dislocation. This is a high energy injury, and the lumbar spine fracture dislocation is associated in this case with transection of the spinal cord. Therefore there is no function below the level of the injury, including nerves to the legs and sacral nerves to the bladder and bowel. The prognosis in this case is very poor.

4. D   Wedge fracture lumbar spine. This is likely to be an osteoporotic wedge fracture. This is a low energy fracture. It is also important to consider other pathological causes such as myeloma or bone metastasis from a primary malignancy.

5. F   Unfortunately the doctor has missed the diagnosis of a C7 fracture. This is because the X-rays did not show the whole of the cervical spine. Adequate trauma X-rays for neck injuries are an AP and lateral showing C1 to the top of the first thoracic vertebrae and an odontoid peg view. This patient has a potentially unstable fracture from a significant hyperflexion injury, and there is now compression of the right 8th cervical nerve root (learn dermatomes!).

6. G   This is a classic case of a neck sprain. The damage to the car suggests that this is a low speed crash, and the delayed onset of pain is crucial in making the diagnosis. Patients with significant neck injuries (fractures or ligament tears) develop immediate pain. A neck sprain requires simple analgesia and neck exercises to prevent more stiffness from developing.

8.

1. G   Realignment surgery. This man is developing medial compartment osteoarthritis in his knee because of his varus deformity. This results in increased load through the medial part of the knee joint and therefore earlier wear. He is too young for a joint replacement but realignment surgery will correct his deformity so that there is less wear on the medial side. This will hopefully slow down the progression of his osteoarthritis, but he may require a joint replacement when he is at a suitable age.

2. H   Arthroscopy. This man has a locked knee secondary to a medial meniscal tear. The meniscus can get trapped in the joint and tears as the knee extends. The meniscus is not very vascular and therefore the bleeding is slow and swelling occurs over 24 hours. An arthroscopy will identify the tear and it can then either be repaired or excised.

3. C   Unicompartmental knee replacement. This man has developed medial joint line osteoarthritis but his knee is otherwise well preserved. A unicompartmental knee replacement is designed to treat just the affected area of the knee. Its advantage over a total knee replacement is that it is a smaller operation and has a shorter recovery time.

4. F   X-ray of the spine. The doctor has not properly examined this lady. The X-ray changes of the hip are very mild and would not explain the severe pain that this lady complains of. Numbness is more typical of neurological pathology, and the fact that the hip has a good range of movement rules out major hip arthritis. This is more likely to be referred pain from the spine and plain X-ray may show degenerative change. Doing a hip replacement in this woman could be disastrous as it is a big operation and would not treat the pain.

5. D   Total knee replacement. This man has had a physical job for many years which has resulted in severe osteoarthritis of the knee. He cannot cope with his symptoms and further conservative treatment is not going to help. He should benefit from a total knee replacement.

9.

1. G   Epidural anaesthesia. The effect of this can last several hours (numb legs) and peripheral vasodilation causes pooling of fluid in the legs which results in hypotension. Other causes of course must be sought before it is assumed that the cause of hypotension is the epidural, but all other parameters are normal in this case.

2. B   Sepsis. This man is in septic shock and requires an emergency hip washout to treat his septic hip. He has risk factors for infection including type 2 diabetes mellitus and steroid treatment (immunosuppression).

3. D   Neurogenic shock. This man appears to have an isolated spinal injury based on his initial examination. This has resulted in loss of sympathetic tone to his legs and therefore hypotension. There is no evidence that he has any other injuries and therefore hypovolaemia secondary to blood loss is unlikely. In patients with spinal cord injury this blood pressure is acceptable and intravenous fluids should be given cautiously to avoid fluid overload.

4. E   Cardiogenic shock. This poor lady is having a myocardial infarction, confirmed on the ECG. This has caused left ventricular failure and therefore pulmonary oedema and hypotension. Thrombolysis is contraindicated here as she is only 4 days post surgery.

5. A   Hypovolaemia. Intraoperative haemorrhage has resulted in hypovolaemic shock and this man's blood pressure has not responded to fluids. He requires an urgent blood transfusion in order to prevent further deterioration. Hypotension within the first 48 hours of surgery is usually secondary to hypovolaemia.

10.

1. A Anterior dislocation. 95% of shoulder dislocations are anterior. This classically occurs when the arm is forced into abduction and external rotation (ball throwing position). Her shoulder will require reduction under sedation in casualty. She should be warned that there is up to an 80% chance of recurrent dislocations in her age group.

2. B Posterior dislocation. Accounts for 2% of shoulder dislocations and is associated with epileptic seizures and electrocutions. It should be suspected when the arm is held in fixed internal rotation.

3. D Hill–Sachs lesion. Sometimes following anterior dislocation of the shoulder the humeral head impacts on the glenoid causing a defect in the posterior part of the head. The articular surface is no longer congruent and so this defect catches on the glenoid in certain positions. This man requires bone grafting to restore the articular surface.

4. B Fracture of proximal humerus. Common fracture particularly in postmenopausal women. Treatment depends on the degree of displacement ranging from conservative to operative fixation or even replacement.

5. E Rotator cuff tear. History of settling injury but persistent weakness suggests rotator cuff tear. Examination findings indicate weakness of supraspinatus. Confirm with ultrasound or MRI.

11.

1. E *Haemophilus influenzae*. This used to be the commonest cause of septic arthritis in infants but is now rare because of a successful vaccination programme. This unfortunate child is not up to date, however.

2. G *E. coli*. This lady has developed a septic arthritis of her hip. This has resulted from haematogenous spread of bacteria to the hip from her urinary tract infection (UTI) and *E. coli* is a common cause of UTIs. Always look for a source when diagnosing septic arthritis.

3. C *Mycobacterium tuberculosis*. Travel to India may have exposed this lady to TB which has remained dormant for many years. This has now become activated, however, and caused collapse of one of her thoracic vertebral bodies resulting in a gibbus (sharp angulated kyphosis). She will need an MRI scan and then bipoisy of the lesion to confirm the diagnosis.

4. A *Staph. aureus*. This is the commonest cause of septic arthritis and osteomyelitis. This girl seems to have developed spontaneous osteomyelitis which will require antibiotics for 6 weeks and surgical debridement of the bone if indicated.

5. B Anaerobic bacteria. This man has an open fracture which is potentially contaminated by cattle manure amongst other things. Anaerobic bacterial and *Clostridium perfringens* (gas gangrene) infection is important to consider here based on the history. The fracture site should be irrigated and debrided urgently in theatre. Heavily soiled wounds should be covered with high dose antibiotics including an intravenous cephalosporin, penicillin and metronidazole. Tetanus prophylaxis should be given if vaccinations are not up to date.

12.

1. A   Salter–Harris fracture. This is a fracture around the growth plate (physis) and these are common injuries in children.

2. C   Pathological fracture. This is a fracture through abnormal bone. The history alone is suspicious of this. This poor man has got lung cancer from smoking and now has metastasis to his right femur which has been painful. This bone is therefore weak and low energy activities such as walking result in fracture. Other primary malignancies that metastasize to bone are thyroid, kidney, breast and prostate.

3. F   Compartment syndrome. This is unlikely to be a fracture because he could initially walk on his leg. Compartment syndrome can occur with or without fractures and this man needs urgent fasciotomies to the compartments (within 6 hours of onset). Absent foot pulses is a very late sign and usually indicates that the limb needs to be amputated.

4. G   Non-accidental injury. The history is not consistent with a healing fracture. Be very suspicious of any fracture in children under 2 years. Take no chances, admit the child and inform the paediatricians.

5. D   Open fracture. Any wound, no matter how small, on the same limb as a fracture should be assumed to be open until proven otherwise. This lady has a puncture wound from when the bone burst through the skin when it was severly angulated. This lady needs urgent debridement of the wound, stabilization of the fracture and antibiotics to help prevent chronic osteomyelitis.

13.

1. E   Nerve conduction study. The distribution of the pain is in keeping with a median nerve lesion. The diagnosis is carpal tunnel syndrome. This is associated with other conditions such as diabetes mellitus and pregnancy. Usually this is confirmed with nerve conduction studies but if the diagnosis is very obvious the surgeon may proceed to do a carpal tunnel decompression without this.

2. B   MRI. This lady has sciatica, most likely from a disc prolapse in her lumbar spine at the level of L5/S1. X-ray may show an obvious cause of the pain such as osteoarthritis but is often unhelpful. MRI will provide detailed images of the soft tissues and vertebral discs. This is also a very useful investigation if sinister spinal disease such as malignancy is suspected. CT is very good at showing detailed images of bones, e.g. for assessment of a complex vertebral body fracture.

3. G   Venous Doppler scan. The leg may just be swollen from surgery, but a total knee replacement puts the patient at high risk of deep vein thrombosis.

4. F   Ultrasound. This is likely to be a wrist ganglion. These are usually diagnosed clinically and excised if they cause problems, but if the clinician is unsure, an ultrasound scan is a simple quick non-invasive test to provide more information. Ganglions are fluid filled and therefore can change size depending on this. In the old days people were encouraged to bash them with a big book to rupture them!

5. C   Plain X-ray. This man may have metastasis to his ulna or radial shaft and a plain X-ray would normally show the diagnosis. Other malignancies that commonly metastasize to bone include thyroid, breast, lung and prostate.

14.

1. B Cervical rib. Occurs in 1 in 200 people and may be bilateral. An extra rib from C7 (may just be a fibrous band) articulates with the first rib or may be free distally. This may cause vascular (subclavian artery) disturbance such as Raynaud's phenomenon or neurological symptoms, normally in the distribution of C8/T1 dermatomes. The T1 myotome supplies the small muscles of the hand.

2. C Pancoast's tumour. An apical lung tumour has resulted in compression of the sympathetic nerves that arise from T1 and run up to supply the eye and forehead. This results in Horner's syndrome (ipsilateral meiosis, ptosis and facial anhydrosis) on the affected side. The tumour is also compressing the T1 myotome.

3. F Radial nerve palsy. The radial nerve runs in the spiral groove on the posterior aspect of the midshaft of the humerus. It is in direct contact with the bone at this point which makes it prone to injury.

4. G Cervical disc prolapse C6/C7. A disc at this level would compress the C7 nerve root causing numbness and/or pain in the middle finger. C7 supplies the triceps and flexor carpi radialis and there is resultant weakness of elbow extension and flexion of the wrist.

5. E Axillary nerve palsy. This chap has sustained an anterior dislocation of his shoulder. The axillary nerve leaves the brachial plexus and winds around the surgical neck of the humerus to supply sensation to the army badge area over the upper lateral aspect of the upper arm, and motor function to the deltoid. This injury is normally a neuropraxia.

15.

1. B Trendelenburg. This man has weakness of his left hip abductors so when asked to stand on his left leg, his pelvis tilts down. This results in a Trendelenburg gait. Bilateral weakness of the abductors results in a waddling gait when the pelvis drops down with each step.

2. E Foot drop. The policeman has purposefully hit the man over his common peroneal nerve to disable him. This nerve is very superficial as it winds around the fibula neck and supplies sensation to the dorsum of the foot and motor supply to the dorsiflexors of the toes and ankle. In order to prevent his toes dragging on the ground he compensates by lifting his foot high. Bilateral foot drop results in a high stepping gait.

3. A Ataxic. This boy has cerebral palsy secondary to meningitis as an infant. There is a loss of balance which is overcome by a broad based gait.

4. D Antalgic. Any painful condition results in an antalgic gait. This is characterized by a reduced stance phase (less time is spent weight bearing on the affected side) during walking.

5. H Spastic. This child has cerebral palsy. Children may display varying degrees of spasticity. Hip adductors contract resulting in 'scissoring' of the legs. The equinus deformity of his feet will also worsen function. He may benefit from complex surgery to correct the deformities.

Index

Note: Numbers in **bold** type refer to figures or tables.